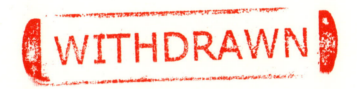

THE LABRADOR MEMOIR OF
DR HARRY PADDON, 1912–1938

MCGILL-QUEEN'S ASSOCIATED MEDICAL SERVICES
(HANNAH INSTITUTE)STUDIES IN THE HISTORY OF MEDICINE,
HEALTH, AND SOCIETY
Series Editors: S.O. Freedman and J.T.H. Connor

Volumes in this series have financial support from Associated Medical Services, Inc.,
through the Hannah Institute for the History of Medicine program.

The Labrador Memoir of Dr Harry Paddon, 1912–1938

Edited by

Ronald Rompkey

McGill-Queen's University Press

Montreal & Kingston · London · Ithaca

© McGill-Queen's University Press 2003
ISBN 0-7735-2505-X

Legal deposit second quarter 2003
Bibliothèque nationale du Québec

Printed in Canada on acid-free paper.

This book has been published with the help of the grant from
the Publication Subvention Committee of Memorial University
of Newfoundland.

McGill-Queen's University Press acknowledges the financial support
of the Canada Council for the Arts for our publishing program.
We also acknowledge the financial support of the Government of
Canada through the Book Publishing Industry Development Program
(BPIDP) for our publishing activities.

National Library of Canada Cataloguing in Publication

Paddon, Harry, 1881–1939
   The Labrador Memoir of Dr. Harry Paddon, 1912–1938/
edited by Ronald Rompkey.

(McGill-Queen's/Associated Medical Services (Hannah Institute)
studies in the history of medicine, health, and society; no. 17)

Includes bibliographical references and index.
ISBN 0-7735-2505-X

   1. Paddon, Harry, 1881–1939. 2. Physicians – Canada – Biography.
1. Rompkey, Ronald II. Title.

R464.P33A3 2003   610.92   C2002-903237-7

Typeset in Sabon 10/12
by Caractéra inc., Quebec City

Dedicated by Dr Paddon to his wife, Mina (Gilchrist) Paddon

Contents

Acknowledgments

Jacques Cartier, one of the earliest European travellers along the Labrador coast, left a lasting impression of it in 1534 with his casual reference to its stark outline as "the land that God gave Cain." This impression endured until the eighteenth century, when George Cartwright, writing in a more factual tradition of travel literature, recorded in his journal, "Although, in sailing along the coast, the astonished mariner is insensibly drawn into a conclusion, that this country was the last which God made, and that he had no other view than to throw there, the refuse of his materials, as of no use to mankind, yet, he no sooner penetrates a few miles into a bay, than the great change, both of the climate and the prospects, alter his opinion." Cartwright, who lived in Labrador year round, recognized its beauty more fully – its sculpted bays and inlets, its miles of untrodden winter white, its skies of aquamarine. He was the first Labrador apologist in the picturesque tradition. The last was Harry Paddon, physician, Victorian, and gardener, one who recalled his initial visit to Lake Melville in 1912 this way: "Here was a Garden of Labrador which during a season of each year could produce vegetables as good as those which would be grown in the Garden of Eden itself." Paddon might also be considered the first Labrador nationalist, the initial to regard its mixed, scattered population as an entity and the first to sentimentalize their homeland as a place.

His memoir consists of 427 typed pages, an elaborate reconstruction from journal-letters circulated to family members in the United Kingdom and articles published in magazines and periodicals. The present edition is based on a copy sent to Methuen & Co. in 1938 under the working title "A Record of Twenty-five Years of Pioneer Medical Work in Sub-Arctic Labrador." Methuen decided against publishing it. Although Dr Paddon's son and successor, Dr Tony Paddon, undertook to make it more appealing, to "round out" sections where, as he put it, his father's modesty "made it so terse as to lack interest," the pressures of a busy medical career made it impossible for him to do so. I am grateful to him for the opportunity to introduce it to a wider readership.

The manuscript exists in a raw state, without benefit of assessor's opinion or copy-editor's pencil, so raw that typographical faults, spelling inconsistencies, and errors of fact abound. These have been corrected silently or referred to in the notes. The style is at times laboured. Even though Harry Paddon was capable of exhibiting a range of rhetorical devices in public and private correspondence, he chose here something more typical of the boy's adventure story, interspersing his prose with literary and biblical allusions that reflect his broad reading and education. The reader will therefore encounter the verbosity, repetitiousness, and incoherence typical of early drafts. These have been left in large part as they are, except for changes in punctuation and paragraph structure executed in the interests of continuity and clarity. Labrador place names, which are spelled irregularly, have been standardized according to the conventions used in *Sailing Directions for Lake Melville and Approaches* (1931) and the *Gazetteer of Canada (Newfoundland)*. Labrador family names have been altered to conform to current practice. General spelling follows the conventions of the *Oxford English Dictionary* and biblical quotations the King James Version.

The editorial process could not have succeeded without the advice and assistance of individuals who generously provided specialized information and direction: Hugh J. Anderson, Melvin Baker, Linda Barnett (Health Sciences Library, Memorial University), Terry Bishop-Sterling, Carol Bryce-Bennett, Catherine Bergin (Wellcome Library, London), Ven. Francis Buckle, Jack Budgell, the late Leonard Budgell, Ruby (McLean) Budgell, Ann W. Caldwell (Massachusetts General Hospital), June Clark, John Crellin, Robin Darwall-Smith (University College, Oxford), Eleanor Dawson, Louise Decelles (McGill University Archives), Larry Dohey (Roman Catholic Archives, St John's), Jack Eckert (Francis A. Countway Library of Medicine, Boston), Susan Felsberg, Earle Gilchrist, Joe Goudie, Linda Hall (Williams College Archives and Special Collections), Susan (Merrick) Hoover, Clare Hopkins (Trinity College Archives, Oxford), Lucy Jardine (Provincial Archives of New Brunswick), Paul Jarrett (Royal National Mission to Deep Sea Fishermen, London), Peggy Jefferson, A.C. Jerrett, Dr Gordon Johnson (Institute of Opthalmology, London), Douglas Knock (Wellcome Library, London), Roger Lescaudron, Karen Lippold (Queen Elizabeth II Library, Memorial University), Gail Lush, José Mailhot,

Julia Mathieson (Anglican Church Archives, St John's), Wally McLean, the late Elliott Merrick, Florence (Goudie) Michelin, Anne Morton (Hudson's Bay Company Archives, Winnipeg), Dr Balfour Mount (Royal Victoria Hospital, Montreal), Peter Neary, Dr Sharon Peters (Faculty of Medicine, Memorial University), John Plowright (Repton School Archives), Carole Prietto (University Archives, Washington University), Stephen Prowse (Medical Library, St Thomas's Hospital), Dr Kenneth B. Roberts, Dr Peter Roberts, Samantha Robins (Dudley Archives and Local History Service), Hans Rollmann, Sen. William Rompkey, Dr Ian Rusted, Dr Nigel Rusted, Chesley Sanger, Doris Saunders, Bella (McLean) Shouse, Rev. Hector Swain, Airi Töyrymäki (Department of Geography, University of Helsinki), Heather Wareham (Maritime History Archive, Memorial University), Patricia Way, Derek Wilton, Susan White (Grenfell Regional Health Services, St Anthony), David H. Wood, and Christopher Youé. I am indebted to them all.

Research assistance was carried out by Darcy Maynard (Department of English), map reproduction by Charles Conway (Cartographic Lab), and photographic reproduction by Sharon Thompson (Photographic Services), all at Memorial University.

I am grateful for access to special collections at the following libraries: the National Library of Canada, the National Archives of Canada, the Centre for Newfoundland Studies at Memorial University, the Provincial Archives of Newfoundland and Labrador, Yale University Library, and the British Library.

I owe an enormous debt to the Paddon family of North West River for their cooperation and for permission to quote from family papers – particularly Dr Harry Paddon's sons, John Paddon and the late Tony, Harry, and Dick Paddon. I also thank Sheila Paddon and Seija Paddon for their helpful comments, as well as Dr Paddon's grandchildren, David, Elizabeth, and Tom Paddon, and his nephew, the late Dick Paddon, Jr, who generously lent me his father's papers. I am especially grateful to Dr Paddon's nephew, Raymond Lloyd, the son of his sister Jessie, and his great-nephew, Richard Lloyd, joint keepers of the Van Sommer papers in the United Kingdom, for their encouragement and for permission to quote from documents in their custody.

I thank Sheila Paddon for graciously permitting me to publish her father-in-law's journal.

Research grants were provided by the Hannah Institute for the History of Medicine and the Vice-President's Research Fund, Memorial University.

R.G.R.
Department of English
Memorial University

Introduction

I talked with him at one o'clock that afternoon, and he was fully rational, but we avoided the possibility of his death, because, though he was too good a doctor not to sense the danger, he still had some hope, and I didn't want his fight to be hampered with worries about his affairs. Though I knew, I never really gave up hope at all. I suppose the human mind simply refuses to entirely accept anything so tragic in one "swallow." Mother was utterly magnificent. She cried a little when the intern came in to tell us, but only a little, after she had said "It was to have been such a happy Christmas," and then she thought of little John, the youngest of us and the least able to stand the blow, and her heart was full, not of her own troubles, but of those of her sons. As she told John the next day, we belong to a family that has much to uphold, and no one made any fuss or demonstration, but you know well – tragically well – the feeling of hopelessness that one feels.[1]

The letter sent from Tony Paddon to Sir Wilfred Grenfell after his father's sudden death on Christmas Eve 1939 constitutes a brief epilogue to a medical career pursued in extraordinary circumstances and performed with uncommon devotion. Harry Paddon was bred for the mission field. Like so many of his late-Victorian contemporaries, he was devoted to a higher purpose, according to the norms of rectitude, honour, and chastity existing in certain European societies before the Great War. By time the war put an end to those norms, Paddon had reinvented himself for service in the Empire, forfeiting the social and professional advancement available to a medical graduate in exchange for the anonymity of Labrador, where his influence reached far beyond the day-to-day clinical tasks of his contemporaries. Why was it to have been such a happy Christmas? Why did the Paddons have so much to uphold? For answers to these questions, let us examine some of the features of Harry Paddon's life.

FAMILY AND EDUCATION

Both sides of his family were devoted Christians. His paternal grandfather, the Reverend Thomas Henry Paddon (1806–87), together with his wife, Anne Locke, the daughter of a Wiltshire banking family, produced five children, all of whom received Locke as a middle name.[2] Susceptible to strong Calvinistic views and alert to "popish" tendencies in the church, Grandfather Paddon accepted the living of High Wycombe in 1844[3] and proceeded to take strong positions on issues great and small, annoying his congregation and his bishop, Samuel Wilberforce, with a succession of petty disputes. The dismissal of his organist on suspicions of "ritualism" is a celebrated instance, for on that occasion the congregation sided with the organist, locking the instrument so that no one else could play it. Potential curates shied away. In 1849, the year following the organ episode, Paddon sent the bishop a sermon preached by one young man containing alleged Tractarian errors, but instead of upholding the vicar, Wilberforce sympathetically advised the curate to depart.[4] When Paddon later applied for a three-year leave on the grounds of ill health, he was refused, and when he continued to harass the curates appointed to replace him, the bishop moved to sequester the living on the grounds of non-residence. Indeed, when Paddon prepared to return in 1856, his parishioners offered him £100 a year to stay away.[5] He remained at Wycombe until 1869, however, at which point he cut all formal ties with the Church of England and took his family to Eastbourne. There he busied himself with a series of hard-hitting tracts like *Thoughts on the Evangelical Preaching of the Present Day* (1872), an exhortation to his fellow clergy against Tractarianism, and for the rest of his career sat as the first incumbent of the new Emmanuel Free Church.[6]

His son, Henry Wadham Locke Paddon (1839–1933), who acquired a commission in the 7th Royal Fusiliers, fought in India in a series of operations on the North West Frontier.[7] When in 1875 Henry met and married Catherine Van Sommer, Grandfather Paddon refused to attend the wedding (perhaps still harbouring resentments against the church) or to settle any money upon his son.[8] A few weeks after their marriage, the couple sailed to India, where two daughters, Jessie and Eva, were born sixteen months apart. When the family returned in 1879, Margaret ("Daisy") was born later the same year, followed by Harry, who was born at home in Thornton Heath, Croydon, on 9 August 1881.[9] Four days later, Catherine died of the malady known as milk fever,[10] and Henry, who had been pensioned the previous January and given the honorary rank of lieutenant-colonel,[11] found himself alone with four children under the age of five. All four remained at Thornton Heath under the care of their father and a wet nurse until early 1883, when the loss of his wife and the upkeep of his children drove Henry Paddon to an asylum in a state of depression. There he remained until his death nearly fifty years later. The children stayed in the care of the Paddon grandparents, but not for long. Despite a legal challenge by Grandfather Paddon, the two eldest became wards of the Van Sommers, who had moved from Eastbourne to Wimbledon Park.

The Van Sommers, descendants of Huguenots who had fled France in the late seventeenth century,[12] were a comfortably conservative Christian family. James Van Sommer (1822–1901), the patriarch, had by then reached the end of a prosperous legal career at New Inn, London, and lived at Cuffnells, a spacious house overlooking the lake on Wimbledon Common. In his household the Scriptures held sway, and the daily round was punctuated by Bible readings and acts of devotion. It began, Harry's sister Jessie recalled, with formal worship:

After breakfast, while still sitting round the table, the bell would be rung at an exact moment; the 4 servants would appear, carrying a form [bench], on which they sat in a row. We all remained where we were, while my Grandfather read and expounded and prayed extempore. His quiet but vigorous voice, never dull, for his mind was upon what he read, was very reverent, and he addressed God as truly *Father*, caring for us individually. So was our day together begun. Before breakfast Aunt Bessie would read the Bible with us in her bedroom. Breakfast was always at 8, and 8.30 on Sundays. What an effort for her to be ready for us soon after 7.30 a.m., when we would say what we had learnt by heart and be taught from the Bible. On Sunday it would be to say a hymn. We also learnt all the Collects.[13]

James Van Sommer adhered to no specific religious denomination but rather espoused the universality of the Christian religion. On Sunday mornings he might be found at a Salvation Army, Congregational, Presbyterian, Baptist, or Church of England service, and he and the members of his family were received at various times into the Christian Brethren at Tottenham. In his last years he published a series of tracts on prayer and Bible reading and spent a good deal of his time spreading the gospel in the surrounding community. Jessie added,

Grandpapa was always giving – fruit or a flower – some wonderful pansy perhaps – which he had grown – oranges, sweets, nuts, to the children of the cottages near our house. His coat tail pockets always had something in them to give away! And other pockets would contain tracts that he wrote himself and had had printed. A favourite occupation was to go to one bench on the Common and then another, sitting there, and then leaving behind him some tract or picture leaflet, to be picked up. Often he would offer personally one of these to some stranger sitting on the same bench and enter into conversation with them. Always, in his quiet way, he was about his Master's business.[14]

Giving was a practice he encouraged in his family of six, two of whom still lived at home. (Daughters Ann and Elisabeth would later go as missionaries to Egypt and West Africa.) In February 1883 he placed the two older Paddon grandchildren, Jessie and Eva, under the care of Elisabeth (known as Aunt Bessie), while the two younger ones remained in lodgings at Eastbourne with their Paddon grandparents and a nurse until, following Grandfather Paddon's death, they too were absorbed into the Van Sommer household in 1888. Bessie became their virtual mother, her earnest religiosity leaving a permanent impression on their lives.

The village of Wimbledon, which began as a gracious London suburb, had developed by the middle of the nineteenth century into an important railway junction. At the time young Harry arrived there, virtually all the land on either side of the railway had been sold for building lots, and the population had increased to over forty thousand.[15] Wimbledon's rapid growth reflected that of London itself, each new suburb expanding with the improvement of rail travel. But Cuffnells, from its position overlooking the Common, was hardly affected by these changes. In summer the house was filled with fragrances from the conservatory. James Van Sommer arose at five to study the Bible and to tend his garden before the gardener himself arrived. From Grandfather Van Sommer the Paddon children acquired not only the habit of giving but of preparing soils and nurturing plants.

Soon after his arrival at Cuffnells, Harry was sent to the Woodbridge Grammar School in Suffolk. In September 1889 he was baptized at Woodbridge. Even at the age of eight he seemed to have a taste for missionary pursuits. During the summer holidays at the seaside in Sherringham, Norfolk, he liked to go to sea for the day with local fishermen, and having declared his desire to be a missionary,[16] he had his first taste of mission work under the tutelage of the Reverend John Taylor Smith of the Children's Special Service Mission. On Sunday mornings Harry and his sisters would distribute leaflets and sing hyms to the fishermen as they sat in their boats. It was as natural as playing.

Yet despite the attention of his aunts and the generosity of his grandfather, Harry felt that he never stayed long enough in one place to call it his home. "I envy my boys their childhood," he wrote later, "looking back on my own with its advantages."[17] At thirteen, he arrived at Repton,[18] an ancient public school that claimed two arch-bishops of Canterbury as old boys. Repton's chapel formed the centre of school life, and the curriculum remained overwhelmingly classical.[19] W.F. Furneaux, the headmaster, summed up the public school philos-ophy at a prize-giving in 1900: "There may be Schools in other countries which equal them in the intellectual teaching which they give, but there are none which equal them in their power of forming character and inspiring affection."[20] Repton formed the whole boy, and Furneaux, headmaster from 1883 to 1900, made striking innova-tions to move his charges outside their sphere. He opened an engineer-ing workshop and, as a hedge against "self-indulgence," founded the Repton Club in the East End of London to arouse an interest in social welfare work. Harry, a self-confessed dreamer, gave his studies only the attention required to succeed but revelled in sports, especially football and cricket. He also liked to engage in public debate and took part in theatricals, playing the lover Lysander in a speech-day produc-tion of *A Midsummer Night's Dream* in 1899 and the servant David the following year in Sheridan's *The Rivals*.[21] That summer, still under the guardianship of Aunt Bessie, he left Repton and prepared to go up to Oxford.

James Van Sommer's will provided £800 for each of the three surviving grandchildren (Daisy died of meningitis at fourteen), to be paid at his death, and he looked after Harry's university expenses by advancing him the interest on his share.[22] Harry took up residence at University College Oxford in the autumn of 1900. He did not adapt well to the academic life, however, for after he sat for his Moderations (the first round of public examinations) in the spring of 1902 his name did not appear in the published results. The tutorial lists show that he had been given an "allowed pass" with a transfer to Modern History, and after a fresh start he appeared in the history lists for 1903. But his name was missing from the history results for summer 1904, when he ought to have graduated. Harry had let the family down. He did not get around to taking his degree until 1906,[23] and in later life his lack of academic distinction was the source of some self-mockery. When Jessie's son Humphrey achieved good results in 1925, Harry commented to Aunt Bessie, "My own degree was one of my humilia-tions: & I can only hope I have been enabled to do something toward graduating in a higher School than Oxford History, & may win a pass, even though others take the Honours."[24]

Oxford behind him, Harry departed at Easter for a fortnight with the North Sea fishing fleet as a missioner of the Royal National Mission to Deep Sea Fishermen (RNMDSF). He returned to the fleet again in August and September.[25] The mission suited his religious tendencies exactly. Although it numbered among its members some clergy and missioners of the Church of England, it strenuously avoided questions of theological affiliation and concentrated instead on working amongst fishermen. Its first secretary declared, "The sympathizers of the Society have always been able to claim that, while never degenerating into a soulless latitudinarianism, the Mission has been broad and common-sense in its outlook ... It has no cut-and-dried formula of doctrine or metaphysical confession of faith; it goes into the field with a wise, prudent, evangelical teaching ... which has been the lifeblood of the Church in all ages."[26] The great accomplishment of the RNMDSF was its pioneer hospital work in the North Sea, especially the fitting out of hospital ships that could remain on station for weeks at a time.

This kind of practical Christianity had also attracted Wilfred Grenfell, whom Harry had heard speak at Repton years before with the same simplicity and Broad Church enthusiasm as Grandfather Van Sommer. At twenty-four, Grenfell had become the mission's first superintendent, soon after he left the London Hospital Medical College. When the mission was invited in 1892 by the fish merchants of St John's, Newfoundland, to find ways of treating the sickness and injury sustained by men engaged in the Labrador fishery, Grenfell was despatched for the summer aboard the Mission ship *Albert*. The following year he returned to build small wooden hospitals at Indian Harbour and Battle Harbour and thereafter undertook the treatment of northern fishermen and their families as his life's work.

Harry became a medical student at St Thomas's Hospital in the winter of 1907 and quickly passed the first set of examinations leading to the conjoint diploma of the Royal College of Physicians and the Royal College of Surgeons, returning to the North Sea in April to preach and take pledges.[27] A keen athlete throughout his Oxford days, he maintained his interest in cricket as a bowler for the hospital club and played at half-back for its football team. In May 1908, we learn from the *St. Thomas's Hospital Gazette*, "When the Old Brentwoods went in again, just before five o'clock, Paddon bowled so well that they were all dismissed for 27. Paddon obtained six wickets for 13 runs, and in spite of a tendency to bowl full tosses his bowling was easily the best thing of the day." Against Upper Tooting, he bowled "very steadily" and against London County "very fine cricket." During the autumn and winter he captained the football team, and the following cricket season, playing against St Bartholomew's for the Inter-Hospital Cup, he came on fresh towards the end and "took four for 20" on the way to winning the championship.[28]

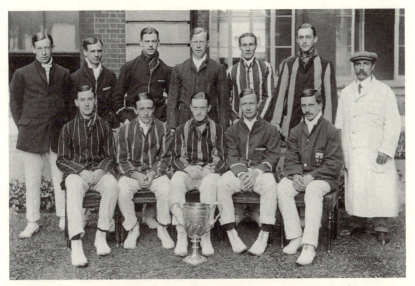

St. Thomas's Hospital cricket team, winners of the Inter-Hospital Cup, July 1909. *Back row, left to right:* H.L. Mann, W. Parkinson, D.M. Gibson, A.F. Morton, H.J.B. Fry, E.H. Walker; *front row:* E.A. Seymour, R.F. Bowis, L. Meakin, F.M. Neild, H.L. Paddon (Paddon Family Papers)

One by one, he sat the examinations leading to his qualification, and in October 1910 passed the conjoint board's surgery exam.[29] The same month, having kept up his connections with the RNMDSF, he returned to Billingsgate for another voyage aboard a Mission ship.[30] For his first appointment as houseman, he served as medical officer in the West Midlands town of Dudley and took on extra duties as assistant house surgeon at the Guest Hospital.[31] In January 1911 he passed the final medicine exam of the conjoint board, and in February received confirmation of his hospital appointment.[32]

Harry now stood on the verge of a conventional medical career. A year later, having been registered as a physician, he resigned.[33] He had accepted an invitation from the RNMDSF to work in the hospital built at Indian Harbour by Wilfred Grenfell. How long he would remain there he did not know. The job suited his missionary tendencies, and in view of the state of public health in Labrador, he would make his training count.

In May 1912 the Reverend Hubert Kirby, Anglican priest at Cartwright, Labrador, had petitioned the colonial secretary of Newfoundland, Robert Watson, for the appointment of a public health officer. Except for Dr John Grieve at the Grenfell hospital in Battle Harbour and Dr S.K. Hutton at the Moravian hospital further north at Okak, there

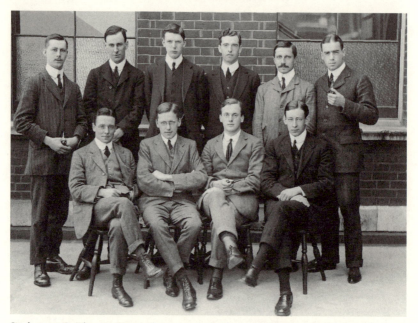

Students at St Thomas Hospital, 1905–10. *Back row, left to right:* F.R. Skrimshir, A.B. Bridges, A.S. Penn, W.B. Laird, H.L. Paddon, H.V. Walsh; *front row:* S.V. Appleyard, C.F. Schuler, M.W. Littlewood, H.L. Mann (Paddon Family Papers)

was no resident practitioner – as Kirby wrote, "no person as far as I am aware directly responsible for the carrying out of the law as regards public health."[34] The same year, the Moravian Church had also petitioned the government, requesting a doctor for the Okak hospital to act as public health officer for that part of the coast. But the government was reluctant to venture into new territory. The attorney general, Donald Morison, advised the colonial secretary that it would be difficult to regulate any expenditures such a person might authorize, "as under the circumstances prevailing on the Labrador coast a Health Officer with advanced ideas might at any moment authorize a very much larger expenditure than would be contemplated by the Government."[35] The assignment of Harry Paddon to the Indian Harbour hospital as well as to winter work in Lake Melville and along the northern coast put the matter to rest.

LABRADOR MISSIONER

Arriving in Labrador at the age of thirty-one, Paddon was up for the physical challenge. He embraced the north and its climate, and with the arrival of winter became "a convinced believer in the future of this lovely region" (p. 50), thankful he had not chosen mission work in Africa or China like so many of his contemporaries. "You soon get used to having your nose full of icicles – they are much nicer than swampy fevers – mists or even London fogs," he wrote in a journal-letter circulated to the family.[36] By the next spring he felt at home, comfortable enough to write his sister, "Every sphere of life must have its disadvantages, but institution life in England, which is the most instructive and varied, means an indoor existence in a town & I reckon that this is quite a deal better than many English practices in the country."[37] The winter had given him the chance to meet his neigh-bours, the small bands of Innu (Algonkian-speaking Montagnais-Naskapi Indians), the Inuit (Eskimo) communities, and the white and mixed population (now called Kablunângajuit in the north or Métis in the south) engaged in trapping and fishing. The lucrative Labrador fishery also brought him into contact during the spring and summer season with thousands of itinerant Newfoundland fishing crews who depended upon Grenfell's hospitals and their shifting assortment of volunteer doctors, nurses, and university students in Labrador and at St Anthony in Newfoundland. Labrador, he learned, remained under the jurisdiction of Newfoundland, but its population of under four thousand enjoyed no democratic representation in its House of Assem-bly and no fixed boundary to distinguish it from Quebec. It had no institution for the maintenance of public order, except what was imposed by the Hudson's Bay Company trading posts, the Moravian Church and its trading posts along the northern coast, and Grenfell's branch of the RNMDSF.

As the Newfoundland fishing crews vanished for the winter, Paddon shifted inland to treat the white and mixed population of Lake Melville. There he encountered the Montagnais Innu who wandered the interior to the south and west, harvesting caribou, fish, and other resources and trapping marten, fox, and beaver. Further north were the Naskapi Innu bands, at some distance from the trading posts but closer to the herds of caribou that traversed the northern part of the Labrador Peninsula. On dog-team patrols to the northern coast Paddon visited the Inuit, descendants of a prehistoric hunting society that had spread across northern Canada from Alaska as far as southern Labrador and north-ern Newfoundland. With European encroachment they had pushed north again. They too hunted caribou, and their livelihood also depended on species of seal and whale.

The Hudson's Bay Company had traded with the Innu as well as with the mixed population since the eighteenth century. In the 1840s, following a decline of trade and the recommendation of its agent, John

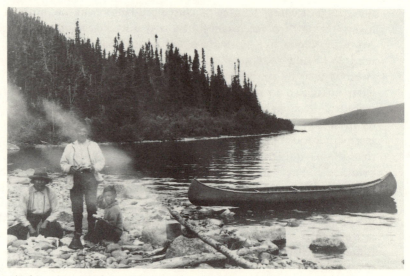

Chief Swashim (Joachim) Ashini (National Archives of Canada PA 148594)

McLean, the HBC had closed its posts north of the height of land. It supplied the remainder from Esquimaux Bay (now Lake Melville), buying out private traders and establishing a chain of posts which, together with the existing posts at North West River and Cartwright, imposed a kind of commercial rhythm on the year. As the post managers' journals show, the small communities at Mud Lake, North West River, Rigolet, and Cartwright were composed of HBC employees, mostly Scots, and former employees who had intermarried with the native population. McLean describes another group of Europeans in notes he compiled in the 1840s: "British sailors, who, preferring the freedom of a semi-barbarous life and the society of a brown squaw, to the severity of maritime discipline and the endearments of the civilized fair, take up their abode for life in this land of desolation."[38] The most influential HBC trader was Donald Alexander Smith (1820–1914), clerk at Rigolet from 1848 to 1852 and until 1862 chief trader at North West River, where he established a model farm and raised cattle (providing a precedent for Paddon's subsequent ventures). Smith took charge as chief factor of the district of Esquimaux Bay for the period 1862 to 1868. Later, as Lord Strathcona, he was one of Grenfell's earliest benefactors in Canada.

The more northern communities Paddon visited were inhabited by Inuit under the religious and cultural influence of the Moravian Church, an early form of Protestantism that had located principally in Germany and England. During the eighteenth century the Moravians had spread their strict form of communal Christianity to Greenland, the Caribbean, Oceania, and Alaska as well as to Labrador. There they had made it their policy to contain the Inuit in what amounted to German communities. Even though the Moravians' first objective was conversion, the Inuit who accepted Christianity were eventually expected to winter at Moravian communities in Nain, Okak, and Hopedale and harvest local resources for exchange at the mission's stores. However, with the appearance on the coast of other cultural groups, notably Newfoundland fishermen, the power of the missionaries had diminished. In Esquimaux Bay, as we learn from W.H.A. Davies, who was placed in charge of the district by the HBC in 1838, the Inuit left because of a shortage of seals:

The Bay was formerly the principal residence of the Esquimaux, from the facilities that it offered for living, the seals frequenting it in great numbers, and remaining in the Bay during the whole winter. But the number of seals has been gradually diminishing of late years, [and] this has caused many of the tribe to leave the place; we must however look to the combined effects of the rum and the vices, imported by the Europeans, for the great diminution that has taken place within the last sixty years in the number of the Esquimauxs belonging to the Bay; even as late as the beginning of the present century, they numbered upwards of 300 – they are now reduced to eight families, consisting of thirty-four individuals, viz.: nineteen males and fifteen females.[39]

Writing in 1872, the French missionary Charles Arnaud lamented, "Quelqu'un qui a passé de longues années avec eux me disait, que pas une femme ou fille était chaste, tout les porte à la corruption, rien qui puisse mettre un frein, pauvres Esquimaux."[40] Both the Moravian physician Dr S.K. Hutton and Grenfell's own physicians recorded the susceptibility of the Inuit to European diseases. Paddon writes of his first extended contact with the Moravians on the coast in 1914: "They frankly admitted that their own pioneers had erred, with the best intentions and quite pardonably, at a time when no one realised the relative susceptibility of these aboriginals to white man's diseases, by encouraging centralisation for purposes of physical, educational and medical service; and they deplore the fact that now, in a generation when these dangers were realised, the Eskimos had become too sophisticated for decentralisation and a resumption of their natural nomadic existence" (p. 115-16).

While Paddon wrestled with administrative problems the first summer, including a shortage of basic medical and surgical supplies, he was encouraged by the presence of a nurse who arrived at the same time. A year older than Paddon, Mina Gilchrist was the daughter of

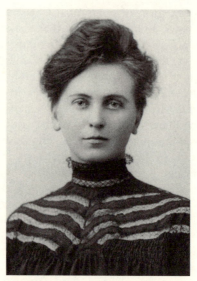

Mina Gilchrist during her nursing
training in Boston (Paddon Family
Papers)

Angus Gilchrist, a New Brunswick mariner and farmer who with his
wife, Charlotte, had settled in Cambridge Parish, Queen's County,
where Mina was born. The family later shifted to Lincoln, a small
town near Fredericton, where she finished her schooling.[41] Determined
to become a nurse, she set off for the McLean Hospital Training School
at Belmont, Massachusetts, an institution founded on the principles of
good character and exhausting work. The McLean course varied
between two to three years, following contemporary trends; graduates
were granted a further year of instruction in medical and surgical cases
at the Massachusetts General Hospital, so that they received a graduate
diploma from that school as well as one from their own. In 1905 Mina
graduated from the McLean and left the Massachusetts General in
1907 to begin a series of contractual jobs in New England as a private
nurse.[42] By doing so, she followed a career pattern more common at
the time than that of a hospital nurse and more remunerative.[43] Like
Kate Austen and other volunteers recruited by Grenfell, Mina went to
Labrador to do something more challenging than caring for individual
patients in private homes.

Paddon, who had never allowed much time for romance, was ready
to marry her by September of 1912, but Mina filled in at the St
Anthony hospital for eight months. They were eventually married at
Indian Harbour on 1 October 1913 by the Reverend Hubert Kirby.[44]

Marriage gave Paddon his first taste of settled family life, especially after the arrival of their first son, Tony, the following year. The couple now began to absorb the broader significance of their task as they moved between the summer station at Indian Harbour and the temporary inland hospital set up in an abandoned lumber camp at Mud Lake. Paddon wrote to his family, "Labrador's social problems, Labrador's industrial disorganisation, Labrador's commercial chaos, Labrador's lack of public opinion, Labrador's lawlessness and need of a prison and reformatory, Labrador's apology for an educational system, Labrador's lack of Representation – are all things which one cannot and should not be blind to although one 'shipped' as a Medical Missionary."[45] Like Grenfell and other colonial physicians before him, he was already looking beyond his immediate practice to the social milieu where illness flourished.

As the resident physician, Paddon developed an affinity for the Labrador communities but came close to leaving when war broke out. During their first furlough in England in the winter of 1914–15, while he brushed up on medical developments and raised money for the mission, he was ready to enlist but abandoned the idea to return to Labrador. At the hospital at North West River, hub of the fur trade, he recruited and screened volunteers for the next few years. "Is it not wonderful the way we have been provided for?" Mina wrote to her sister-in-law. "I have felt all the time that it would be so. I feel very strongly that it is right for us to be on the Labrador and right for us to have children and after we have done what we can, we should be content to leave the rest to God without worrying."[46] By now Mina was as dedicated as Paddon himself, and their joint decision to stay in Labrador involved a lifelong commitment unmatched by any other members of Grenfell's staff except Dr Charles Curtis at St Anthony. To cover the territory sufficiently, they continued to divide their efforts between Indian Harbour and Paddon's winter tours of the coast. Just before Christmas 1915, a second son, Harry, was born.

In the autumn of 1919, following the devastating Spanish Flu epidemic, Paddon left his family at Swampscott, Massachusetts. He substituted for Grenfell on a lecture tour of New England, New York, and Canada with a plan to build a residential school for orphaned children. As the tour progressed, however, he realized that as someone directly engaged in the well-being of the population, he was not delivering quite the same message as his leader, a charismatic speaker who liked to entertain audiences with exciting tales of northern adventure, illustrated by lantern slides of icebergs and polar bears. Instead, Paddon had much to say first hand about the difficulties of survival. That spring, as he toured the United Kingdom, he received word of the RNMDSF board's decision to reduce its annual grant to £1,000 – even if he raised more for the society himself. After twenty years the RNMDSF had lost its enthusiasm for Grenfell's expensive overseas venture. Paddon felt betrayed. He realized he no longer spoke for the London board, but for the trappers, fishermen, traders, and aboriginals he treated day by day.

He continued to be frustrated by the absence of democratic representation and basic government services. In 1917 he had written forcefully to Richard Squires, the colonial secretary in St John's, to recommend the appointment of a district commissioner, the kind of local authority often found in other British colonies. He concluded,

The coloured races of Egypt & Nigeria are administered by first rate men. Sir Frederick Lugard [in Nigeria] has reaped the harvest of years of able patriotic service during this war. I realise Labrador is not of such strategic importance as African colonies: but I don't believe the least populous, the least productive, the least strategic, the least anything that is British deserves taxation without representation, & bogus exploitation without employment, to say nothing of a collection of summer tripping officials whose services are certainly not in proportion to their remuneration, & resident ones of whom the less said the better![47]

His idea of the appointment of a permanent official was not a new one. In 1905, after a tour of the Labrador coast, the governor of Newfoundland, Sir William MacGregor, had made similar observations and suggested the appointment of a minister or parliamentary secretary. The "proper development" of Labrador could not take place, he argued, unless one of these solutions were adopted – at the very least, an annual visit by a minister of the Crown.[48] Yet the kind of district officer Paddon had in mind was something different: a familiar figure in British overseas administration – decorous, resolute, and usually possessed of a public-school education, someone who would exercise leadership in local matters and encourage the middle-class values of regular habits, productivity, and self-control – someone like Paddon himself. The government, however, would not consider exercising this level of authority over such a small, shifting population.

Paddon also found himself disagreeing fundamentally with the policies of Grenfell and the board of the International Grenfell Association (IGA), the network of fundraisers founded in 1914 with branches in the United States, Canada, and Britain. He reported to his sister in 1919, "We have won over my beloved chief from treating Labradorians as an interesting group of tragic individuals who can only be saved by bringing them *out* of their country. He now realises that they are worth giving a chance to, *in their own country*; which is *well* able to support them, if only they are given fair play."[49] By this time he and the Reverend Henry Gordon, the new Anglican priest at Cartwright, had raised enough money to build a residential school at Muddy Bay. When Grenfell paid the school his first visit, Mrs Gordon observed, "I felt that it had made a very deep impression upon him, and sown the seeds of a rather different attitude of his Mission to the question of local education."[50] Unfortunately, Grenfell left the direction of policy to his board, who shared his former views, and most of them lived in the United States.

Paddon returned from another furlough in June 1920, leaving the family at Malet's Bay on Lake Champlain. There Mina gave birth to a third son, Richard, and acquired the services of a governess to take care of the three boys. A year later, nearly a decade after Paddon's arrival, the family took up residence in the first wooden hospital at North West River, where Paddon started to cultivate a nearby tract of land for his own use and the encouragement of local people. He was beginning to see some progress in the battle against nutritional diseases, for as he observes in his memoir, "It is the house not built with hands that outlasts any structure of timber or even of concrete, and we now had a centre both for local development and also wide radiation of ways and means of building up public health and welfare" (p. 143). In January 1924, his optimism received a major blow when the hospital burned to the ground as he lectured in the United States. Despite this discouragement and the IGA's inclination to abandon North West River and consolidate its services at St Anthony, he struggled to have it rebuilt. He did so by October after a strenuous fundraising effort.

The Paddons now needed to decide where their sons, who had so far been educated at home, should be sent to school. Should they be sent to the United States, or to England, where they could reconnect with their British cousins? For practical reasons, the United States was chosen since Mina could live there for a time and communicate more readily with North West River. Consequently, in the spring of 1927, Paddon rented a four-bedroom house at Stockbridge, Massachusetts, where Mina lived off and on for the next four years. First Tony and then Harry entered the Lenox School, a new institution founded in the Berkshire Hills by three Episcopal clergymen, while Dick remained in the public system. (Their fourth son, John, was not born until June 1927.) No stranger to boarding schools, Paddon was delighted with the moderate fees and the dedication of the masters. "They are splendid fellows," he reported to the family in England, "sympathetic with boyhood in a way that I must confess I never experienced, though things may have changed since... I am thankful to have it as a stand-by for

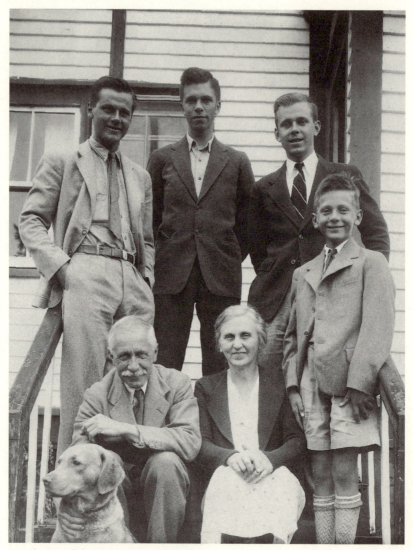

A gathering of the Paddon sons at North West River, c. 1933. *Back row, left to right:* Harry, Dick, Tony; *front:* Dr Paddon's dog, Sinbad, Dr Harry Paddon, Mina Paddon, John (Paddon Family Papers)

our boys' development; and hope they may contribute something to the high traditions the staff seek to establish and maintain."[51] Dick too would go to Lenox, and Paddon remained impressed by its mixture of academic and non-academic training, especially its attention to religion and its progressive attitude to what he called "boy life." But Grenfell (who received a knighthood for his years of devotion in 1927) criticized this preference for American education, and when Paddon's sister also questioned the decision, he erupted:

For Sir Wilf & his wife, who have ample means, and who turned over their children to an American grandmother anyhow; and who deliberately chose the most exclusive rich men's sons' school in America *when he had a brother a schoolmaster in England,* to hold up his hands in amazement at my "preference for American education" is palpably absurd. I love the dear man: but I know him far better than ever you will. He also has numerous friends and connections in Canada. He can get free scholarships for all his children in any English-speaking country. So why did he choose Groton and stand amazed at my choosing Lenox as the best solution of a difficult problem?[52]

In the summer of 1927 Paddon saw one of his desires fulfilled: namely, the establishment of a permanent boundary between Labrador and Quebec by a decision of the judicial committee of the privy council of Great Britain. This decision opened up the possibility for further economic development at a time when Newfoundland was threatened with bankruptcy. However, the future of Labrador still remained in some doubt, even though the terms of reference for negotiation had been fixed since 1922, for the prime minister of Newfoundland revealed in 1925 that he was prepared to sell the territory to Canada for $30 million as long as Newfoundland fishermen retained access to the coast. He was refused, even when he cut the price in half. When arbitration began again in October 1926, Canada and Newfoundland remained fundamentally at odds over one crucial matter: the definition of *coast.* Canada argued that the coast granted to Newfoundland in previous treaties consisted of a strip of land along the littoral. For Newfoundland, the coast of Labrador encompassed the watershed area. Even when a decision overwhelmingly favouring Newfoundland was handed down in March 1927, the story did not end. For the next decade, as Paddon reflects in his memoir, Labrador became the subject of considerable speculation in timber, minerals and hydroelectric power, an expectation expressed in the "Ode to Labrador" he wrote at about this time:

Thy stately forests soon will ring, Labrador, our Labrador,
Responsive to the woodsman's swing, Labrador, our Labrador.
   And mighty floods that long remained,
   Their raging fury unrestrained,
Shall serve the purpose God ordained, Labrador, our Labrador.

In 1931 the Newfoundland government under Sir Richard Squires again offered to sell Labrador to Canada, and again the offer failed. The shifting fortunes of Labrador account to some degree for the insecurity and anxiety expressed in Paddon's memoir as he concluded it in 1938.

Also in 1927, during a period of separation from the family, he developed a second plan for social reform: a "cottage sanatarium system" for the treatment of tuberculosis. Similar to his plan for boarding schools, which he envisioned as a chain of "cottage" residences instead of dormitories, he had in mind a chain of log houses with staff and patient quarters, each self-sufficient with goats, a supply of cod oil, chickens, gardens, and industrial work for the production of fishing nets, toys, needlework, and weaving. The HBC was expected to assist with the administration, and Paddon had found a generous New England donor to help finance it. Just as he got started in November, however he found himself a patient at St Anthony and had no choice but to abandon the medical service at North West River, leaving it in the hands of Kate Austen, his Australian nurse.

At St Anthony, Paddon was treated for the first of a series of illnesses brought on by years of sheer toil and exposure to his patients. This time he suffered excruciating pain from a shutdown of the kidneys which might have developed into a serious case of stones if it had not been caught in time. In November he confessed to his sister, "I am a lot better now, but the chemistry of the body, especially of the kidneys, has been all upset by 4 influenzal attacks (associated with severe exposure) in the last 12 months; and I still have to depend on medicine, & may have to do so for some time."[53] The sojourn at St Anthony gave him a chance to observe how the other arm of the Grenfell Mission was developing in Newfoundland, in contrast to his own sphere of influence. As he recuperated with the family in Stockbridge at Christmas, he had time to reflect on the hospital's overwhelmingly American style:

St. Anthony is an American colony. I spent 5 weeks there, and studied it from chimney tops to basement. The medical officers have been American there for over 20 years. Just as U.S.A. is nominally a Democracy but really an Oligarchy, so St. A. boasts 1/2 a million of real estate in an area where there is no more than 4 months' employment in the 12 for the great majority of the men & has rigid caste barriers. Further, after 37 years of work, not a single native holds any better position than an artisan's. While we are 20 years younger I have had 3 native members of staff in the last 2 years; & my whole policy is based on progress towards self-dependence. At St. Anthony, take away I.G.A. and the people must clear out or go on govt. relief. At N.W. River my ideal is to build up a local machinery, with the salaried jobs increasingly held by natives, which will eventually be able to "carry on" if death or age removed myself or any successor.[54]

Paddon's St Anthony sojourn reinforced what he already knew – that his vision was radically different from that of the IGA board and Dr Charles Curtis, the medical superintendent. He felt even more at odds with his colleagues.

As he entered his fifties, Paddon acknowledged his diminishing capacity for an itinerant practice and his impatience with the annual fundraising tours. He was no longer the thirty-year-old athlete newly arrived at Mud Lake. However, when his sister hinted at retirement, he replied, "I assure you, I love the wilderness life by far the best; but Sir W. is about played out, and I must do what my employers ask of me."[55] Only he or some other medical colleague could make the necessary connection between the work and the subscribers, most of whom resided in the United States, and although he did not possess Grenfell's rhetorical skills, he had developed his own style of communicating with audiences and knocking on corporate doors. He also acknowledged something he could no longer ignore – he was not staying up to date professionally. He had chosen the broader role of social reform in 1917 when he refused an offer to replace Dr John Mason Little as chief surgeon at St Anthony, and community development did not leave him much time to stay current. What he could do was farm and open up land for cultivation. In 1932 he wrote with some satisfaction,

Here, some 200 miles north of Belle Isle Straits, we have produced, this year, almost exactly three tons of potatoes; a quarter of a ton of cabbage; more than a quarter of a ton (nearer half) of beets and carrots: and hundredweights more of peas, Swiss chard, turnips, radishes, and rhubarb. Four tons is a conservative estimate of our garden produce for a single season while we still have but little well cultivated land. We can produce thousands of gallons of fresh milk annually; thousands of eggs; pork and (with experience in curing) bacon and ham. We have put up over half a ton of native berries; have simply eliminated canned fruit and imported jam from our requisitions. We have successfully preserved salmon, grouse and rabbits; and are experimenting with cod-fish, smelts, caplin, and some seal products. Apart from cereals, beverages, and condiments, we can and will live by the land and the waters. And this is "that God-forsaken wilderness" of ignoramuses and cynics.[56]

The farming program formed part of his vision for resisting nutritional diseases and relieving the starvation brought on by the Great Depression and the decline of the fishery. As Newfoundland slid closer to

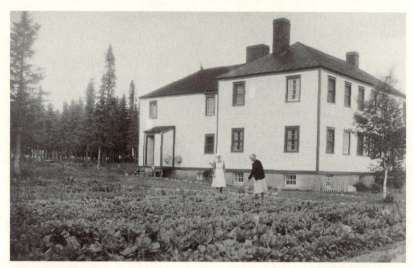

Hospital garden at North West River (Faculty of Medicine Founders' Archive, Memorial University)

financial ruin, he wrote to the colonial secretary with a proposal to consolidate communities. This proposal brought him directly in conflict with the HBC.

According to Ralph Parsons, the HBC fur trade commissioner, Paddon had devised a strategy to consolidate the coastal settlers in order to create an interest in farming and give access to food depots to be supplied by government and administered by the Grenfell Mission. Quoting W.O. Douglas, manager of the HBC fur farm at Muddy Bay during the period 1930 to 1932, Parsons claimed that Paddon "also had hopes of being appointed Commissioner for the Coast."[57] Such a plan was anathema to the HBC, who counted on trappers to remain close to their traditional fur paths. "You know that their natural occupation is hunting," Parsons wrote to the Roman Catholic missionary Father O'Brien, "and if you take them away from their present locations and trapping grounds, where they can at least obtain a few foxes in ordinary years, and assemble them in villages, where it is impossible to find work of a productive nature for them to do, the result I fear will be disastrous."[58] At this time the HBC had suffered losses for eight years, and Paddon's scheme would not have helped them recuperate. Parsons suggested instead that the HBC take responsibility for poor relief and predicted that it could do so at a considerably lower cost. Neither plan was attempted, for a few months later the British parliament appointed a commission with legislative and executive authority to govern Newfoundland, and early in 1934 these officials took office with wide-ranging powers, including responsibility for health and public charities.

In 1935 Grenfell retired as the mission's figurehead. For Paddon he had been a benevolent but erratic friend with whom he frequently differed. "He is a born autocrat, in a way," Paddon wrote to his sister, "although he likes and respects those who stand up to him. But he is a person of no settled policies, and of frequent changing impulses, and very impressionable."[59] What kind of leadership would emerge in Grenfell's absence? That summer a delegation of the IGA board held a series of meetings with the commissioners to clarify its area of jurisdiction under the new regime. Meeting at St John's, the two sides agreed on matters related to customs duties, education, home indus-tries, and health, but the IGA also wanted well-defined areas of respon-sibility; it sought government support for its schools as well as a reduction of its overall medical program, fearing it would run into debt. The income from its investments had declined as a result of a reduction in the value of currency. Donations had also fallen off.[60]

In effect the Commission of Government gave the IGA jurisdiction for medical work in Labrador from Blanc Sablon to Indian Harbour and for most of the northern peninsula of Newfoundland. For its part the IGA agreed to proceed as before but promised in addition to supply publications of the Department of Health to its institutions and submit its medical reports before it released them to newspapers and mission magazines.[61] By this means, while acknowledging the importance of the mission's work, the commission delicately brought the IGA hospi-tals under government control for the first time, and such changes made Paddon uneasy. Would he, senior in terms of service, supervise Charles Curtis, who had managed the clinical side? Or would Curtis, more advanced surgically, supervise Paddon, even though Curtis had seldom visited Labrador and had frowned upon the community devel-opment program? In the end it was Curtis who became executive officer of the IGA.

The Paddons turned to building a house after nearly twenty-five years of marriage, and their cottage reverted to the teachers of the Yale School. As they took up residence, further anxieties arose over the future of North West River. The Commission of Government, eager to develop a third pulp mill, gave Bowater-Lloyd, the British paper pro-ducers, the right to build a mill and township in Newfoundland and expected it to start operations by the end of December 1940. At the same time it promised to grant a timber licence covering three thousand acres of Labrador territory and an exemption from royalties until 1945.[62] Paddon was alarmed by the changes that might inevitably follow, changes brought home dramatically when his son Harry was

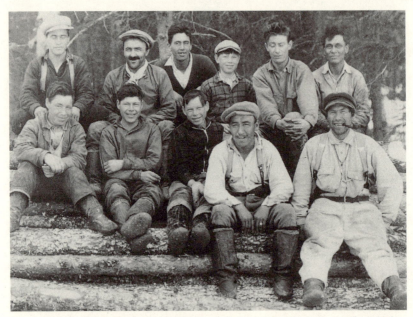

Woodcutters at North West River, 1935. *Back, left to right:* Frank Best, Judson Blake, Saul Seaward, Howard Blake, Isaac Rich, Bob Best; *front,* Irving Blake, Dick Blake, Tom Blake, Alvin Blake, Gilbert Blake (*Them Days* Archives)

engaged to help construct a base camp down the road from where he lived. Paddon wrote nervously to the relations in Britain in April 1938, "It was rather like listening to our death sentence, as we heard by Radio the Commissioner for Natural Resources, in St John's, reading out the general terms of the contract about to be signed ... If they are to supply their own medical and educational services, what need for us any longer?"[63] Fearing that a township might emerge in or near North West River, the Paddons considered leaving, even though Tony, who had entered medical school with the intention of relieving his father, would have had to alter his plans as well.

At length the government released Bowater-Lloyd from the agreement and provided for the expansion of the existing mill at Corner Brook; yet Paddon remained fixed on the possibility that his life's work would be wasted. During this period of uncertainty, he began his memoir, and the sense of impending change accounts to some degree for its polemical tone. He also expressed his anxieties privately to Grenfell, fearing that the board of the IGA and its executive director, Cecil Ashdown, might lease the mission property for the proposed townsite to help balance the shrinking budget. Lady Grenfell replied reassuringly,

Sir Wilfred and I feel very doubtful about leasing Northwest River property to Bowater, Lloyd & Company, and I know that Sir Wilfred has written strongly to Mr. Ashdown about it and has received Mr. Ashdown's assurance that nothing is settled. I don't think it has anything whatsoever to do with funds being raised in America or elsewhere. I don't see why that should make the slightest difference. I believe it is an attempt on the part of the Directors to lessen the budget, as they are finding it increasingly hard to raise the necessary maintenance funds now that Sir Wilfred is unable to lecture.[64]

But Paddon was not mollified, and he continued to speculate about where such a townsite might be located as well as what services it might provide for the employees. "Meanwhile," he wrote in the mission journal, "it remains to be seen where these invaders are going to settle, whom they are really going to employ, and how far they will replace the facilities we have offered."[65] He also let the Grenfells know about his plans for a book,[66] plans he had put aside in draft while he and Mina moved into their new house.

In the autumn of 1939 they left for the United States with the intention of holding a Christmas reunion in Pennsylvania, travelling together for the first time since their marriage. Tony would arrive from the Long Island College of Medicine, Dick from Trinity College, Hartford, and John from boarding school. (Harry remained in Labrador.) On the morning of 23 December, Paddon, Mina, and John left New Haven by train en route to Haverford, where they would stay in a house loaned by a Grenfell worker. But Paddon suddenly developed a chill with all the signs of impending shock. Thinking he had sustained another attack of influenza, he decided to complete the journey after Tony joined them at New York. As soon as he reached Haverford, a physician put him immediately in hospital, and even though everything possible was done to relieve him, he sank rapidly and passed away at 7 P.M. on Christmas Eve, suffering from diffuse peritonitis which had apparently arisen from an acute intestinal infection he did not have the strength to resist. At the time, there was no treatment for it.

The funeral took place at St Mary's Episcopal Church, Ardmore, on 28 December, followed by cremation.[67] Mina was inconsolable but steady. On Boxing Day she wrote the relations in England, "From now life will be a duty, not a joy."[68] Despite his own anguish, Tony insisted that he had much to uphold. "Ever since I have been old enough to think," he continued in his letter to Grenfell, "my heart has been utterly bound up with Labrador, and though my knowledge of it is yet very slight, I think my background will prove of great value. For it is my wish to carry on his work, as it was his wish that I should."

As these events unfolded and the IGA board again contemplated the future role of the North West River hospital, Curtis wrote to Ashdown to warn against closing it. Having visited North West River himself, he could appreciate what had been accomplished there and subsequently recommended reducing it to a nursing station with Mina in charge, at least until the war was over. "As I have written to you many times before," he said, "we cannot abandon this station and we must keep the agriculture and child welfare work going, and I know Mrs. Paddon is a very good executive."[69] Mina ran the station for the remainder of the war and for her accomplishments was made an officer of the Order of the British Empire. Tony enlisted in the Royal Canadian Naval Volunteer Reserve as a medical officer. Upon his release, he returned to his father's hospital and remained there until he himself retired in 1977, completing a combined practice of sixty-five years. From 1981 to 1986 he held office as lieutenant-governor of Newfoundland with jurisdiction in Labrador, where his father had struggled to attract government attention of the most basic kind. In 2001 the Parliament of Canada made a constitutional change adding the word *Labrador* to the name of the province.

PUBLIC HEALTH CONDITIONS

What were the principal threats to public health in Labrador during Dr Harry Paddon's tenure, and how did the Grenfell Mission respond to them? Statistics published by the Newfoundland government suggest that when Paddon arrived in 1912, the colony was experiencing a public health crisis of unprecedented proportions. The report of the Commission on Public Health, published the same year, showed that while infant mortality produced the highest death rate (roughly fifteen in every hundred births), the gravest potential threat was presented by pulmonary tuberculosis, which existed at a rate twice as high as in the British Isles.[70] Between the ages of twenty and forty-five, two-thirds of all deaths in Newfoundland were attributable directly to this single manifestation of the disease, such that broad measures for its control were set forth in the Tuberculosis Act of 1912. By the 1930s the threat of TB had acquired the urgency of a plague, and the language of the Health and Public Welfare Act of 1931 projected the kind of fear and paranoia associated with plagues before and since.

Historically, plagues have been regarded not just as scourges of societies but as judgments, health being associated with order and self-control, disease with poverty and depravity. As Susan Sontag has observed, TB has been associated with poverty and deprivation, with "thin garments, thin bodies, unheated rooms, poor hygiene, inadequate food,"[71] and thus the victim is twice victimized. It is not surprising, therefore, that the Newfoundland act not only called for a tuberculosis public service but detailed stringent measures for the treatment of individuals. It required every medical practitioner to report the names of the infected and made the failure to do so an offence. Physicians were also required to notify public authorities within twenty-four hours if an infected person vacated living quarters, so that those quarters could be disinfected. And as for the infected themselves, it became an offence to spit or secrete bodily fluids that might endanger the lives of others. No consumptive was permitted to handle food in the workplace, and infected children were forbidden to attend school. Not surprisingly, people in Labrador were reluctant to come forward to be treated, and Newfoundland fishermen, whose livelihood depended on a share of the catch, refused to go home once they were diagnosed.

Tuberculosis occurs most frequently in the lungs. But it may also occur in the intestinal tract, the lymphatic glands, the bones, the joints, the skin, and the brain, enveloping the whole person to such an extent that all the body's organs degenerate and the patient literally wastes away from long, chronic illness. For this reason it was known popularly in the first half of the twentieth century as "consumption" or "white plague." The cases discovered by Dr Paddon usually had been infected through proximity in crowded housing conditions or in close quarters aboard fishing vessels. Those with lowered defences from malnutrition also succumbed. Since no antibiotic for TB was available in Newfoundland until the late 1940s, the orthodox treatment, wherever possible, was to install patients in a temporary outdoor lean-to (p. 31) or send them home for bed rest and ample food. That is why Paddon insisted on sending otherwise productive members of fishing crews back to Newfoundland and, where there was no alternative, amputated tubercular limbs, making it difficult for trappers and fishermen to work. A broader strategy, one with no clear results, involved programs for the improvement of social conditions as well as aggressive public education – the insistence on personal hygiene, household cleanliness, and attention to diet.

Before the arrival of streptomycin, one other treatment of TB was linked to a belief in the efficacy of cod-liver oil, both as a topical application and a dietary supplement. It must be remembered that the benefits of cod oil had been widely accepted since the 1840s and that Newfoundland had produced it for export early in its therapeutic history. The London physician Arthur Leared wrote in 1855, "The utility of Cod-liver oil in a great variety of diseases is now so fully established, that the mode of its administration is a point of corresponding interest."[72] The beginning of the Vitamin Age added impetus to belief in the benefits of cod oil when it was shown that it contained the fat-soluble vitamin A. By the 1930s, with its status assured, further interest was shown in its use as a preparation for wounds, particularly tuberculous lesions. Paddon followed the discussion in the *British Medical Journal*, including a leading article on 16 May 1931 that laid to rest any doubts about the inferiority of Newfoundland cod oil for the treatment of TB and rickets. At one point he conducted a modest experiment with one of his own patients (p. 235).

The second medical preoccupation in both Newfoundland and Labrador was what Paddon calls "nutritional disease," particularly beri-beri, a phenomenon familiar to physicians in rice-eating cultures such as Indonesia, where it received its name, but not to physicians in the north. Beginning with a loss of feeling in the legs, the onset of beri-beri produced swelling in the lower half of the body and sometimes heart failure. Normally, only severe cases were admitted to hospital: that is, those involving paralysis of the limbs or dilation of the heart. Otherwise, the symptoms might be so widespread as not to be linked to beri-beri at all. For example, in Newfoundland and Labrador, the seasonal syndrome known to physicians as "Newfoundland stomach," characterized by prolonged constipation, irritability, indigestion, itching and burning sensations, and general lassitude, was also caused by vitamin deficiency, not by severe beri-beri. Indeed, the first case of beri-beri recorded in the northern colonies, detected by Dr Cluny Macpherson in 1903 or 1904 at the Battle Harbour hospital, was so rare that Grenfell dismissed the diagnosis as absurd. However he rapidly came to the same conclusion when presented with the evidence.[73] During Paddon's medical training, his textbook had attributed beri-beri to "bacilli" and recommended removal of the patient to an uninfected locality (p. 14). Just as Paddon was seeing cases of it himself, researchers discovered that it stemmed not from infection but from a deficiency of thiamin (vitamin B_1), a nutrient required at a level of only one part in a million parts of diet if all other nutrients were present. Surrounded by so much of it, the Grenfell Mission began a long campaign to study the causes and develop a plan of action.

Paddon claims that Dr John Mason Little, during his tenure at the St Anthony hospital (p. 14), laid the groundwork for research with a paper published in the *Journal of the American Medical Association* in 1912. Little found that at certain times of the year, when the diet was reduced to white bread and tea, beri-beri appeared in northern Newfoundland and Labrador – in other words, if white flour were substituted for rice, the same conditions prevailed, as manifested in symptoms such as night blindness, urine retention, tingling feelings, or numbness. Once the diet changed, these symptoms quickly disappeared. But if a further malady such as a cold were added, the symptoms advanced rapidly. "There are many isolated communities in which the diet is restricted and in which tuberculosis is rife, to which education for the prevention of tuberculosis is being brought,"[74] Little observed. It would be a simple matter, he thought, to add to the information distributed about TB some further advice advocating the vitamin benefits of whole-wheat flour. Public education was part of the solution.

In 1914 Little wrote more extensively in the same journal, basing his conclusions on experiments conducted at the Harvard Medical School with Richard Ohler. Ohler had discovered that chickens fed on a diet of white bread developed a staggering gait and died of paralysis, just as they did in the winter in northern Newfoundland and in Labrador. "Although in recent text-books beriberi is still classed among the infectious diseases, the infectious theory of the disease has been given up," he reported.[75] Of five thousand out-patients at the St Anthony hospital, Little listed 220 cases of beri-beri, including six deaths from heart failure. With such a high incidence the Grenfell Mission required a broader policy for its treatment, and in September 1915 Little held a small symposium aboard the hospital vessel *Strathcona* at St Mary's River, Labrador, attended by Grenfell, Dr John Grieve, Dr Beeckman Delatour, and Paddon. Little read both papers and set out a strategy for the treatment of malnutrition, including nutrition surveys, laboratory work, and the encouragement of kitchen gardens.[76]

One of the first to confirm Little's analysis was Dr V.B. Appleton, an instructor in pediatrics at the University of California. Appleton spent the autumn, winter, and early summer of 1919–20 on the Labrador side of the Strait of Belle Isle to examine the diet and the incidence of dietary disease. For comparison he made a similar study in June 1920 on the Newfoundland side. In Labrador he found only isolated cases of beri-beri, while in Newfoundland there were over a hundred and as many cases of xerophthalmia, an affliction incorporating a range of signs produced by vitamin A deficiency. The difference in diet was slight but significant: even though the Newfoundland subjects were more prosperous, they had no canned milk or vegetables, and their supply of fresh fish stopped two months earlier.[77] Even slight variations in diet brought about by seasonal habits could produce different deficiencies. Consequently, during the summers from 1920 to 1924, nearly thirty nutritionists under the direction of Dr William Emerson, founder of the nutrition class movement in Boston, were brought north from colleges in the United States. Two nutritionists remained full time throughout the winter as part of the mission's new "child welfare department" created by Marion Moseley in 1923.[78] The following year Moseley turned it over to Elizabeth Criswell, who remained until 1928, when the initiative was terminated and Criswell turned her attention to public education at North West River. She remained at the North West River school until 1932.

Further research on nutrition was carried out by Dr W.R. Aykroyd, an Irishman who first became interested in deficiency diseases as a house surgeon at the General Hospital in St John's. In 1928 Aykroyd published a paper on vitamin A deficiency in Newfoundland with particular attention to night blindness, then regarded as the most common consequence, and treated it with cod liver oil. Little had regarded night blindness as an early sign of beri-beri, but Aykroyd found that it could occur in otherwise sound individuals. "During the next few years," he jested, "an attempt will be made to prove every disease of unknown origin a vitamin deficiency."[79] In the winter of 1928–29, Aykroyd, who became a nutritionist, went to St Anthony to study cases of beri-beri he expected to appear the following spring, and his article in the *Journal of Hygiene*, based on an examination of patient records for the period of 1912 to 1928, was the most extensive study to date. Most cases of beri-beri, he confirmed, were admitted in April, May, and June after winter supplies had run out, and it was he who first suggested that they were directly associated with poverty, not necessarily with diet: "The association between beriberi and poverty is so close, that, in examining a suspected case of beriberi, a very useful short-circuiting question is to ask whether the patient was successful at the previous year's fishing."[80] For beri-beri to appear amongst a population on a diet of white flour, he maintained, the supply of other ancillary foodstuffs had to fall below the lowest European standards. And since the Grenfell Mission's advocacy of whole-grain flour over the previous fifteen years had produced no effect, he recommended that the solution lay not in altering entrenched habits but encouraging vegetable gardens and livestock – even to the extent of giving the poorest families their own livestock, seeds, and farming implements at government expense.

As Aykroyd finished at St Anthony in 1929, Helen Mitchell, director of nutrition research at the Battle Creek Sanitarium, and her assistant, Margery Vaughn, arrived for eight weeks to conduct a nutritional survey on both sides of the Strait of Belle Isle. What they found startled them. Of the fifty dietaries collected in twelve communities, the fare available to most families consisted of a barrel of white flour a year for each adult, molasses, salt pork, salt beef, butterine or oleomargarine, beans and peas, and a generous amount of salt cod and tea. The nutritive shortages were most apparent in minerals and vitamins, and clearly local gardens were needed. The nutritionists were also surprised by the lack of clinical evidence of disease but detected more subtle signs, "an ill-defined lack of 'pep' and ambition, chronic under-nutrition, and a low resistance to various diseases such as tuberculosis, all of which may be due to the poor food eaten."[81] As a result of this survey Vaughn was stationed at Flowers Cove, Newfoundland, during 1930–31 to encourage gardening and dietary reform through baby shows, cooking demonstrations, health talks, and good-teeth campaigns. By this time the Grenfell Mission had taken more serious steps to encourage agriculture, and Grenfell had engaged the services of Professor Fred Sears of the Massachusetts Agricultural College, who made annual visits beginning in 1928. "To receive personal visits from such an authority, who showed a strong and sympathetic interest in individual struggles with soil and parasites, lent undoubted encouragement to many who needed it" (p. 236), Paddon observes.

During the period embraced by the Paddon memoir, the mission promoted one further study with broader implications when in September 1939 it made its records and its patients available to David Steven and George Wald of Harvard University. Once again, night blindness, an affliction widespread within the general population of Europe and the United States, was the subject, and the scientists were looking for a connection to vitamin A deficiency. This study involved two groups of schoolchildren between the ages of six and seventeen, one group of fifty from the Grenfell orphanage who received two and a half times the normal dosage of cod liver oil and a second group of seventy-eight from the Grenfell school, who received no vitamin supplement at all. This comparison revealed no significant differences, for the visual thresholds of the two were close, corresponding to normal results obtained elsewhere. Another group of 280 subjects from the general population was also tested, including eighty-eight patients undergoing treatment for nutritional deficiency and seventeen with beri-beri. For these, the application of brewer's yeast (containing thiamine) made no difference to their adaptability to light. This experiment confirmed the link with social conditions already made by Aykroyd.

Although so much attention is given to the lingering problems of tuberculosis and malnutrition in Dr Paddon's memoir, none of the effects is presented as dramatically as the onset of the Spanish Flu in 1918–19. On 31 October 1918 the HBC post manager at North West River wrote in his journal, "Almost all of the people in N.W. River are stricken with a sickness which is supposed to be Spanish Influenza. John Blake, Sr., is dying and also John Bird's little girl has been sick these five days. Abe & Mrs. Ewing have been sick but are over it." Nearly three weeks later he added, "Allen Goudie & Judson Blake arrived from Mud Lake today & brought the news that John & Donald Michelin's wifes had died during the past week and also that the whole of the people of Mud Lake were stricken down with the same sickness as was here."[82] Then came what Paddon calls "a long, wild nightmare" (p. 159), one that fell short of a complete disaster only because some of the medical staff, including Mina Paddon, were not infected.

It came without warning, a strain of influenza so lethal that a victim could die within hours. As Paddon shows, it manifested itself at first through high fever, shivers, coughs, muscular pain, and sore throat, the normal symptoms of the flu. Then patients would rapidly develop dizzy spells, indifference to food or drink, and breathing difficulties. The body haemorrhaged, the lungs filled, and patients drowned in their own fluids. In less than twelve months, three waves appeared around the world. During the first wave, in the spring of 1918, mortality was not unusually high. But the second, the one that hit Labrador in the autumn, was one of the most devastating of any disease in recorded history. It followed the trade routes and shipping lanes across the globe, and the rapid movement of armies during the Great War hastened its transmission from one continent to another. By the time it exhausted itself, it had infected as much as half the world's population, not distinguishing between young or old, rich or poor, healthy or sound.[83] It was especially devastating for families welcoming sons home from the battlefields of Europe, for these men innocently brought the virus with them and killed their own relatives. (It touched the president of the United States, Woodrow Wilson, who was negotiating the peace in Paris in the spring of 1919.[84]) In Labrador, many of the young and healthy were fortunate enough to be away at their traps, but they returned to discover whole families and sometimes whole communities wiped out. Approximately one-third of the Inuit population was lost.

HARRY PADDON'S MEMOIR

From these details, one may see why Dr Paddon's memoir should not be read as conventional autobiography – as life history that somehow defines the writer – but as a narrative of northern adventure experienced by an itinerant doctor going about his district in challenging circumstances. Read this way, it resembles northern memoirs such as Peter Freuchen's *Arctic Adventure: My Life in the Frozen North* (1935), which was available at the time of writing and may have served as a model. In the opening pages, Paddon appears before us as an innocent abroad, victimized by an unscrupulous travel agent. However, once installed in Labrador he becomes our interlocutor, ready to discourse on such varied topics as the plight of the aboriginal, the behaviour of the sled dog, the construction of the komatik (or sled), the voraciousness of the black fly, the failure of government, the dishonesty of the merchant, and, of course, the prevalence of disease. Strange and exciting events give rise to dramatic episodes: storms, frosts, thaws, disasters, drownings, accidents with firearms, cases of madness, escapes and close calls, mysterious phenomena and unwelcome apparitions, plagues and pestilences. Beneath all this runs an *apologia* for Labrador at time when its future is cast in doubt.

We might wish that Paddon had been less self-effacing in these pages and more candid on personal topics such as married life or changes in religious outlook; but such a reading assumes that he is the subject, not Labrador. Instead of revealing to us his inner life, Paddon represents himself as an agent of change in a territory disparaged by observers and ignored by successive Newfoundland governments. This kind of self-writing falls within the broad domain of the memoir, as a literary form that concentrates not so much on the author as on the events and circumstances the author considers extraordinary or important for his or her own purposes. The memoirist is a participant with a moral vision, one who revives the past, sometimes inaccurately, to create an impression or advance an argument. The value of the work, then, lies in its representation of a world physically remote from our own or inaccessible because of its political or social exclusivity. "The memoir is never a presentation of history," writes Marcus Billson; "it is a representation of history, sometimes an argument, always a personal interpretation."[85] Thus, unlike autobiographers, who reconstruct their lives out of a sense of personal accomplishment, memoirists acquire significance from their imagined role in a field outside their lives.

Yet the impulse to write does require a sense of history, for the memoirist knows the past is unrepeatable and that there is a responsibility to interpret it lest it be forgotten or misunderstood. Regardless of how events might have actually occurred, they must be charged with excitement, selected for their dramatic quality. As an organizing principle of this memoir, Dr Paddon has chosen the trope of construction, and each episode contributes to the perceived pattern of his career as builder. Part 1, "Survey," describes his arrival in Labrador, the early pioneer years divided between Indian Harbour and Mud Lake, and the outbreak of the Great War. Part 2, "Foundations," relates his efforts to build a hospital at North West River and the founding of the Labrador boarding schools. Part 3, "Construction," outlines his strategy for child welfare and the beginnings of his agricultural schemes. At the conclusion, Paddon is no longer an innocent abroad but a seasoned Labradorman, eager to show that despite physical challenges and disappointments, much can be accomplished.

Memoirs, especially political ones, are also written out of a sense of public crisis. The stability of a community or a nation appears threatened. The future looks bleak. A people or a culture may be perceived to be passing away, and its passing is lent significance because of some apocalypse the memoirist anticipates over the horizon. As Dr Paddon proceeds up Lake Melville for the first time in 1912, we hear the first note of impending crisis: "When would Labrador's day come, and could the local people be prepared to play a worthy part in the development of their country instead of seeing it exploited at their expense?" (p. 26). Although he probably did not ask such a question at the time, he inserts it here, writing within the circumstances of the 1930s, when Labrador figured as a "wild card" in Newfoundland's negotiations with Canada prior to the imposition of commission government.[86] As a region ready for industrial development, it seemed open to whatever scheme the Commission of Government could contrive once it assumed power in St John's.

Despite his years of service, Paddon possessed limited power to influence events. Had he lived another year, he would have witnessed at Goose Bay the construction of an international airport bringing wage labour and industrial values to Lake Melville for the first time. Representing Labrador at the National Convention in 1946, the Reverend Lester Burry, United Church minister at North West River, was summoned to offer advice to the British parliament on what form of government Newfoundland should pursue. Had Paddon lived another ten years, he would have witnessed the electoral representation he so earnestly sought as well as numerous industrial and political developments that altered the face of his beloved Labrador forever. In his preface he writes, "I can only hope that this manuscript, if it achieves publication, may reach at least some with kindred tastes or interests" (p. 4). After sixty-five years, it now has the opportunity to do so.

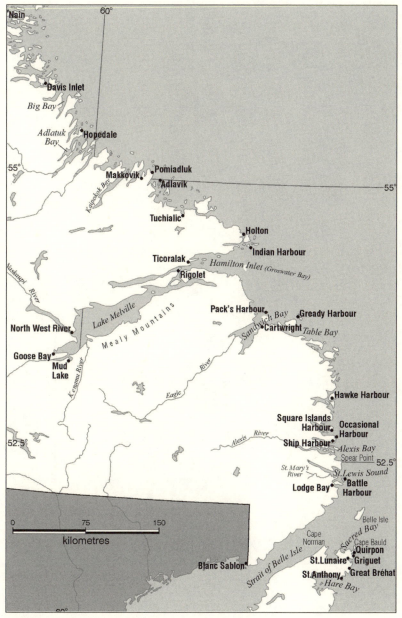

Labrador coast

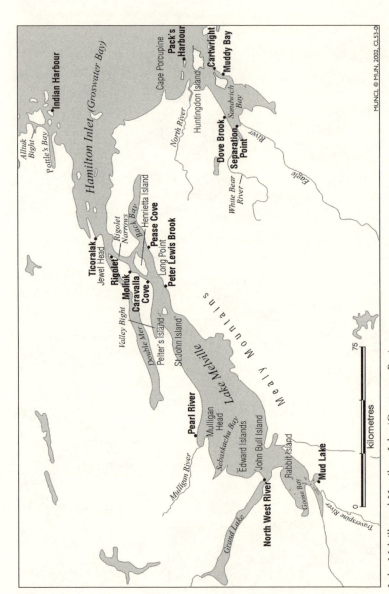

Lake Melville and Hamilton Inlet (Groswater Bay)

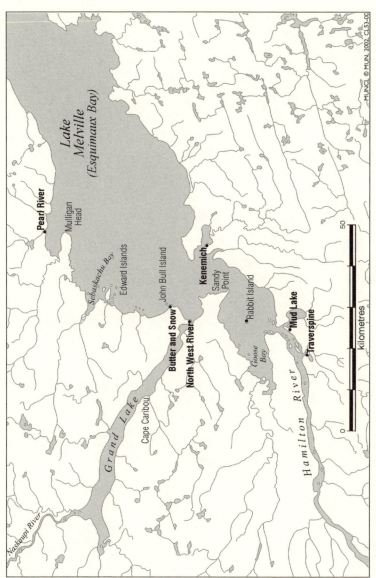

North West River and vicinity

THE LABRADOR MEMOIR OF
DR HARRY PADDON, 1912–1938

Preface

The purpose of this book is first to portray something of the interest, the adventure, the pathos, and, thank Heaven, the humour of frontier medical practice during a quarter of a century in sub-arctic Labrador, with its small, scattered and mixed population; secondly, to put on record something at least of the Labrador that has been but which is even now about to disappear to a great extent before the relentless advance of Big Industry. At the outset I would make it clear that I have no wish to suppress or camouflage the fact that for over twenty-five years I have worked as a member of Sir Wilfred Grenfell's medical mission staff or that it is to him, my superintendent and friend, that I owe much of what my career has meant to me. None the less, what follows is not planned to be a "missionary book" for very definite reasons.

In the first place Sir Wilfred himself, as is very right and proper, has presented that theme in the autobiography *A Labrador Doctor*, and it is at least not my intention to be guilty either of poor plagiarism or vain repetition; and in the second place, while I lack his justification for attempting an autobiography, there was naturally no room in such a work for much that I would try to perpetuate. It has seemed to others besides myself that there might be room for a work which, besides including the two main themes mentioned above, should also offset to some extent the impressions conveyed in such derogatory catchphrases as "the land that God gave to Cain" or "a god-forsaken wilderness, unfit for human habitation," or again, "a land of cod, dog, and fog," and set down the other side of the story, which stands out in such vivid contrast and is far more true than these superficial witticisms or pessimisms so freely applied to Labrador in print.

The mission field, like every other aspect of human association, has included good, bad, and indifferent: leaders and followers, athletes, adventurers, organisers, and administrators of a high order. It is only necessary to mention, in alphabetical order, such names as Gordon,[1] Sir Wilfred Grenfell, Sir Henry Holland,[2] Dr Albert Schweitzer[3] – at once doctor of divinity, philosophy, music, and medicine – and C.T. Studd,[4] to make this point convincingly. Such men have gone ahead of governments and trading adventurers and often ahead of explorers of note to bring onto the map remote corners of the earth, and the quest has satisfied aspirations other than religious.

I believe in God, despite problems of pain, and I believe in man, despite war and strikes and intolerance of every kind. I hold that the trinity of faith, hope, and love has done far more for humanity than the triple alliance of gas, guns, and tyranny; and I see more hope for civilisation in the application of the Golden Rule than in treaties, whether vengefully imposed or dishonourably violated. But I am also devoted to the sea and boats, to human contacts in other walks of life than that in which I was brought up, to beauties of nature and to animals and to social aspects of medicine outside of the operating room, ward, or laboratory. I can only hope that this manuscript, if it achieves publication, may reach at least some with kindred tastes or interests.

When I first saw its rugged, surf-beaten, and ice-rubbed shores in 1912, Labrador was perhaps the least known as well as the most thinly populated of British dependencies. Its chief contributions to the world's markets were uncertain quantities of salted cod-fish, also salted salmon and trout, seal and whale oil, and raw fur. Not even were its geographical boundaries clearly defined, which alone was a fatal bar to honest commercial enterprise. Its people were unrepresented though taxed (in customs duties at least) – a state of affairs unknown, I believe, anywhere else in the British Empire. Its inhabitants were entirely dependent on missionary enterprise for educational facilities and almost entirely so [for] medical service, the only exception being a single doctor who travelled on the Labrador mail steamer during the open water season. Moreover, a large proportion of this man's time was spent on board between St John's and the Labrador coast, with no opportunity of service, and even this appointment was not regularly filled.

In 1938 a great transformation is already in progress. First and foremost, the boundary line was definitely settled in 1927. Secondly, a chilled salmon industry has largely replaced the salted, with better remuneration to the catcher, at less cost in time and preliminary outlay.[5] Potentially important developments in the cod fishery are still perhaps in the experimental stage. A great herring industry for the manufacture of both oil and chicken meal is on the eve of birth.

In other directions the great timber reserves are at last being tapped, the mineral resources are being intensively investigated, immense water powers have been surveyed with a view to possible harnessing; and the possibilities of domestic reindeer herding, successfully accomplished in Alaska and widely copied later in Canada, are also under consideration. A great meat belt north of the wheat belt may yet extend across the great moss tundras on the northern limits of timber lands from the Pacific to the Atlantic, including Labrador. Almost in a night this "God-forsaken wilderness, unfit for human habitation" has become a Land of Promise, beckoning to Capital and challenging adventure. But where China's millions absorb invaders, Labrador's few thousands must be swamped by any considerable influx of population, and before the woodsman's axe and the miner's blasting, the face of primaeval nature will be made unrecognisable. Is that which has been to be buried in complete oblivion? Has the inside story of a country newly come onto the map no interest for the public of the bigger communities which are going to share in its resources?

In covering over 25,000 miles by dog-team and probably twice as much in small craft, varying from a thirty-foot open motor boat to a forty-ton crude oil-burner or a hundred-foot steamer, I have naturally seen deeply beneath the surface. The results of the contacts between the two native races and the invading whites, with all their implications, have been vividly driven home to me. And having read the publications of pioneer missionaries, explorers, ethnologists, botanists, ornithologists, and geologists, I would fain attempt the addition of the family doctor and long-time resident to the scanty bibliography of Labrador. In making this attempt, my one regret is for what must be omitted, for so much and so many that have loomed large in my horizon must be relegated to the background and either omitted or but casually mentioned – my superintendent and friend, my colleagues – of attainments and achievements greater than mine; shorter-service workers and many volunteer helpers; friends of the best that ever a man had, whose faith and works and bounty have counted for so much in anything worthwhile that has been accomplished. To these (and they are many) I can but pay this brief impersonal tribute and assure them that if unnamed or but briefly mentioned, they are by no means forgotten.

Harry L. Paddon

PART ONE

Survey

I

From London to Labrador
via Newfoundland

It was a bright June day of 1912 as SS *Tunisian*[6] cleared the tortuous channel that affords access to the Mersey and Liverpool and emerged into the Irish Channel, outward bound for Quebec and Montreal. Behind was England and all that England had meant for nearly thirty years – home and preparatory school, Repton and Oxford, St Thomas's Hospital in London, and finally fifteen months as house surgeon, then medical officer at the Guest Hospital, Dudley, in the Black Country [industrial Midlands]. "Slumming" in London during university vacations and a series of holidays out among the North Sea trawlermen as a relaxation from the hospital grind had afforded contacts with those in other walks of life which were not without value.

And now, with the above background, I was embarking on a chosen but still rather nebulous career in Labrador, the least known perhaps of British dependencies, a career that had been determined by a single hour's contact at the impressionable age of sixteen with a magnetic personality [Wilfred Grenfell]. How far was the long preparation to prove an asset in what lay ahead? And what defects, revealed by the acid test of practical experience when standing on one's own feet, were later to be regretted? On board were 350 young emigrants from Dr Barnardo's homes about to become budding citizens of Canada, fellow adventurers whose future was even more of a mystery than mine, though it concerned them less at the moment.[7]

To embark for St John's, Newfoundland, via Quebec may well seem a needlessly circuitous route to take, as indeed it was, and it was accidental rather than designed. North Sea wanderings had resulted in a preference for small vessels and a small group when at sea, and this preference had led me to seek passage on a two-thousand-ton tramp steamer. Unversed in the ways of tramp steamers, it had come [to me] as an unpleasant shock when her announced sailing was postdated eleven days. As there was no direct passenger steamer sailing for St John's in the immediate future, my impatience and inexperience had made me a ready prey for a passenger agent with a flair for extemporised fiction. With glib words and graceful gestures this gentleman assured me that there would be no difficulty at all about leaving the *Tunisian* at Rimouski, where the St Lawrence pilot came aboard, and in a moment of unholy inspiration he added that communications between Rimouski and St John's were easy and frequent. I accepted his assurance and he my passage money, and I was committed to 3,000 miles of extra travel, which eventually landed me in St John's a few hours later than the next passenger boat from Liverpool would have done and also just missed my connection at St John's. But by the time that the cup of disillusionment was drained, the agent was at a very safe distance, and there was nothing to be done about it. Experience is proverbially a costly commodity. While *Tunisian* was no modern ocean greyhound or leviathan, her movements seemed lethargic to one used to the lively kick of trawlers, and the chief thrill of the voyage was my first sight of a big iceberg somewhere off the southern coast of Newfoundland.

Any student of history, however humble, especially if his studies were subsidised by a perusal of Gilbert Parker's *Seats of the Mighty*,[8] could get some interest from a visit to the historic city of Quebec, but my time there was limited to a few hours. The magnificent situation of the Hôtel Chateau Frontenac, as well as the panorama seen from its windows, the Heights of Abraham and the Montmorency Falls, were fleeting impressions. Neither Wolfe nor Montcalm had a chance for a midnight appearance, nor was there even time or inclination to recite Gray's "Elegy."[9] Nor did two nights and one day in a train on the Intercolonial Railway[10] leave the traveller much of an authority on the maritime provinces of Canada, though some spice of rather doubtful flavour was added to this stage of the journey by running short of funds in a strange country with not a single acquaintance to turn to, which caused further reflections on imaginative passenger agents. A choice between a sleeping berth for the second night or breakfast on arrival at Sydney, Nova Scotia, was settled in favour of the latter, as it is proverbially best to face trouble on a full stomach, so I broke my fast royally and set out to get money or take the consequences. My nearest funds were in the Bank of Montreal at St John's, and it was a relief to find a branch of that institution in Sydney. A telegraphic communication with St John's soon replenished the pocket book.

A sweltering day in Sydney was made more tolerable by a leisurely swim, and that evening I embarked in SS *Bruce*,[11] of something over one thousand tons, for a night run across the ninety-mile Cabot Strait. Next morning we landed in Port aux Basques and after the usual customs formalities set out [aboard the Reid Newfoundland Railway] on a thirty-hour run across Newfoundland.[12] Here, at last, one had time and opportunity to feel really abroad and to assimilate worthwhile impressions of new surroundings, and the trip across Newfoundland had both interest and charm. For the first seven hours the track follows the west coast as far as physical features allow. Then, skirting the lovely Bay of Islands, it takes a plunge from Humbermouth right into the heart of the country. The basin of the Humber River is well wooded, and since 1912 the International Paper Company has wrought great changes in this region with their big pulp mill and power plant at Corner Brook and their extensive logging operations.[13]

It was verily a case of up hill and down dale. At times, as we climbed, the attainment of the summit by the labouring engine seemed open to doubt. Again, as we careered down hill with a gay abandon, the derailing of the train from its narrow-gauge track seemed to be at least a possibility. Anon, as we traversed great mossy tundras, there was an instinct to look for a herd of wild caribou fleeing from the invading train. More timber varied the scene at times, chiefly spruce, fir, birch, or larch, and low mountain peaks supplied a canvas for the afterglow of the setting sun. We skirted great lakes, island-studded, and followed or crossed streams that made any angler long to cast a fly into their pools. When night came, it brought at once a sense of regret and of relief – of regret that so fascinating a moving picture should be interrupted and relief at an interval in such a series of new impressions. The "lure of the Labrador" was still an untested catchphrase,[14] but the spell of Newfoundland was already a reality.

The night was short-lived, and the new day found us skirting the east coast. The forests around the Exploits River were already being worked, and the Grand Falls of Newfoundland – to be distinguished from the far greater falls of that name in Labrador – were already harnessed: cargo after cargo of paper for newsprint was going across the Atlantic for the Northcliffe Press in England. Bonavista and Trinity Bays each had their beauties, and Conception Bay contains Bell Island with its great iron mine. (Bell Island must be distinguished from Belle Isle, which guards the straits of that name at Newfoundland's northern extremity.) Crossing the narrow isthmus which unites the Avalon

Peninsula to the rest of Newfoundland, we had a view of Placentia Bay, which indents the south coast, and crossing the Avalon Peninsula, reached the capital city of St John's about noon, only to learn that ss *Prospero*[15] had sailed that very morning for northern Newfoundland and southern Labrador.

The hospitality of St John's is proverbial, and I have experienced it on several subsequent visits, but at the time referred to I knew no one there and was chiefly concerned to get to my journey's end. My predicament was shared by two fellow passengers on the ss *Bruce* and on the train, a nurse and a medical student from the United States who were both bound north in search of new experience and adventure as volunteer workers for the summer in Labrador.[16] We were informed that the choice lay between a rather indefinite stay of anything up to a week in a St John's hotel or an attempt to head off *Prospero* at Exploits, at the mouth of the river above referred to. To do this we must leave by train again that same afternoon, change at Notre Dame Junction shortly before midnight and take a branch line train to Lewisporte, where we must join a steamer, ss *Clyde*,[17] which would carry us to Exploits. It all sounded rather speculative, but again impatience won, so that our stay in St John's was limited to about four hours.

The chief features that attract the notice of a visitor to St John's are the magnificent landlocked harbour, somewhat flask-shaped with the narrow neck bent on the body at almost a right angle. The narrow portal is impressive, with Signal Hill frowning down on the side and another considerable eminence across the channel, a veritable marine gulch. Even this channel is further narrowed by a reef with a light on it. The land around the harbour, while less precipitous, is very steep, the roads ascending to the crest zig-zag fashion, while there are short cuts for pedestrians by steep flights of steps. The buildings, largely of timber construction, seem to strain towards the summit from which government buildings of grey stone look authoritatively downwards. The environment is picturesque, consisting of undulating hills, woodlands and small lakes or ponds, with many country houses. Four o'clock that afternoon saw us once more on our travels, and the next three days and nights were a mixture of nightmare and a Mad Hatter's tea party[18] in which the majority of the guests were always moving on without getting much satisfaction.[19]

Notre Dame Junction, Lewisporte, and ss *Clyde* ran to schedule, merely depriving us of a night's sleep between them, but at Exploits the elusive *Prospero* had once more slipped us. More kindly optimists appeared and rushed us aboard a half-decked launch almost before we could get our breath, pointing out that *Prospero* had many ports of call and we were almost bound to overtake her. Unfortunately, Neptune had something to say to that and staged a hard westerly wind and rough sea. So long as we kept well under the land, all was well, but when it became clear that only a short cut across Green Bay would enable us to overhaul our quarry, it was a question if our little craft could live. The captain of the *Clyde*, dodging from port to port behind us, thought not. "If they keep that course, that's the last of them," was his grim comment when he saw us putting out from under the land. However, we were not bent on suicide. When heavy water began to come aboard and the engine to complain of an undue admixture of brine with gasolene, we scurried back shorewards. As there was nothing else to do, we rejoined *Clyde*. When she reached her turning point at Tilt Cove, *Prospero* was out of sight, and we found ourselves still about a hundred miles from St Anthony, which was our first objective, in a village with no hotel but a disused copper mine. However, we found a friend-in-need in the local doctor. He had a small, decked power boat in which he visited his far-flung patients. He could not charter her for a two-hundred-mile round trip which might prove to be of indefinite duration, but he did tell us of a decked boat which might be hired from La Scie, a village five miles away but accessible by telegraph. And when an affirmative reply came, he kindly offered to send us out in his boat to join the other in sheltered waters, which would save valuable time. Needless to say, we thankfully accepted.

Our new liner proved to be a tubby thirty- to thirty-five foot craft with a single-cylinder engine, which was innocent of any silencer and did its work amid a series of deafening explosions. Her crew consisted of an ancient mariner who looked as if he had just buried his last friend and another cheery optimist who united the functions of engineer and cook and who assured us there was "lots of grub aboard." He drew roseate visions of a fifteen-hour run on a perfect night with St Anthony in sight on the following forenoon. Little did he know of the absorbent capacity of my two fellow passengers, lately reduced to a similitude of two volcanoes in full eruption on the stormy waters of Green Bay, with two aching voids to fill at the first safe opportunity. Nor did he anticipate the in-wind, dense fog, and heavy drift ice which all materialised within three hours of his rash prophecy. We fled incontinently into the nearest harbour. Next morning we dodged ice for a few brief miles in fog, wind, and rain, ere seeking shelter in the landlocked haven of Fleur de Lys, where we were penned till after midnight. Then, when the sky cleared and an offshore breeze sprang up, the ice started to move out and the ancient mariner announced a move; the engine baulked and kept baulking, and before our sleepy eyes an ardent optimist was transformed into an embittered pessimist for the space of three hours. Suddenly, Fleur de Lys awakened, man, woman, and child, by a shattering explosion which became a barrage dealing insomnia with every revolution. Our gallant launch chugged and banged her way out of the harbour. When day dawned, it was actually fine and calm, and we made St Anthony by six in the evening.

Here I was to be the guest of Grenfell of Labrador – a lineal descendant of Sir Richard Grenville of Elizabethan days, who was immortalised by Tennyson in "The Revenge" for pitting his one little ship against fifty-three Spanish galleons[20] – and his wife. Dr Grenfell retained all the fighting qualities of his illustrious ancestor but expressed them differently. An athlete of note while at Oxford, at rowing, football, and boxing, he had also acquired a master mariner's ticket in addition to his medical diploma.[21] A sportsman with rod and gun as well as nature lover, writer, and caricaturist, lay preacher, and justice of the peace, ready at any time to launch out with unabated enthusiasm into any new venture that would further his aims, this lovable, erratic genius – and genius surely always is erratic – had devoted his life to practical philanthropy, not the signing of big cheques but the solving of big human problems, including the supreme one of making self-doubters believe in themselves: a man who was bound to make enemies but whose friends were legion and to be found in all walks of life.

After the experiences of the last few days, which had not included one good night's sleep since leaving the *Tunisian*, a few days of cleanliness and other creature comforts were no unwelcome prospect, with added interest associated with the hospital of St Anthony. A bath and a tasty meal soon removed any clouds from the mental horizon, and that same evening found me in the out-patient department, meeting what was to me a new disease.

I still have my old textbook of medicine (of which a new edition had come out in 1908) when I began to walk the wards of St Thomas's, and when I turn up beri-beri, I read, "It has been attributed to unsuitable food, but the cause is not yet really known."[22] And in the paragraph devoted to treatment, "There is no specific remedy for this disease. The *essential thing* (the italics are mine) is removal to an uninfected locality."[23] And what a change thirty years later! In 1908 the term *vitamine* had not been invented, I believe.[24] I certainly never remember meeting it in training days. But in 1912 the stocky, quiet assistant doctor who largely ran St Anthony Hospital while his restless chief ranged the coast by boat and dog-team or campaigned for funds at a distance had already launched out into research work at that humble shack in northern Newfoundland which was elaborated in the leading institutions of two hemispheres. This was Dr John Mason Little, at once a brilliant surgeon and a truly scientific physician.[25]

It is now known [in 1938] that so far from flight being the best treatment for beri-beri, it is more readily eradicated right in its strongholds than any other serious disease, if only the economic and dietetic problems can be adequately dealt with. It has taken legislation divorced from politics [*The Health and Public Welfare Act, 1931*] to deal what may be hoped is a death blow to beri-beri in Newfoundland. Among the poor of that island community, white bread with salt fish and tea formed quite an unduly large proportion of the food intake. A ration of brown flour with the addition of leguminous vegetables such as peas and beans would alone be adequate safeguard, and small-scale agriculture is better still.

In the same way, sunshine plus cod-oil, with which latter commodity Newfoundland fairly flows, will eliminate rickets which causes so many crooked limbs and deformed chests, and the person who was thus protected against beri-beri and rickets need not fear scurvy, especially if the native berries are added to the vegetables. And, as recent polar expeditions have abundantly proved, raw fish or meat is even more effective as a cure or protection against scurvy than fresh vegetables. Nutritional diseases, then, are the last things that should trouble the inhabitants of Newfoundland or Labrador, though they are the most prevalent diseases, except consumption, if not outpacing the "white plague." Thus, before I even set foot in Labrador it was borne in upon me that the basic methods to be employed in a fight against nutritional diseases must be educational in character: teaching ignorant, prejudiced victims to use the very remedies with which they were surrounded, yet which they largely neglected.

The population of Newfoundland was largely of Cornish and Devonshire stock, I believe, with all the British tenacity and hatred of change inbred. Because of these qualities they could face Neptune's legions in home-made schooners undaunted or jump from a moving steamer onto a floating ice-pan at the great seal hunt in early spring, migrate annually *en famille* from their homes in Newfoundland to rude shacks away north in Labrador for one third of each year, wrest a living from sea, ice, and soil and also from forest or mines, without any settled profession or make any sacrifice to help neighbours in distress. Yet just because of these qualities, a small, insular, proud community with very inadequate educational facilities was lagging far behind more developed continental communities in matters of health and hygiene. To try to tell fisher-folk how to live in a different way was to make enemies and arouse opposition. Example must speak louder than precept, and the mills of God must grind slowly.[26] Reformers cannot afford to be impatient.

Such was my first evening at St Anthony Hospital. The next morning was spent in the operating room. *Prospero*, as usual, had landed a group of patients, both medical and surgical, and there were still a few of the latter awaiting treatment. I was appointed anaesthetist for the day. The first case was an operation for tubercular shoulder, done by Dr Grenfell. A young fisherman and a family man was faced with the loss of his job and his life unless the diseased bone was removed and a "false" joint created. The agile debater and restless man of action showed a deliberation and thoroughness that came as a surprise if he were too hastily judged by first impressions. The second case was that of a young girl with a malignant tumour of the thigh, of a size seldom if ever seen in more developed communities, where it would always be detected and dealt with in an earlier stage. Smoothly and rapidly, Dr Little removed the useless, cumbersome, and painful limb. Unfortunately in such a case, cure was extremely improbable as there was almost certain to be a secondary growth somewhere, but at least a period of comfort and also of hope was assured.

As there were still three days before any northward-bound steamer was expected, Dr Grenfell suggested my taking a little medical cruise to neighbouring ports in his steamer *Strathcona*,[27] a generous gift from Baron Strathcona, once Donald Smith of the Hudson's Bay Company in Labrador. The stretch of coast to be covered is known as the French Shore, and the names of the ports explain the title: Bréhat, St Lunaire, Griquet, Fortune, Quirpon.[28] When a patient, on being asked where he lived merely replied "Ha Ha," he was apt to be suspected of a warped sense of humour, a man to whom a real joke might be fatal if he saw it; but there actually is a village with that name [Ha Ha Bay] on the French Shore.

Steam was soon up and the little steamer, 110 feet over all, backed away from the wharf and headed down the harbour. Looking back on St Anthony, a village with about six hundred inhabitants, its setting became noticeable [to one] for the first time amid so many new sights and ideas. In shape the harbour was not unlike that of St John's, with a flask-like body and a narrow neck set almost at a right angles to the flask, but there the likeness ended. The immediate surroundings of the harbour were less steep from the waterside, and the village being small the surrounding country was more in evidence. There was considerable vegetation but no timber of any size, the trees or shrubs being chiefly dwarf fir and alder. The nearest timber of commercial importance was in an area in Canada Bay, fifty or more miles to the south, but wood enough for a good deal of fuel could be cut in Hare Bay, just to the south of St Anthony. Cape St Anthony is a bold headland, but the hills were not impressive. Its proximity to the Strait of Belle Isle, distant less than twenty miles – which straits are the real home of fog – means that St Anthony is somewhat often visited by unwelcome fog banks.

The distance between harbours was short, and we were soon at work. Some outpatients usually turned up as soon as we entered the harbour with the invariable query, "Is you coming ashore, doctor?" Apart from the interest of seeing first hand how these people lived, it is, of course, only too true that the most serious cases are often the slowest to seek a doctor, and many opportunities are sure to be lost if there is no house-to-house visiting. And the above truism was well illustrated on this occasion, for at one house I saw a young expectant mother. She had a headache and her vision was a little blurry, and there was a little dropsy [swelling] of the feet and legs, and she had noticed that her eyelids seemed a little puffy in the morning, but some at least of these things had been associated with previous events of this kind [pre-eclampsia],[29] and she had always got through all right. However, after a brief but frank interview, she came on board *Strathcona* and back to St Anthony and was saved [by delivery] from the results of one of the most dreaded complications of her condition. This case alone made the trip worthwhile, but we collected four other cases requiring hospital treatment. Truly, this interesting work was the natural complement of the institutional service.

On returning to St Anthony the night before ss *Home*[30] was due, there were several other things to take note of in a final look round. First, Dr Grenfell considered it unthorough treatment to patch up a human body only to return the patient to the very condition of which he was already a victim, and therein surely lies a valid criticism of much institutional work. To try to meet this problem locally, there was a Department of Auxiliary Industries,[31] alike for housewives eager to increase their contribution to the family budget and also for those unfortunate B2 and C3 citizens[32] who cannot pursue such arduous occupations as fishing and trapping and who are no attraction to employers of labour, if such appear. There was also a sawmill at work, it appeared, in Canada Bay, with the idea of employing able-bodied men who had failed in fishing or other means of livelihood to an extent that left their families short of necessaries.

Another new enterprise was in prospect where a young volunteer from New Zealand[33] was experimenting with the productive capacity of this northern soil. The object of this experiment was to develop a further aid to economics and health. And twenty-five years later, a fine herd of cattle as well as pigs are in evidence, also vegetable and flower gardens and greenhouses. A tannery, co-operative store and a haul-up slip on which schooners and small steamers are under repair all through the open water season are further instances of practical therapy, at once preventive and curative. When the time came for these early timber shacks to be replaced by modern buildings of reinforced concrete, it was a local contracting team that did most of the work. A one-time Labrador cod-fisher and trapper [Ted McNeill][34] was the mastermind with Labrador mason and electrician and northern Newfoundland plumber and carpenters.

In this close association of medical with social service, I believe that Dr Grenfell has been very much of a pioneer, in versatility at least. I remember that in my training days at St Thomas's Hospital I was rather vaguely aware of the Almoner Department which followed up some medical cases of the hospital in the district, but I think that the stately and efficient Lady Almoner would have been considerably astonished if a medical student had evinced any interest in her department, and as she was often attended by a bevy of attractively gowned maidens she might have scented a wolf in sheep's clothing. In various visits to the United States I have visited mental institutions where occupational therapy was practised, alike for the physical and mental well-being of the patients and the practical economics of the institution which, in some cases, produced much of their own food and equipment. In this respect, *so far as I have seen*, the United States had taken a long start of Great Britain. But this was the first time that I had seen any such combination, and I was much impressed with it.

On July 5th I left St Anthony on the *Home*. She touched at the same ports that we had visited in *Strathcona*, but she carried no doctor and was only supposed to provide passenger and freight service. The northern peninsula of Newfoundland, long and finger-like, ends in two promontories, Cape Bauld and Cape Norman. Passing Cape Bauld eighteen miles out from St Anthony, we headed out into Belle Isle straits, shaping a course for Battle Harbour, then called the capital of Labrador, with an estimated population of one hundred. Happily, the straits were free of fog, which was well as there was a lot of loose pan-ice and many bergs in sight. The captain told me that he had counted 133 of these white monsters at one time from the bridge of his vessel during a recent trip. It is well to give them a wide berth, as they have a playful habit of turning turtle and disintegrating, with most destructive results for any incautious mariner who might be caught in such an upheaval. In fog the odds are on the iceberg. Today, however, the sun shone gloriously, and the sea was a lovely blue.

Sixteen miles out from Cape Bauld on our starboard side was Belle Isle. The person who named that forbidding-looking mass must have been weary of the sea and very hungry for any kind of land. There are two lighthouses on the easterly and westerly points, but none would live there from choice, I imagine. A few schooners hang on in a poor summer anchorage for a time while "fish is in." Away to port was a line of blue-looking cliffs, the Labrador coast, with the straits proper separating it from the northern and part of the western coast of Newfoundland. As we approached, the uniform blue colour and rather shapeless outline took on more varied hues and configurations. Schooners under sail were to be seen here and there. Towards sundown we entered enclosed waters and soon made harbour. The siren blew, and for the first time I heard the "Labrador band," a full-throated chorus of long-drawn, wolf-like howls from a pack of husky or Eskimo dogs. A few minutes later we landed on Labrador soil.

2

"Down North" along the Labrador
Coast in a Newfoundland Icebreaker

Interesting and instructive as the little visit to St Anthony had been, I had clearly to face the fact that I had witnessed both talent and facilities which could never be mine further north. At Battle Harbour, however, was another Grenfell hospital of more modest dimensions and equipment, where there was more to be seen that might be reproduced further north. The medical officer in charge there was Dr John Grieve,[35] a burly Scot whose chief interest outside medicine was classical music, though Battle Harbour afforded little opportunity for cultivating this taste. He was also a great raconteur with a quick sense of humour.

The little hospital stood on the lesser of the two islands which formed the narrow harbour. A fish merchant's premises were rather intimately related to those of the medical institution, due to the fact that the fish firm had been there first and owned the land.[36] A small Church of England edifice and a score of settlers' houses completed the capital of Labrador, with the addition of the one all-year wireless station north of Belle Isle straits at that time. Half a dozen extra wireless stations were operated during the open water season. The summer floating population of Battle Harbour varied according to the movements of King Cod. Eskimo dogs ran everywhere uncontrolled, and the first thing to strike the mind of anyone interested in public health was the problem of a safe water supply on this small island. Despite an obvious effort to fence off a rocky collecting basin on the summit, whence a pipe sloped steeply down to the hospital, water for drinking purposes had to be boiled to be safe. There was not a tree to be seen, and firewood had to be transported from the mainland by boat. Frankly, I was not attracted by Battle Harbour except for one thing: outside the harbour were many ugly and dangerous reefs which produced most spectacular breakers in rough weather.

Perched on a hilltop, I was fascinated to watch part of a round in the age-long battle between King Neptune's created warriors and the rocky defences of the Labrador coast. In endless, unhurried onslaughts the attack was pressed home, but the defenders' outposts met it, hurled back foremost assailants in a wild, eddying confusion that often foiled those following behind. In such places it was only a shattered relic of the shoreward surge that reached the cliffs. But reserves were endless in this war of attrition. Elsewhere, such outer bastions were lacking, and granite and trap-rock cliffs met the full fury of the assault. With the aid of the winter frost and the resistless expansive power of ice, fissures were slowly but surely widened till a landslide occurred. It was rather in the less resistant sectors, where the sea whirled sand and shingle about so contemptuously, that the very fury of the waves was building up a rampart which would eventually rise triumphant from the greedy waters.

While nature supplied so splendid a spectacle for a leisure hour, the little hospital offered plenty of professional interest. There was much less surgery, naturally, than at St Anthony, but I soon saw that Dr Grieve was prepared to tackle quite formidable work. Particularly do I remember the case of a veteran fisherman, a victim of the lack of dental facilities in the neighbourhood of his home. The irritation of jagged, carious stumps persisting through many years had eventually resulted in cancerous changes in the jaw, and only drastic surgery offered any chance of recovery.

While at Battle Harbour, I met a nurse [Mina Gilchrist] who was waiting to travel north with me to work that summer at Indian Harbour, where there was another small cottage hospital on an active fishing centre at the mouth of Hamilton Inlet, the greatest of Labrador fiords. But now the wind chopped round again and blew from the east, bringing back the fog and drift-ice. None the less, ss Sagona[37] nosed her way into the anchorage one afternoon, and we embarked on the last stage of our travels.

The Sagona proved to be a rather tubby steamer of about five hundred registered tonnage. She was crowded with a late consignment of fisher-folk and early summer tourists. As soon as the freight for Battle Harbour was out, we left for a four-day battle with ice and fog. At first there was at least novelty in watching an icebreaker at work. There was an enormous field of ice, hundreds of square miles in area, and for nearly sixty miles northward from Battle Harbour we were exposed to the full weight of ice, as there were no islands outside us except when we turned in to make some harbour. The pack was pretty tight. Small pans were thrust unceremoniously aside until some worthier foe was encountered in a pan perhaps hundreds of square yards in area. Then the rounded bow rode up to the enemy, which split asunder with a sullen grinding. At times the contest was so unequal that *Sagona* would have to back astern to gain fresh momentum. Numerous bergs were also in evidence. Every few miles *Sagona*, as if bent on self-destruction, would head for the grim cliffs until, rounding some great buttress, another harbour would open up, then a greeting blast, a reply from the "Labrador band," a rush alongside for mail or freight or news of the fish or perhaps a few patients for the ship's doctor, then a laconic "Freight's out, sir," and up anchor and out for another round with the ice. It soon grew monotonous, though there was some interest in the increasingly marked Eskimo appearance of the Labrador men as we proceeded northward.

On such a trip, anything humorous is a godsend. On one occasion (not on this trip but on a similar one), a captain new to the route had the misfortune to ground his vessel on a rock at the entrance of a seldom-visited harbour. As the agitated mariner alternately ported and starboarded his wheel with the engines full speed astern to work her off, he was driven almost to homicidal fury by the antics of a fair passenger with more charm than perception. Pirouetting gaily before him, she chanted, "Oh, I'm just crazy about this! I wouldn't have missed it for the world." If the captain's face was read aright, he was calculating his chances of escaping capital charge if the lady ended her song in the water.

Manifestly, to escape from a crowded vessel even for half an hour is a coveted privilege, and equally obviously the captain does not like to be kept waiting by dilatory passengers when he is ready to leave. There are few wharves north of Belle Isle straits capable of accommodating a mail steamer, and the ship's boat which takes ashore disembarking passengers and mail for that particular port can take few "joy-riders." On one occasion, a gentleman of considerable tonnage succeeded in getting ashore to visit friends, and the departure blast found him still under the hospitable roof. In full view of the irate skipper, he emerged and started to walk the quarter of a mile or so to the wharf, where a motor boat awaited him. This did not at all suit the angry autocrat on the bridge, and the siren boomed an ultimatum. The walk became a reluctant elephantine trot, and whenever this showed signs of relaxing, the siren stimulated the offender to fresh efforts at the risk of apoplexy. A pulseless wreck flopped into the motor and with a last desperate effort climbed the companion ladder and collapsed on deck. Even the captain felt that further eloquence would be wasted.

Despite several extra "fishermen's boats" in spring and autumn, the rush north and south cannot be dealt with in strict accordance with maritime regulations. The men must get to the fishery or their families will go short of necessaries, in many cases, for the following winter, and the demoralising and expensive dole will run riot; so plimsoll marks[38] disappear below the surface and are forgotten, and fisher-folk throng decks, holds, alleyways, saloon tables, and benches in quest of rest or warmth and some means of preparing food. The galleys and supplies are overtaxed, and worst of all, water is apt to run short. In an extremity, I have seen the ship's boat rowed to the mouth of a brook and filled with water as full as was safe, the crew necessarily standing in the precious fluid for the return journey. At such times, drinking is a luxury and washing almost a crime. I have also known what it is to pray devoutly that a certain "happy event" might be delayed till the expectant mother could be removed from the over-crowded steerage quarters to *anywhere ashore.*

Few things could be more unwelcome on such a cruise than an alarm of fire, which I have experienced on two occasions. On one of these an undoubted oil cask was discovered blazing cheerfully on the outside, it being an old-fashioned wood cask. The ship's pump choked for the occasion, and the captain, since more robust methods proved ineffective, grew positively polite. "Couldn't *someone* just pour a bucket over that cask?" he pleaded. Finally, this was accomplished, and then it transpired that the cask did not contain oil at all.

On the evening of the second day, a powerful aroma which forced its way through the fog heralded our approach to the whale factory at Hawke Harbour[39] long before it was discernable to sense of sight. The oily water and abundant refuse made the harbour a most undesirable one to linger in, but for our sins we were condemned to a whole night there as well as a long evening. A large consignment of freight, added to the density of the fog and uncertainty of making another port before dark, decided our fate. An elderly fellow passenger who modestly claimed to be the champion salmon fisher of the world produced rod and tackle and proceeded to whip the waters of a small rapid stream that connected the harbour with a large pond. The trout were there and hungry, and the angler soon filled his creel, but when part of his catch appeared on the supper table, the memory of those foul waters and copious refuse resulted in an unwonted affection for the ship's dietary.

The next morning, we had the thrill of the voyage in an alarm of "man overboard!" Fortunately, it occurred when we were in harbour, incidentally at a time when few people were yet out of their bunks. One of the firemen had an acute maniacal attack and plunged over the side. The mate, who was no swimmer, pluckily raced down the companion ladder, pushed off into the deep water, and managed to flounder at the surface with the frenzied man in his grasp till both were fished out. We now entered sheltered runs inside islands, and so far as ice was concerned, we were only occasionally handicapped when emerging for a few miles at a time into more open water, but the fog still bothered us. For over a hundred miles the old catchphrase a "land of cod, dog, and fog" seemed to have considerable justification, but turning westward from Gready into Sandwich Bay, for twenty miles or more we had a glimpse of a different Labrador.

Rounding a point, we entered the beautiful landlocked harbour at Cartwright. Major Cartwright was a trading adventurer who operated on the Labrador coast during the last quarter of the eighteenth century.[40] He was connected with the family of the Earl of Sandwich, after whom he named the bay.[41] Conferring his own name on what was to become the chief settlement, he called the chief island Huntingdon Island, also after the family of his kinsman, and he also named Paradise the second city of this little empire. He had considerable losses through American privateers in those days of Anglo-American hostility. He left behind him a journal, interesting if frank, which was published.[42] So part of Labrador, at least, has an aristocratic background.

It was a refreshment to have pierced the fog belt and to revel in sunshine once more and feast our eyes on trees and grass in their freshness. We had also emerged from a cod zone to a salmon zone. The salted produce of these days has been largely replaced by the chilled product and also the tinned. In this new venture, the Governor and Company of Gentlemen Adventurers Trading into Hudson's Bay, now known as the Hudson's Bay Company, had been at least the local pioneers, and it was here that "The Company" had the southernmost of a series of posts in this region. Like Battle Harbour, Cartwright had a little Church of England edifice, but the village was neater and the surroundings more picturesque; also, the local Labradormen were far more convincing in appearance than those whom we had lately been seeing. Birds, Davises, Learnings, Browns, and Pardys seemed to be the chief clans, and some of the elders were either English or of English parentage, which latter category included many of the younger generation. Lethbridge, Painter, and Macdonald were other family names which were not unfamiliar in the Old Country. One of the English members of this community was a shipwright, and the standard of carpentry averaged higher in Sandwich Bay than in any other group on the Labrador coast.

We had now seen something of the catchers of cod, whales and salmon. The trout fishery was not a highly developed or organised pursuit and was not much in evidence. There still remained fur-trapping and seal-catching or hunting. There was nothing in Labrador to compare with the great annual seal hunt in ice-breaking steamers, of which a fleet usually left St John's about March 10th, and seals were killed by the hundreds of thousands in some seasons. But some varieties of "bay seals" were annually killed in thousands in some districts of Labrador. The market for seal oil has fluctuated very greatly, the fat being almost worthless to the hunter or fisher at times. King Herring had yet to be crowned and is only now approaching his coronation. Besides these predatory industries, there were still waterpower, timber and mineral resources, and reindeer herding to be investigated.

Sandwich Bay, while not the best timber area, at least held out hopes that Labrador forests were not altogether a myth. But if Sandwich Bay was something of a revelation after the surf-beaten and ice-rubbed granite shell of Labrador, which we had been tied to for three days, Hamilton Inlet was to be a far fuller one. Cartwright has changed markedly since 1912. The village has grown, and two schools and a cottage hospital now offer facilities to the local population. A floating salmon factory anchors there summer by summer. It was there that the first airplane to land in Labrador came down on the harbour ice one early spring afternoon,[43] and it was there too that the Italian air squadron under General Balbo made their landing.[44]

It is into Hamilton Inlet that the great Grand River watershed empties itself, a system with falls that dwarf Niagara for height and which has in relation to it the greatest reserve of timber that the country has to offer, as well as mineral resources which are only today undergoing any intensive investigation. This great fiord indents the Labrador coast to a depth of nearly 150 nautical miles. It is divided into two basins, the eastern one being approximately fifty miles in length, with a twenty-mile mouth narrowing down to a few hundred yards in the Rigolet Narrows. Here the traveller might well think that he was at the head of the inlet, but passing through the narrows Lake Melville opens up with a length of about seventy miles and a maximum width of over twenty, and with glorious scenery. Rigolet was then the most westerly steamer port, and it was thither that we went the following day, anchoring off another of the Hudson's Bay Company's posts. HBC is sometimes taken to mean Here Before Christ. While not quite so old as that, the company had already passed the 250th anniversary of its charge in 1912.

Hamilton Inlet is the most cosmopolitan of the Labrador bays, as traces of both the native races are to be seen there as well as markedly different types of settler stock. And topography differs as widely as ethnology as one passes from the kind of coast already described, first to patches of scrub timber and then on to real forest lands. The biggest mountain range, if not quite the highest peaks in the country, are also to be seen in the Mealy Mountains, on the south side of Lake Melville. Seven peaks exceed three thousand feet, and two approach within two hundred feet of four thousand. Away north, in the regions of Cape Mugford and Eclipse Harbour, a few peaks exceed four thousand feet. The whole inlet is really the Grand River estuary, though the Naskaupi River system also makes a goodly contribution to the outflow. Reduced salinity of water had been recorded as far east as a point twenty-five miles outside Rigolet.

Even in 1912 a premature lumber venture was just petering out at the mouth of the Grand River, one of three that have failed. Every country on the eve of development is the happy hunting ground of some knaves and some fools as well as honest visionaries who are in a little too much hurry, and Labrador has had its share of all these types as well as of some who have been unduly pessimistic. Here were romance, latent power, and raw material both in nature and human nature. When would Labrador's day come, and could the local people be prepared to play a worthy part in the development of their country instead of seeing it exploited at their expense?

Rigolet offered a tragic and eloquent commentary on the contact of white with native races. Here were the southernmost survivors of the Labrador Eskimos, and a truly pathetic relic they were – not "merry brown folk in dancing kayaks and picturesque native costumes" but listless, tuberculous-looking, European-clothed specimens of a race almost exterminated by white man's diseases and white man's interference with their natural means of livelihood. As a final touch, a number of them had been allowed to be exported for exhibition purposes to Chicago, and what they acquired and brought back with them had not helped towards the survival of the race.[45] Added to that the contributions made locally by visitors from Newfoundland and elsewhere, and their doom was sealed.

They had adopted to a great extent white man's food, white man's raiment, white man's dwellings, and white man's diseases. Aggregated instead of nomadic, they were simply "cannon fodder" for any epidemic that came along. Already riddled with venereal disease and tuberculosis, smallpox and scarlet fever, measles and influenza had all taken their toll. There was probably not enough healthy blood stock left to recuperate the race, however carefully nursed, for the future. Fusion seemed the only alternative to extermination, and what of the fusion? Having interbred with them, often for his pleasure, the white man stigmatises the produce as "tainted stock," and while he cannot disclaim a large share of physical responsibility, any other claims have certainly been largely ignored.

Of course, the first impression, like all first impressions, needs some dilution. Many settlers, domestically inclined, had no choice but to marry native women, and many marriages have been faithfully observed and have resulted in happy and prosperous homes.[46] None the less there is much truth in the above and a very real debt of honour to be liquidated according to preconceived and traditional ideas of British justice. The potentialities of the mixed stock will be abundantly illustrated later on.

I have since discussed the above problem not only with Moravian missionaries, whose viewpoint might be considered a prejudiced one, but with such dispassionate judges as officers of the Royal Canadian Mounted Police, and I have also read much of the literature available on the Eskimo race. The two outstanding publications that have come to my notice have been the internationally recognised and highly scientific Eskimos, by Kaj Birket-Smith, and the deeply interesting volume on Eskimo folklore and habits [Eskimo Folk-Tales], written by the late Knud Rasmussen, who travelled right across Eskimo land from Greenland, of which he was a native of Danish-Eskimo parentage, to Siberia. The conclusion to which I have been driven after such study as this is that in their uncontaminated state the Eskimos are about as near to Utopia as anything that the world contains, and I say that while professing full belief in the essential Christianity of Christ, sincerely and intelligently applied to modern times and problems, as the one hope for civilisation. But has Christendom much to boast of as compared to the despised Eskimo?

Polygamy, yes, and "free love," but these are not confined to the Arctic Circle; nor is divorce probably proportionally common there as compared to some sections of civilisation. Infanticide, yes. But does not the superior white man limit offspring to suit economic conditions, if not for the less worthy reason? Elimination of the aged and infirm, yes; but euthanasia is being widely advocated in other regions with far less excuse than in the Arctic. What pleasure of life is left for a sightless, feeble member of a community that depends on mobility for existence? If paganism needs diluting with Christianity, surely Christianity, as it is widely interpreted, needs diluting with a little common sense and honesty.

The Eskimo's taste in food is not as ours, but we do not live in the Arctic, and he might think caviare and Gorgonzola cheese at least as open to criticism as some of his delicacies at which we look askance. The sterling virtues of honesty, loyalty, and self-sacrifice have been recorded by those who really know the Eskimo, in examples which, while they would not put good white men to shame, would do any white man credit. Surely anyone with a sense of justice and reason can see that it is something of a toss-up for which the individual cannot be fairly blamed as to whether the instincts of the Arctic or of a more temperate zone will predominate as a mixed stock, and if equally balanced, what is the inevitable result?

Is not the fairer way to approach each individual with an open mind and a helping hand, to look for, encourage, and develop the more promising traits and to try to find the best solution for those who are groping in a bottomless morass, with their hereditary instincts at variance with their environment? That there are a number capable of responding to such treatment and of pitting their brains as well as their muscles against the brighter, if not the brightest, of civilisation's products can again be demonstrated convincingly. In all too many cases, however, initiative is lacking. Without the faintest conception of the value of money, these victims have forsaken their natural mode of life for an existence which has neither filled their pockets nor caused them to prosper in body or mind.

At Rigolet, too, we met other natives of Labrador and loved them not. These were vast hordes of hungry mosquitoes and sandflies, the former happily not malarial. These welcomed a fresh infusion of bloodstock with an enthusiasm that was truly diabolical. The bald head of a veteran Labradorman who rowed some of us ashore was almost invisible because of them, but his anaemic scalp was but the taking-off place for a raid on the newcomers. The mosquito sleeps not, it seems, and his slogan, or rather hers (for it is the ladies that do the biting) may be taken as a warning or an added aggression according to the mood of the sufferer. The sandfly does retire for the night, but by day he is too intensively and vilely occupied to worry about a slogan. It is said that in "the good old days," when Eskimos and Indians conducted their quarrels unchecked by the peace-loving white man, a favourite penalty for warriors who were rash enough to be caught instead of being killed was to strip them and leave them to the winged pests. Besides the insects mentioned, there is an animated airplane that, Shylock-like, demands his pound of flesh.[47] He is locally known as a "bulldog" or "stout" and is really a deer fly. If I seem unduly poetic in regard to insects of Labrador, the reader is cordially invited to come and see. The above will then seem to be very inadequate prose. It was a blessed release when *Sagona* blew for a night run to Indian Harbour, our destination.

Apart from digressions, this chapter has portrayed the voyage on an icebreaker rather from the captain's viewpoint. The overcrowding, the shortage of water, the exuberance of passengers, the excursions ashore, and any fire alarms – these all add to his burden. In regard to navigation especially, he knows that he is being rakingly criticised by a number of more or less expert judges, including some whom he knows to be about his equal and many who are convinced that they are his betters.

Before closing the subject, one more anecdote may be added. It was October, and the old *Meigle*[48] of about seven hundred tons was southward bound with over five hundred people on board. These were mostly fisher-folk bound home from the fishery. It was stormy weather, and a voyage which should fill one week bade fair to exceed two. It had been simply impossible to avoid the overcrowding. At port after port men, women, and children thronged aboard. "We have our fish made. We have nothing to eat and nothing to burn, and we've got to come." Such was the story constantly told. Bad weather held us up two days in our harbour and two more in another. Food was short as well as water. It was imperative to lose no chance of getting ahead, but it was rough. [As we were] leaving one harbour, the fo'c's'le was crowded like the rest of the deck. *Meigle* had shipped no green water all day, but now, just for once, she dived deeply into a wave. I was but a few feet from the captain at the time, and never shall I forget his face as he waited for the expected cry of "man overboard," and it might just as well have been a dozen. But no one was washed off the deck, though how many suffered subsequently from the cold autumn ducking, with limited facilities for changing wet clothing, cannot be said.

It was a perfect night as we left Rigolet for a run of between forty-five and fifty miles. As we were due to arrive in the small hours of the morning, it seemed to be hardly worthwhile to go to bed, and as it turned out, to have done so would have meant the sacrifice of one of the most beautiful scenes that I have ever witnessed. Still in the first half of July, the hours of darkness were but few. Sunset hues still lingered in the sky in what was hardly less than twilight, and the blush of dawn was to appear almost before the last of this glow had vanished. There was no wind, a clear sky, and a bright moon. In the still, watery mirror, promontory and island, hilltop and woodland were so clearly reflected as to convey the sense of floating inverted in an aerial fairyland, and tonight of all nights the Aurora Borealis staged a benefit performance. Multicoloured streamers flamed and writhed, faded and flamed again. The dawn came after four memorable hours. Slowly, crimson turned to gold, and shortly before *Sagona* blew what was for us her final blast of arrival, the sun rose above the watery horizon. It was a fitting climax to a voyage full of new sights and experiences.

3

Cottage Hospital Experiences at Indian Harbour, Labrador

We stood upon the rocks at Indian Harbour, I for one feeling more at sea than ever I had on *Sagona*. Our party consisted of the nurse [Mina Gilchrist] and myself for medical staff, a student volunteer worker for general utility, named Reeve,[49] two maids from Newfoundland who had worked at Indian Harbour hospital the previous summer, a third maid, a Labrador woman hastily picked up at Rigolet, and five patients reaped during the later stages of our journey. To arrive after an aesthetic but sleepless night before four in the morning with a party of eleven, at a place that no one but two maids knew anything about and which had been shut up for about eight months, was a little bewildering.

A portly little man of middle age came forward and introduced himself as the local fish merchant, Mr Charles Jerrett.[50] He told us that a large consignment of supplies of various kinds for the hospital and staff had come by a previous *Sagona*. These he had kindly landed and warehoused for us pending our arrival. In his wake followed a lean Labradorman [John Rich], who had been appointed watchman for the hospital premises by my predecessor in view of certain unfortunate occurrences there between one and two years previously. He had been directed to come out to Indian Harbour from his home before any vessels arrived from the south and to stay on the premises till our arrival. He and his wife and two small children had spent several weeks in a minute, single-roomed outhouse. He had done poorly the previous winter with fur and had been unable to bring adequate supplies with him, and so far as I could make out, the family had subsisted largely on mussels gathered from the harbour rocks. He was to receive a stated sum for his services and was anxious to get off to his summer fishing place. This man conducted us up a walk of rough-hewn plank to the hospital, which stood, still inhospitably shuttered, nearly a hundred yards back from the shoreline on rising ground. He also showed us a shed in which reposed a supply of coal and firewood.

It was a good thing that there was a long day ahead of us. Fires had to be lit, a meal prepared, rooms scrubbed and aired, also bedding found and aired, patients washed and disposed of, supplies of all kinds located and unpacked as required. Happily, the nurse took everything "in her stride" with complete composure, and Reeve and I, with what was left of the Labradorman, waded into the freight, manhandling bales of dry goods, hardware, food and drugs, and carrying them on hand-barrows up the long ascent to the hospital storehouse. We learned that a fishing skipper's wife did the hospital laundry for a stated sum per season, and as our predecessors had shut up shop in a hurry when they left the previous autumn, there was work for the laundress right away. To add to our task, patients dropped in from time to time, in some cases largely to look over the new doctor, I think. At one stage of the proceedings, Reeve and I felt that we must swim or die, but the presence of ice-pans in the harbour did not incline us to prolong this interlude.

Fortunately, none of the cases that had come was very serious. One little chap had an abscess the size of a tangerine behind his ear, which needed careful investigation to exclude mastoid disease, but he did not seem acutely ill, and it turned out to be no more than a superficial abscess. On him we did a minor operation the next day. As I had been informed that a fourth-year medical student from the United States was coming to be my assistant by the following *Sagona*, I naturally preferred to avoid any major surgery, unless in case of emergency, till we were reinforced by his arrival.

Our plant was primitive in the extreme. A square building, almost flat-roofed, about thirty feet by twenty-six, had to do duty for staff and patients. There were two floors. On the ground floor were a tiny staff sitting and dining room, a kitchen, out-patients' dispensary, doctor's bedroom, and one other small room which Reeve had to share with my assistant when the latter arrived. Overhead were the nurses' room, maids' room, two small wards with five beds for men and three for women, a small operating room, and a linen closet. There was no plumbing at all inside.

Semi-detached from the hospital was a small chapel for the doctor, who also acted as parish priest. And on the back of the latter was a little lean-to structure, canvas roofed, with three beds for tubercular male patients. From the early days of the season we were chronically overcrowded, and I confess that it did not seem to me very practical

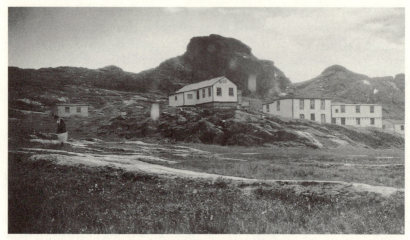

Medical staff bungalow, hospital, and adjoining chapel at Indian Harbour, c. 1914
(Faculty of Medicine Founders' Archive, Memorial University)

religion to invite people to be preached to on Sundays but reject all
but a very few if ill on weekdays. One of the first changes to be made,
as soon as we had the means, was to transform the chapel into hospital
quarters, have the other part of the building for staff only, and build
a new chapel at a sensible distance from wards and operating room.
Furthermore, all our water supply for drinking, cooking, washing, and
surgical purposes came from a puncheon sunk in a swamp which was
fed by surface drainage water. True, there were no dogs here or any
buildings or any regular source of contamination above this makeshift
well, but makeshift it certainly was and something to be readjusted on
the first possible occasion.

   The surgical equipment was in keeping with the other facilities –
wood and ebony-handled relics of Noah's ark, which soon made a new
shoal in the harbour, as I had brought some instruments of my own.[51]
Within two years, there was to be a staff-house and semi-detached
hospital, as planned, with accommodation for twenty-four patients
instead of eleven. There was also to be a reservoir and water system
with baths for staff and patients as well as the new chapel. But let it
be at once admitted that I was extremely fortunate to get the where-
withal to make these changes. Such was our plant, and owing to a
brief breathing space, the next day gave us an opportunity to become
acquainted with our little island domain. On a glorious afternoon we
ascended to the summit of the island, where at an altitude of three
hundred feet we surveyed the landscape and seascape.

To one used to Wimbledon Common and Richmond Park, to the Surrey pines at Weybridge and the woodland scenery of the Thames Valley, to the meadows and parks of Oxford and also the parks of London as well as the beauties of Derbyshire in the neighbourhood of Repton and the Trent, the complete absence of trees was very noticeable, though the sea compensated for much that was missed in the landscape. Looking at our own island first, which was about two square miles in area, the immediate impression of its low, rocky eminences, its swamps and low-lying areas of rock and grass was a bit disappointing, yet as it was fitted into a wider panorama it gained in attraction, and subsequent exploration revealed at once the hardihood and also the opportunism of nature on this sub-arctic coast, nearly two hundred miles north of Belle Isle straits. Almost at our feet lay a deep gulch *with a southerly exposure*, which afforded a vivid contrast to much that lay only a few yards away, for here, protected by the rocky walls from all the colder winds, grew a surprising profusion of ferns. A few hundred yards away, again on the south side of a rocky ridge, we discovered quite a plantation of wild iris. Sedum or "stonecrop" luxuriated in many spots. We also found wild violets and many other flowering plants or ground vines; thus, table decorations were to be had for the picking. But that was not all that concerned the table. There was food not for the eyes alone. An abundance of edible berries grew there. There were cranberries, blueberries, and bakeapples [*Rubus chamaemorus*], which were something like a coarse yellow raspberry in appearance but which grew singly on small plants instead of bunched on canes. There were also what are locally called blackberries [*Empetrum nigrum*], though they are nothing like the bramble products found elsewhere but grow on a vine resembling miniature spruce in its foliage and so thickly that the berries are often faceted as to their surfaces by pressure. On the bigger island across the harbour were to be found some wild currants, and these abound in many more inland regions, as do wild raspberries. There are also two other varieties of blueberries and at least three further edible kinds.

Further auxiliaries to the catering department were to be found in numerous edible fungi and a rather celery-like plant called Alexander. Add to these dainties cod, salmon, trout, ducks and geese at certain times, mussels and clams, flounders and herring, smelts, and eggs which were to be had in abundance from fishermen's wives, who brought chickens north with them, and it will be seen that there was no fear of starving, even apart from imported tinned goods. I have mentioned a few of the more familiar plants, and I bragged for many years of the achievement of a nurse who collected sixty-eight different varieties of plant life from our little island in her spare time till a professional botanist came along and exceeded the two hundred mark. "You can eat everything in Labrador except the rocks," said a visiting scientist to me some years later, and he was not far wrong. This man had come to make a study of macroscopic and microscopic life in both fresh and salt water in these latitudes and was a little provoked to find that the distilled water which he had imported all the way from New York was rather less pure than the surface drainage water in our new reservoir. This may seem rather a material discussion [related to material comfort], but its relation to health problems is obvious. The question fairly leaped at one: "Why all this nutritional disease?" And the inescapable answer was "ignorance and laziness."

Our little island, then, was by no means devoid of practical interest as well as being the foreground of a panorama that grew on one the longer it was studied. The narrow harbour running due east and west was usually animated by the presence of schooners as well as the first "rooms"[52] and stages used by the "planter"[53] fisher-folk ashore. I have a photograph of seventy-five of these craft, lying at anchor with sails up to dry their canvas on a calm and sunny day; and on one October afternoon when there was a lull in work and the sun was unseasonably warm, I have reclined on the hillside for the space of three hours and watched over eighty of the graceful birds of passage careening to a spanking northerly breeze, foaming along the five miles of Cut-Throat Gap to Indian Harbour and rounding up neatly to anchor. Almost as though at the bidding of a magician's wand, the sails came down, the anchor splashed, and the chain rattled, and the speeding hull lay at rest.

Evidence of glacier action abounded on the rocks, ripple marks left by the ice resembling those of waves on the sand. Again, superimposed layers of dark trap-rock lying on the paler granite spoke of the same resistless force. The formations are very old, Laurentian or pre-Cambrian, I believe.[54] I am no geologist, but when many years later I stood beside an archaeologist on the deck of a boat which was cruising in the neigbourhood of Cape Mugford, Dr Tanner[55] (who is from Helsingfors in Finland), who is used to reckoning in terms of aeons, saw the work of nature over an estimated period of 1,500 millions of years spread out before his eyes. Raised beaches up to an altitude of nearly four hundred feet above present sea level were noted on this cruise, testifying to the antiquity of the formations.

Looking further afield, eastward, there was a group of islands, and to the southward of those the open ocean with icebergs almost always visible. According to the weather and clouds, there was a great variety of colour to be seen in the water: grey, green, blue, ultramarine, black, and also the crimson and purple of the sunset hour. A third island closed the harbour at the eastern end, cutting the channel into two arms, neither navigable for the mail steamer. Southward, fifty miles away, could be seen the high land of Gready outside Sandwich Bay. Westward, the great inlet stretched away for forty miles before turning southwest to Rigolet, and at sixty miles or more the higher peaks of the Mealy Mountains often shone white above the lower foothills. To the northward were more islands beyond which projected the mainland in the northwest. As the summer gave way to autumn, the somewhat sombre hillsides of these outer islands were to be lit up by a glow of berry vines changing colour, adding greatly to the scenic effect. Such was our domain and its prospect, but we were soon to pay for our little breathing space.

On the third day, a gigantic young fisherman came slowly up the woodwalk to the dispensary. A few days previously, he had slipped from the rocks into the icy water of the harbour while launching a boat. He was too busily occupied to change his clothes immediately and had contracted pneumonia. He had fought the cold to the limit of his endurance, thereby further handicapping himself in what was to be a hard fight for life. It was the worst case of pneumonia that I have ever seen survive. It was eleven days before the crisis came [when the pneumonia reached its peak, not the normal ten days], and the drain on his vitality was just too great. It was a nightmare of a time. The nurse and I shared or alternated vigils while the raging fever necessitated frequent cool sponging and the pulse and respirations grew more and more alarmingly rapid. There were no such refinements as cylinders of oxygen to subsidise nature's efforts. To loosen the hard cough, aid the embarrassed heart and lungs, maintain nutrition, and secure all possible rest were the chief services that we could render. At one time a rapid fall of temperature raised hopes, but it proved to be a "false crisis," and the thermometer soon showed the horribly familiar elevation. At last it seemed that the end must be near, and the old father whose mainstay the young man was came to pay what might well be a farewell visit. But in that very hour a change came, and the patient felt it before we could detect it. It seemed like the ravings of delirium when an apparently almost moribund patient, instead of whispering of pearly gates, burbled of a desire for apple pie. Within a very short time the real crisis was manifest, and while the process represented a period of considerable risk after so severe an attack, once the patient started on the right road he never looked back. Twenty-five years later he is still a familiar figure at Indian Harbour, summer by summer, and it is the old father who has long since disappeared from the scene.

While *Sagona* was lying at Rigolet on the voyage north, I had been much interested in a trim, white-painted auxiliary ketch named *Yale*.[56]

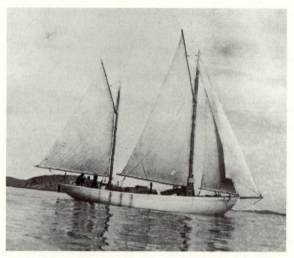

Mission ketch *Yale* (Faculty of Medicine Founders' Archive, Memorial University)

She had been presented two years previously by a group of students of the well known university of that name to act as a tender to Indian Harbour hospital, tucked away as it was on a remote island and with such few and infrequent communications. *Yale* could fetch and return patients between the hospital and outposts or hamlets never visited by the steamer. To eke out her costs of maintenance, she had a contract to carry mail as well as any chance passengers between the steamer port at Rigolet and the headwaters of Hamilton Inlet to North West River, where were trading stations both of the Hudson's Bay Company and their rivals, Revillon Frères,[57] and also to Mud Lake, at the mouth of Grand River, where a premature timber venture was nearing its end but a sawmill was still at work. After we had left Rigolet for Indian Harbour, she had completed her mail trip and returned to us with some patients. She had since left again to connect at Rigolet with *Sagona* and had taken our first group of in-patients homeward. While I was more than keen to take a trip in her to the head of the inlet to see the people up there, including the Montagnais Indians, who spent some weeks of each summer at North West River, and to see the new scenes and (it was to be hoped) to see *Yale* really put through her paces, it was impossible to leave Indian Harbour at present. *Yale* had brought some surgical cases, and I only awaited the arrival of my expected assistant by *Sagona* to get to work on them. *Yale* carried a crew of three. These were first a Labrador skipper and a pilot, Fred Blake; a second Labradorman, a cook-sailor, Sam Pottle; and a

Newfoundland lad, Will Simms, who tended the auxiliary engine and relieved Fred at the wheel when required.

We were sitting at dinner one day when the maid burst in full of excitement. "*Yale* is wrecked but no lives lost!" I hurried out and found Fred Blake in the kitchen. He had just rowed twenty-five miles or thereabouts in *Yale*'s dory. His story was that in thick fog the little vessel had run on a reef, ever since known as Yale Rock. While the disaster had occurred in comparatively sheltered waters, there had been a fairly heavy swell, and the crew had had a hard time getting the three women and two children, returning patients, to the nearest island, which was three quarters of a mile away. A shelter had had to be extemporised from some spare sails and oars, as the island was small and quite devoid of any buildings or woods. As it was known that the Hudson's Bay Company's steamer *Nascopie*[58] had gone into Rigolet shortly before, Sam Pottle had borrowed another dory from a chance schooner fishing about four miles from *Yale*, and he had rowed into Rigolet on the chance of getting a pluck-off for *Yale* as *Nascopie* came out of the bay, but the steamer had already left before he arrived.

All too early in my new career, I was faced with a problem quite outside my previous experience. The salvage of boats was a matter that had not concerned me at all. Even if I could go, I could give no expert advice. The fishery was at its height. Time was money, and it was quite hopeless to organise a relief expedition from Indian Harbour. Reeve was the only recruit that I could send, though Mr Jerrett kindly lent grapnels and rope which would be of use. *Yale* was immensely strongly built. Her frame was of oak and teak and her hull of double pitch pine. A deep iron keel of two tons weight protected her planks from contact with rocks (unless she was laid far over), and three tons of cement ballast gave valuable support from within to frame and hull. Fred had mentioned that she was not leaking, but the fact that she had grounded at high water, on a tide that was particularly high because of a southeast wind and full moon, added to the difficulty of salvage. However, the crew won. Taking out everything that could be removed and working waist-deep at low water, they drilled through the keelson, hauled down wood casks under the bulge of the hull, each cask being able to raise from half to three quarters of a ton, and set out anchors and grapnels far into deep water. Then, on another high tide, they triumphantly winched her off with her own little hand-winch, very little the worse for wear.

Before Indian Harbour saw *Yale* again after her delayed trip up the inlet, *Sagona* had come and brought my assistant, not a fourth-year medical student but a fourth-year college student who was thinking of taking a medical course. It was a rather embarrassing situation for us

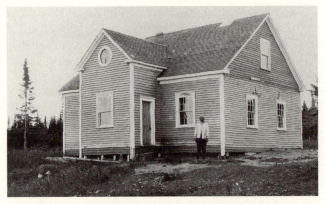

Revillon Frères residence, North West River, c. 1925
(*Them Days* Archives)

both, but apart from a certain amount of inevitable handicap to the work, neither Frank nor I found any cause to repine over another's error, for a friendship began which time has only strengthened, and that summer had a certain value in shaping the destiny of one who has since risen to a very responsible position.[59] The air cleared, we faced the situation and set to work.

The first case was an abdominal operation on a woman [Priscilla Groves] in the prime of life, in excellent health, and apart from a natural deliberation, everything went smoothly. The second case was her little foster-son, Johnnie Lloyd, a delightful, lisping boy of six who was as good as gold. Twenty-five years later, both are dead, the woman of aneurysm and the boy a victim of a Labrador winter blizzard, lost when travelling alone by dog-team. He suffered from double hernia, and his case too was a success. This early experience gave us both confidence and also our neighbours.

A little later, there came a more formidable case that would have been much easier if X-ray had been available. It was a case of renal stone, which caused some anxiety but finally terminated favourably. Then came our first setback, not at the expense of a patient but in a mishap to me. This was the incurring of a nasty septic infection in my right hand. Besides the pain and loss of sleep involved, I could do no surgical work. Frank had to be my right hand, doing my ward dressings and any minor surgery in the out-patients department. The inevitable abscess was slow in forming, and impatience resulted in premature explorations for pus without results. Finally, worn out with pain and lack of rest and fed up with directing incisions on my own hand, I gave Frank a lecture on the anatomy of the hand, took a general anaesthetic

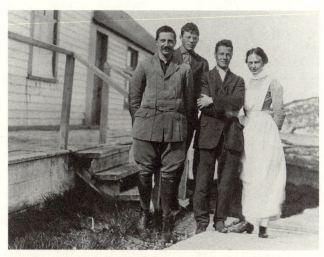

Dr Harry Paddon, Frank Babbott, Austin Reeve, and Mina
Gilchrist at Indian Harbour, 1912 (Faculty of Medicine Founders'
Archive, Memorial University)

administered by the nurse, and went to sleep hoping for the best. Frank
did his job well, and convalescence at last began. For another week or
more, Frank had to carry on as surgeon, and it was just such an experience that was needed to enable him to decide that medicine was his
desired career. Twenty years later, I was to attend the installation of
Frank as president of a well known medical school in the eastern United
States which has made real strides under his administration. Before she
died, the woman referred to above told me that her one clear memory
of her operation was that on coming out of the anaesthesia she realised
that "the young doctor" was keeping marauding mosquitos off her face.
That was like Frank. He might not be able to do an operation at that
time, but he would always find something to do for a patient's comfort.

   The in-patient work did not provide all the thrills. I can still vividly
remember one schoonerman walking into the dispensary carrying his
right ear in his right hand, although the organ was still united to the
scalp by a long strip of tissue. Caught with his weather eye closed
when running before a following wind with both big sails squared out,
one on either side, "wing and wing," the foresail boom had gybed
across the deck and caught him on the side of the head. Most fortunately, he escaped without a fractured skull, but the ear was simply
swept away and left hanging. The crucial point now was whether the
tag that held the ear to the scalp contained the necessary blood supply
to maintain the vitality of the organ. Happily, it did, so it was a simple

matter to sterilise the area and stitch the ear back in its proper place. A few days later, a grateful and happy patient sailed away northward.

One other case of that summer seems worth recording because it illustrates the dual problem, medical or surgical and also social, that so many of our cases did present. A young Labradorman was admitted with one of the varieties of club-foot. The great muscle-tendon at the heel, the most powerful in the human body, was contracted, and the heel was drawn up towards the calf of the leg. [His] condition, an attack of scurvy, [was due to] the associated debility and inactivity, in which case the more powerful flexors are always apt to cause deformity at the expense of the extensor muscles unless suitable precautions are taken.[60] The scurvy was due to lack of initiative and also of knowledge, with failure to use the very facilities which nature so abundantly offered. It was a simple surgical operation to correct the deformity but not so simple to make over the inner man. The lad had got into other trouble as well, bringing him within the reach of the law, and badly needed to get right away into new surroundings and to make a fresh start. As it happened, a prosperous man who lived away north needed a young assistant and was willing to take the convalescent patient. He, however, refused to go. When given an ultimatum that if he persisted in refusal we were through with him as soon as he was landed at Rigolet, he still remained obdurate. So he was finally warned and then discharged, cured.

A few months later, when making a dog-team patrol, I found him attempting a parasitic existence at the expense of a kind-hearted neighbour. But even a worm will turn, and the involuntary host had had enough of him and suggested that he should return to us. To this I returned an unqualified refusal. When a plea was attempted on religious grounds, the obvious retort was that it is laid down in Holy Writ that "if any man will not work neither shall he eat."[61] This man had no dependents, and there was simply no excuse for his being a parasite. If he refused to make any effort to live, the world would certainly be no poorer for his absence. If this sounds hard, surely it is simple truth that there is no greater injury that one man can do to another than to rob or relieve him of self-respect. With a single individual, the issue seems clear. It is when there are women and children to suffer for their sins that the parasite has administrator or philanthropist to some extent at his mercy. And in this case the mailed fist proved effective. His bluff called, the parasite became a self-supporting citizen more years than not, and such periods of depression as there may have been were at least brief. If a defective man tries, much may be forgiven.

That summer was also to know the bitterness of failure. Encouraged by visible successes among neighbours and kinsfolk, a stout, elderly woman presented herself suffering from a serious pelvic condition. I knew perfectly well that the necessary operation needed greater facilities than I possessed, largely because of the patient's stoutness and a weak heart, a case where speed was needed but was difficult to achieve. I tried my best to make her see this and to persuade her to go where there was a bigger team, but she would not consider going further from home. To go away as she was meant much suffering and shortened life. I did not expect her to live a year without an operation. On the other hand, while the surgery must be done under considerable handicaps at Indian Harbour, there was a fair chance of a complete cure, and the patient was more than willing to take the risk. So we operated, and in the last minutes of what should have been a successful operation, she collapsed and succumbed. To have to conduct the funeral service was not a light penalty for failure. Happily there were no children. I was, of course, sorry for the husband, but he soon married again.

There were also touches of comedy without which a medical career would be a depressing one. In the autumn, a homeward bound schooner anchored in the harbour, and a boat brought ashore most of the little ship's company. Of these, one member was tenderly borne up the wood-walk by the rest. "He's a wonnerful sick man, doctor. His legs is so weak he can't hardly walk. We had to do most everything for him, and he hardly gets a wink of sleep at nights." The patient looked extremely comfortable and well fed. It was admitted that there was little wrong with his appetite, and it was not altogether surprising that he was wakeful at night, as he did a considerable amount of sleeping by day. I had no doubt that he was a malingerer, but it is always best to make as sure as possible before accusing a man of shamming, and it was obviously impossible to convince his benefactors that their philanthropy was misplaced by a bare statement to that effect.

So the patient was taken to the dispensary, stripped, thumped and "sounded," and generally fussed over, all of which strengthened the first impression. He was then told that some conditions, especially of the heart, are more readily detected after a little exertion. If he would cooperate by ascending the hill behind the hospital and then returning to the dispensary, further examination might reveal something at present obscured. The patient, flattered by all this attention, agreed to the suggestion. As soon as he was fairly under way, encouraged by shouts to further exertion, the audience was summoned. Eyes bulged, senses reeled, words failed, and then simply poured. Meanwhile, the star performer reached the crest, turned, and saw what awaited him. His descent was a longer performance than the ascent and met with no applause. In grim silence, he was seized, marched down to the waterside, projected into the boat, and returned to the ship, which soon got under way. Something told me that one member at least of that schooner's crew would do his full share of work for the rest of the voyage south.

As a relief from stress when stress there was, nothing was a better relaxation on a fine evening in the sunset hour than to scale the rather menacing crag that almost overhung the little hospital and watch the play of colours in sky and water. Indian Harbour was ever a great place for sunset effects. There was another feature that I have not yet mentioned. When viewed from the right angle, this crag presented a remarkable silhouette of an Indian's head, though I do not know if that had brought the name to the harbour. Headdress, aquiline nose, and fairly well marked chin were all complete, and the effect was intensified when twilight or moonlight left the foreground indistinguishable and threw the profile into sharper relief. And in addition to the head, the continuance of the ridge made a very fair representation of a recumbent body with hands folded on the breast under a blanket and knees drawn up. Generations of mortal fisher-folk might come and go and the Labrador Indians and Eskimos might pass away, but the silent guardian of Indian Harbour, the relic of an ice-age of remote antiquity, still keeps his endless vigil while time shall last or until some great earthquake or the slow but relentless efforts of winter frosts shall mar or destroy that proud profile.

And the northern lights. At one time, a whole sector of the sky was ablaze, as it were, with the vivid crimson glow of a great forest fire, at another time with those writhing, multicoloured streamers; and once only but never forgotten, a great globe of empurpled light, which broke like a wave and foamed across the sky, gathered itself together and broke and foamed again. One group of scientists used to say that these lights, which come nearer to the earth in these latitudes than anywhere else, never approached within sixty miles of the earth's surface. I am prepared to swear (and to call witnesses to bear me out) that I have seen these lights within six hundred feet of the sea level and far below the summit of hills charted at six hundred feet.

Nor has Indian Harbour been altogether devoid of historic interest. It was from here in 1909 that Peary[62] despatched his message announcing the conquest of the Arctic and the attainment of the North Pole, the most northerly of the summer wireless stations then being close to Indian Harbour at Smokey Tickle. During this same summer of 1912, we were to receive a visit from Peary's companion and successor in

United States Arctic adventure, Commander Donald MacMillan.[63] To Indian Harbour again in 1914 came a power schooner carrying a unit of the famous Royal Canadian Mounted Police force. A captain, a sergeant, and a private[64] had been despatched to round up the Eskimo slayer of a white man in far north Canadian territory. It was a manhunt that lasted two years, and the police got their man. But the slayer was acquitted, and this case provoked considerable discussion, one school maintaining that no white man would now be safe amongst those Eskimos and the other that equitable judgment is the best type of British justice. I think that history has since vindicated the verdict. On various occasions, too, Captain Bob Bartlett,[65] the veteran arctic captain of Newfoundland, has breezed into Indian Harbour in his power schooner [*Effie M.*] *Morrissey*. And in 1924, it was to Ice Tickle, right alongside Indian Harbour, that the first round-the-world fliers from the United States made their final trans-marine hop from Greenland to North American soil, and Indian Harbour was the headquarters of the American naval squadron that waited on the aeronauts.

Enough has surely been written to show that the position of day and night nurse, combined with that of housekeeping, was no sinecure for one woman [Mina Gilchrist] at Indian Harbour in 1912. I had been promised a second nurse "when the work justified the request," and I had long ago sent out an SOS. Communications are slow on Labrador, and the brunt had already been borne when relief came. When at last we knew that an assistant was due on the imminent *Sagona*, there was something of a lull in activities in hospital, and I determined to seize the opportunity for that trip up the inlet in *Yale*. Besides any patients to be seen, there was a further need to plan for the winter. Thus far, there had been no resident doctor between Battle Harbour and the far distant Okak Moravian Mission centre in Eskimo territory.

For the coming winter, Dr Arthur Wakefield[66] of London Hospital, a freelance who had already spent a winter in makeshift quarters in Cartwright on one occasion, was to join up with me for a common headquarters at Mud Lake if we could get permission to use the buildings of the expiring lumber company, and as Dr Grieve was to be out on furlough, one of us would patrol by dog-team to Battle Harbour and the other northward as far as Nain. Mrs Wakefield[67] would accompany her husband into winter quarters, and a nurse [Laura Coates][68] would complete the party.

4

Up Hamilton Inlet to the Garden of Labrador

After six or seven rather strenuous weeks ashore, it was a great refreshment to be afloat once more, and as it turned out I could not have chosen a much better time to see what *Yale* was really worth as a seaboat. The run to Rigolet was uneventful. It was later that I learned that the islands off both shores of this eastern basin of Hamilton Inlet and the sheltered waters that they help to enclose, as well as the marshy lands of the mainland, are a vast natural nursery for migratory birds such as might delight the heart of Grey Owl[69] or Jack Miner.[70] It was true that they were not an officially protected preserve, nor were they altogether unviolated, but the amount of disturbance offered no threat of extermination to the vast hordes of geese and ducks of various kinds. Of course, the majority go farther north to breed, and only a modest toll is taken for food from those that remain in the inlet.

A few miles from Rigolet is a small island [Smith's Island] that has since become of local historic interest. It lies but a few hundred yards off the south shore. The intervening water is a fairly rapid tideway and exposed to all but southerly winds. One day in early spring, a sheet of new ice formed and froze onto the thick shoal ice which had been there all the winter. The danger of venturing on "young ice" is well realised because of more than one tragedy, and the younger generation had been duly warned by their elders at the little hamlet of two households situated on this part of the shore. But on that particular morning, the men were all away in the only boat that was caulked and ready for use, and the temptation to go fishing on the young ice was irresistible to two boys. And that very morning, the wisdom of the elders and the rashness of youth were terribly illustrated, for the young ice broke loose with a flood tide and a strong wind and went drifting out into the tideway. Too late the pair realised their danger, and their despairing shouts were heard by the women and children ashore.

There was no boat of any kind available except a cranky, leaky little "flat"[71] built for tending nets just offshore in smooth water. She had not been used for two years, and her seams gaped wide. Nevertheless, a rescue party was made up of two women and a girl, the women to row and the girl to bail with a ten-pound butter tub. The flat reached the ice safely and the boys were taken aboard. Of course, the added weight put additional seams under water, and the leakage increased alarmingly. The final touch that sealed their doom was added when the makeshift bailer suddenly disintegrated and the water rushed in unchecked. Before the eyes of all those left ashore, the flat foundered, and one after another of the five victims disappeared, struggling and screaming to the last.[72] The men returned to find their homes decimated as with a pestilence. The heroic self-sacrifice of the three would-be rescuers was fittingly commemorated with a memorial cross which stands on the summit of the little island and flings its challenge to passersby.

Thanks to the wireless station at Smokey Tickle, which could usually give timely warning of *Sagona*'s approach, we did not have long to wait at Rigolet. Meanwhile, a stiff northeaster had sprung up which rapidly increased to a full gale of wind. At least it was fair in direction for our run up Lake Melville. When the steamer arrived and we secured our mail, it was soon a case of up anchor and away for a real sail. Neither Fred nor Will was afraid to carry sail, and jigger, mainsail, staysail and jib all went up without a single reef in any of them. For ten miles above Rigolet, we had to pass through the Narrows run, and from hills several hundreds of feet in height which rose from the north shore great squalls of wind leaped down onto the surface of the run, whipping up whole acres into the whirling spindrift. Had such a puff reached our sails with unabated force, disaster must have followed, but by keeping well over to the south shore Fred avoided any damage. Our portside anchor was frequently submerged as *Yale* careened, but with the leverage of her deep iron keel at work, there was no fear of her capsizing. If only her planks were kept from contact with rocks in a heavy sea, *Yale* was almost a lifeboat.

Rigolet, like Cartwright, was a salmon fishing centre, and all the way up the run were little summer dwellings at intervals. The north shore was well wooded and the scenery was picturesque, but it was a terrible region for flies of the baser sort. At the western end of the run, little Eskimo Island cut an already narrow channel into two narrowed arms. I was told that on Eskimo Island no less than four hundred Eskimos died during a single epidemic of smallpox.

Emerging on the wider waters of Lake Melville, [we found] the wind was less squally, but there was still plenty of it, and we reeled off the miles in delightful style. From ten to fifteen miles above the Narrows, a chain of islands runs right across the lake, dividing it into two unequal basins, the larger being some fifty miles long with an extreme width of over twenty miles. With mountains up to nearly four thousand feet high on the south side and hills exceeding seventeen hundred feet on the north shore, it is a great place for wind, and the short lop, aggravated by a certain amount of tide, is more smothering to small vessels than any ocean swell. As we pointed up from the Narrows, astern of us was a long cul-de-sac stretching away for nearly thirty miles to the eastward. Subsequent investigation convinced me that this was the remains of the original estuary of the Grand River watershed, which used to run out to the sea through what is now the strand shore, between the eastern basin of Hamilton Inlet and Sandwich Bay. The age-long battle between salt water and fresh has silted up a bank which has become an isthmus joining a long peninsula to the rest of the mainland. This isthmus is over ten miles in width, consisting of low-lying marshes, ponds, and wooded land. This view has been since confirmed by a scientific investigation, the results of which were published.[73]

The scenery of Lake Melville was glorious. Besides the mountains, real forests contributed their quota and the islands also. The loftiest, St John Island, is a great mass of rock, rising almost sheer in places for nearly eight hundred feet from the water, with wooded and grassy coves around the base. With a smaller island, it forms a narrow and very lovely harbour.

The islands left astern, it was like going out to sea again, except for the shortness of the lop, a point of land far ahead on either bow but nothing directly ahead for some hours except white-capped waves. As we had not left Rigolet till well after noon and the approach to North West River is tortuous amid dangerous shoals, we turned into a deep bight on the north side to make a straight-shore anchorage about thirty miles from North West River. The wind had dropped considerably with the sun. The following day we made North West River in the forenoon, steering through the narrow channel that crosses the bar by marks on the land. The river channel is barely half a mile in length, being merely the narrow outlet of the whole Naskaupi system which rises on the height of land from Lake Michikamau, which adjoins another large lake that gives origin to the greater Grand River. Above the short channel mentioned are two lakes joined by a short rapid: first Little

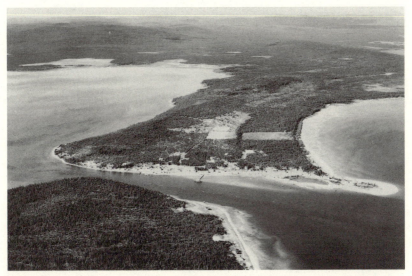

North West River and approaches to Little Lake, 1935 (Yale University Library)

Lake, three miles in length, and the Grand Lake, forty miles long. And so I beheld the lovely hamlet which within three years was to become our headquarters for medical work and social service and where much later again our own home was to be built. The hamlet was to develop into the most prosperous and productive village on the whole coast north of Belle Isle straits, pending the coming of Big Industry, and might well become the leading port of the Labrador of the future. Where now was the land that God gave to Cain or a "God-forsaken wilderness unfit for human habitation"? Cod and fog are far away. Here was a Garden of Labrador, which during a season of each year could produce vegetables as good as those which would be grown in the Garden of Eden itself.

The place fairly gripped you with its beauty. Spruce, fir, larch, and some aspen poplar, with an occasional mountain ash and great beds of alder, supplied the woodland and features of the landscape. The woods came to within a few rods of the water's edge, but a good strip of grassy bank was available on either shore, and there was usually a breeze either up or down the channel and the bay outside. It was one of the best places as regards insects anywhere on the coast. The daytime temperature was altogether too hot for the mosquitoes, which only emerged in the cool of the evening, and so long as one kept in the sun there was almost assured immunity. In the woods or swampy places, however, there was trouble in store for rash adventurers.

The bay was about ten miles wide at the head of Lake Melville. On the south side, Sandy Point run led on westward to Goose Bay, the final basin of any size in the inlet, and into the near end of Goose Bay opened the mouth of Grand River. Both shores were densely wooded, and behind the foothills of the south shore rose the Mealy Mountains, which followed the inlet to its extreme limits westward and extended beyond them. The afterglow of the setting sun, especially when snow lay on the mountains, was a spectacle worth seeing. On the north of the river was the Hudson's Bay Company's post, where Donald Smith had been a clerk of the company before he achieved fame and earned a baronetcy as a prime mover in the inauguration of the Canadian Pacific Railway. Below the post, which included agent's house, handyman's house, store and warehouses, the bank was usually occupied for most of the summer by anything up to two hundred Indians, the Montagnais, a surviving sub-tribe of the great Algonquin race. Being more nomadic than the coastal Eskimos, they had survived the contact with the white races better; none the less, the "white plague" was active amongst them, and as the trappers of white or mixed stock increased and multiplied and spread further and further into the hunting grounds which the Indians considered to be their birthright, life became for them more and more a dire struggle for existence. There was resentment, occasional raiding of hunters' tilts or huts, and rifling of caches of food, also appropriations of traps and stoves by the Indians which roused the white man's ire. There never had been bloodshed, while there had been attempted starvation and pursuit of raiders with loaded rifles. On the whole, however, there was a wide degree of tolerance and sometimes real friendship in time of stress, and not all on one side. On the south bank stood the rival fur-trading post of Revillon Frères. The agent, Monsieur Thevenet, while of French birth, had lived in Canada and had fought in the Boer War on the British side.[74] His assistant was Monsieur Lescaudron, an ex-sailor of the French navy.[75]

The Indians were Roman Catholics, Jesuit fathers having been the first missionaries to them, and ranked as Canadian subjects though frequenting this spot of supposedly Newfoundland territory. On leaving North West River, it was their custom to travel across to the Gulf of St Lawrence, where was an Indian agent of the Canadian government.[76] The Indians having already left, I had to postpone my first meeting with them indefinitely. After a visit to the two posts and after treating one or two cases, we left for Mud Lake.

The wind was still from the northeast, and we romped across the bay to take Sandy Point run. We now entered a maze of sandy shoals outside the mouth of Grand River. A giant tree, towering above all

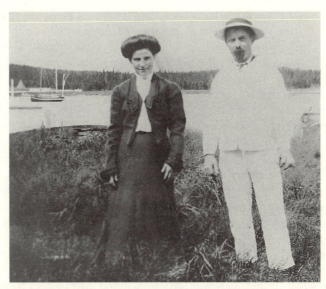

Harriet Pardy and Joseph Lescaudron with Revillon Frères vessel
Roméo in the background, c. 1920 (*Them Days* Archives)

others in that neighbourhood, had to be kept in line with a little peak
on a line of hills to go through one part of the tortuous channel. Then
we swung off northwest to pass Rabbit Island and turned southwest
into the river mouth. We crossed the stream diagonally, following the
opposite shore fairly closely for a time, and turned into a narrow
channel leading out of the mainstream, where we anchored between
a small island and a point around which opened another channel
leading into Mud Lake. *Yale* could only traverse this on high tides, in
autumn or spring, so we had about three-quarters of a mile to row
into the settlement. Ahead of us lay Mud Lake, a sheet of water about
fifteen square miles in area, but we had to turn off into yet another
channel which flowed around an island on which stood Grand Village,
the headquarters of the Grand River Pulp and Lumber Company, just
going into liquidation.[77]

Two paddlewheel tugs were resting on the bottom for their final
disintegration, as were two enormous lighters. A sawmill was still at
work sawing up the last of the cut logs, the lumber to be sold locally.
A young Nova Scotia man came forward to receive the mail. I then
learned that an epidemic of scarlet fever had visited Mud Lake. The
epidemic was over, but sequels remained in the shape of running
ears and enlarged tonsils. During the previous winter, the company
had kept a doctor there, and there was a dispensary still fairly well

supplied, so I got quickly to work. I then inspected the buildings which were to be our winter quarters, a block of three small cottages being the most promising, in one of which was the dispensary. The island was well wooded originally, though it had been largely denuded by the lumbermen, but the surroundings were beautiful. It was a most fertile spot, consisting entirely of alluvial washings of the great river close by. A visit to the "lake shore" revealed a little group of quite attractive Labrador homesteads. On the island, the buildings were rather standardised shacks of rough lumber and shingles for employees of the company. It seemed as if we were to have some very interesting and charming neighbours for our winter at Mud Lake. The lumbermen had introduced horses, and there were also two cows and some fine hay meadows and some nice garden plots.

As we emerged from Sandy Point run on our return journey, my attention was called to a tall smokestack belonging to a defunct lumbermill at a place called Kenemich, on the south side of the bay and in sight of North West River. This mill had been a far bigger structure than that which was still working at Mud Lake. It had had a capacity of 170,000 feet per day and had cost $70,000. It worked just for one single week before the crash came. The wrecking of a supply ship was the final straw. The mill had boasted electric light and telephone, and the foundation beams were sixteen-inch square in size, cut locally. In a store were lumbermen's jackets, boots, shirts and blankets under the charge of an incorruptible Scot, Malcolm McLean, who guarded them unpaid year after year.[78] It was only when marauding squirrels ate their way through the wood walls and started to destroy the dry goods that it at last became possible to persuade the caretaker that this was abandoned property, from which he was fully entitled to recover what he could of sixteen years' overdue wages.

Having called at North West River again for mail, we chugged down Lake Melville in glorious but all too calm weather, our auxiliary engine only affording rather funereal progress. The "lure of the Labrador" was no longer a meaningless catchphrase for me. Despite the visible failure of two premature enterprises, I was henceforth a convinced believer in the future of this lovely region, with its great water system and its forests besides possible minerals.

Within twenty-five miles of Indian Harbour was a defunct copper mine, and there was abundant evidence of iron. Rumours of gold needed to be accepted with reserve, of course. Then there was the evidence of the responsiveness of the soil and also of the feasibility of cattle, and if cattle could flourish, poultry could too. The lumbermen had kept pigs. Mud Lake had shot its bolt for a time, at any rate, and it was comparatively inaccessible as compared to North West River.

A two-thousand-ton tramp steamer had just been able to pass the bar of Sandy Point run to ship lumber off Rabbit Island, but vessels of any tonnage could reach North West River. A favouring wind that night speeded up our return to Indian Harbour, and our round trip of three hundred miles had taken only a little over three full days. An extra nurse made a great difference, though Frank had had to leave by the steamer that brought her. She turned out to be my fellow traveller [Alice Metcalfe] between St John's and Battle Harbour on the rather hectic trip of two months previously.

Tension eased and the rush reduced, there was leisure to summarise the medical experience and impression of those early weeks. First, as to the general run of cases. In any industry there is apt to be an occupational type of disease or disorder, and the cod fishery offered no little scope for these. I have already referred to the dietetic deficiencies in the normal life of many Newfoundland fishermen, and if this was the case at home it was liable to be intensified when away at the fisheries, except for the abundance of fresh fish when "fish is in." But a number of fishermen came to the Labrador in anything but first-rate condition and were liable to go from bad to worse. So we were seldom without some case or cases of beri-beri. Again, the very nature of the work, splitting and cleaning endless cod, strongly favoured septic infection of cuts and grazes from knives and bones. In the rush of the week's work and with very defective facilities for strict cleanliness, these were apt to be neglected till they assumed painful and disabling proportions. An inactive member of a fish crew is not popular. To get his share of the proceeds, he must do his share of the work. There was no system of workmen's compensation or insurance. Hence, the victim of such circumstances often held grimly on till he was compelled to desist, by which time burrowing pus not infrequently threatened (if it had not already destroyed) the vitality of one or more finger bones. Yet another occupational affliction was the extremely uncomfortable tendency to boils, chiefly where rough oilskins chafed wrists or neck. Neither fishermen, skippers, nor merchants, for the most part, seemed to have any idea of the value of prevention by antiseptic cleansing of the hands as a routine and prompt disinfection of a cut or of the importance of early treatment when infection had obviously occurred.

If you blamed a shareman,[79] he probably blamed his skipper or the merchant. You could hear two or three sides to almost every story without really getting anywhere, except to final amputation perhaps. The men were there to fish, first and always, and Sunday was the only day they had any time to be ill. The fact that malingerers were not unknown, of which illustration has already been given, no doubt added to a problem already more than sufficiently complex. Furthermore, the free use of surface drainage water by groups of fisher-folk always held out the possibility of a typhoid "carrier" causing an outbreak. In over a quarter of a century, I have met but one case of typhoid in a Labrador patient, whereas it has been by no means uncommon amongst Newfoundland fishermen in that time.

The nature of the occupation, involving long hours in open boats in all weathers, as well as in buildings far from weatherproof, also made the common cold a formidable affair at times, even leading on to pneumonia. Here again, the rarity of pneumonia among Labradormen as compared to Newfoundlanders, even allowing for the difference of population, has appeared to me to be marked. Besides these well-known conditions, there were various disorders of the digestive apparatus not amounting to disease, and skin complaints were also very common. A great scarcity of dentists in Newfoundland outposts and their complete absence in Labrador naturally meant a good deal of trouble, and enlarged tonsils and adenoid growths were also common. But worst of all, a real menace to public health and economic welfare was "white plague" or consumption. On this again, occupational rigours had a marked influence.

There was also the element of tradition to be reckoned with in the fishermen, as well as a great relative ignorance of disease, as compared with the London cockney, and deplorable attachment to quack medicines. Compared to the glib cockney, educated by teaching rounds in the surgical and medical wards where his case was freely discussed, the Newfoundlander was almost inarticulate about his diseases. "Bad head," "bad side," "bad back," "bad stomach" (which often meant lungs), and "bad legs" were common in unenlightening medical histories. The rest must be found out by eyes, hands, stethoscope, and laboratory methods as well as by leading questions. The cockney had been apt to fire off the family and individual history for two generations or more, almost without drawing breath. Reverting once more to occupational considerations, many "bad backs" were simply the result of working in cramped positions for long periods, but the amount of Dodd's Kidney Pills taken by people with no more kidney disease than I had was appalling.[80]

There was also a pathetic faith in plasters and liniments, the latter being freely drunk, and this among people who admitted that they had been spending precious dollars on these palliatives and painkillers for periods of many years. Working in cold water while hauling hard on heavy twine produced many cases of strained muscle tendons of hand and wrist. These were comparatively easy to relieve and cure, despite anything that the patient might do, within limits, of course. There was in many cases a rooted objection to the knife which offered the one

chance to a poisoned finger or even a limb. Poultices were greatly
overworked – and such poultices! A sticky mess of molasses and
soaked bread often confronted the surgeon who was in a hurry to treat
a closed or discharging abscess, and such preparations as "dragon's
blood,"[81] a gummy, crimson preparation, also added much labour in
cleaning up the skin for incision. To spend twenty minutes in explain-
ing the elements of massage or the value of rest and elevation in certain
conditions instead of just slinging out pills and plasters seemed to many
of my patients sheer callous neglect, and it was sad to hear victims of
beri-beri describing as "dog food" the brown bread which was going
far to restore them to health and which would also have gone far to
prevent their disease. Sometimes the family doctor in Newfoundland
was blamed because a man had come to the fishery who should have
stayed at home, and I can only hope that those gentlemen remembered
that there were two sides to some of the stories which they were
doubtless told about me.

One day a Newfoundland fisherman walked into my dispensary with
a distinctly limping gait. On investigation, [I found] he had a great
abscess presenting in the left groin which was the size of a large orange.
It was clearly not an acute septic condition but a chronic tubercular
process. For any possible cure, complete and prolonged rest were first
essentials as well as surgical interference. When this was explained to
the patient, he ridiculed the idea. He had come north to fish, with the
consent, *as he declared*, of his doctor at home. If he did not fish, he
could not support his family for the following winter, beyond which
he seemed quite incapable of looking. Could I help him to fish in
reasonable comfort? It was quite impossible to let him go away like
that, which he evidently intended to do if he could get no satisfaction
from me, so within a few minutes about a pint of pus was evacuated,
dressings applied and more provided for the future, and a grateful
patient walked comfortably out of the room and went aboard his
schooner to go on north. But how long was he to live?

Another case was the following. A planter fishing from a room
within a furlong of the hospital came one morning to have a septic
finger treated. He also had masses of tuberculous glands on either side
of his neck and a "graveyard cough." He obstinately refused even an
examination of his lungs with a stethoscope, and any rest from fishing
was not to be thought of. But when I elicited the fact that he shared
a bunkhouse with five other men, three of whom were married, sharing
of course the common eating and drinking utensils, it became much
more than an individual problem. An attempt to get him to realise his
social duties and responsibilities produced only resentment, and he
angrily demanded to be released. By this time I was angry too, although

sorry for him, and I detained him till his skipper could be sent for. When he came, I put the matter to him:

"Jim, you and I are good friends, and I have no wish to interfere with your fishing or this man's liberty, except in so far as I am bound to. He has enough disease in him to kill not only himself but all his fellow men who share the bunkhouse with him and three families into the bargain."

Jim gasped. "But doctor, he's one of the best and strongest men I have."

The skipper was a first-rate man, intelligent, honest, kindly, but simply uneducated in matters affecting tuberculosis and public health. The cough to him was just a cold, and the lumps in the neck seemed to be doing no harm, and the man was a good fisherman and a willing worker and that was that. I then suggested that a lean-to be erected on the back of the bunkhouse to provide separate sleeping accommodation and that special eating and drinking equipment be provided for the patient. When Jim promised this, with one or two additional precautions, I believed that his promise would be faithfully kept, and the man departed. I am sure Jim thought I was in error *for three weeks but no more*. The patient went rapidly downhill and died. Probably, I had hastened his end by destroying his hope, but it was done to save a number of others from sharing his fate, if possible.

I certainly have not overdrawn the picture of 1912, as any well informed person familiar with the places and conditions dealt with would readily admit, but at the same time a movement in the right direction was taking place in the appearance of NONIA – not a star actress or prima donna but the Newfoundland Outpost Nursing and Industrial Association, started, I believe, by Lady Davidson, wife of the governor of Newfoundland of that time.[82] This organisation has wrought a great change in many places and people.

Summer gave way to autumn, and the equinox came and went with the traditional gales. The fish moved out into deep water, and "making" rather than catching fish became the order of the day. For this process, the split cod, which have reposed in the fish stage heavily salted all the summer, are brought out, washed out with sea water and then spread to dry on the rocks. If rocks ever run short, open stages made of small spruce or fir trunks and called "flakes" are used for this purpose. The summer sun is too hot and burns the salted fish. Three days' drying produces the quickest recognised cure, known as "Labrador slop." Other cures up to a week or more are required for "shore fish."[83] If rain threatens, every available man, woman and child works on the "bawn,"[84] piling the fish into circular "bulks" which are covered with tarpaulins. Special steamers or square-rigged schooners collect the fish for export either to St John's or direct to Italian, Spanish or Grecian ports.

Schooners came speeding south, the "well-fished" ones with very little freeboard. Opportunism was needed to take every good chance to get south without undue risk. In the spring, fog and ice are the chief terrors for the schoonermen, in the autumn, equinoctials. One anecdote will illustrate the ice problem of navigators of unprotected vessels. I have heard Sir Wilfred Grenfell relate how a little squadron of these vessels was nosing a way through a fairly loose pack when a shift of wind packed the ice more tightly. One vessel was nipped between two heavy pans so severely that her seams started. To avoid foundering, the crew were compelled to jettison their precious salt to bring the damaged planks above the waterline. Her ribs were also damaged. Seeing her condition, other schooners butted their way alongside, buoyed her up and succeeded in working her into the nearest harbour. A Newfoundlander can do almost anything with an axe and a tree, and she was hove down and repaired. Then, to save her losing time by returning for more salt, each of the salvaging vessels contributed a quota of its own. Such is the freemasonry of the sea.

One spring a great field of ice drove the main portion of the northward-bound schooner fleet into harbours, where they were penned for three weeks, but about a dozen of the leading vessels had got ahead of the ice and passed on north. They, in turn, were penned in by another icefield. They thought they would try at least for a meal of fresh fish, but it turned out that an immense school of cod shared their limited expanse of water. In ten or twelve days, every one of these vessels was filled to capacity, and just as the other schooners began to arrive they were ready to go south and come back for a second voyage that season.

The time arrived to close Indian Harbour down for another winter, but before our party broke up there was one thing of vital importance to me to be settled. Could the association of three months between my nursing colleague [Mina Gilchrist] and myself be prolonged into a life partnership? Her answer was an affirmative, though there was an eight-month separation to be faced first.

5

Autumn Cruising –
Into Winter Quarters

For the open water season each year, *Yale* was to me what a motor car is to a country practitioner with a wide extent of country to cover in other lands. The car must be understood and kept in a reliable condition, and the doctor must familiarise himself alike with main roads and byways in his district. And if this is true of more developed countries, what about a deeply indented coast hundreds of miles in length, the haunt of rocks and shoals, gales, fog, downpours of rain that would not disgrace the tropics, and untimely blizzards of snow – a coast, moreover, that was very poorly charted?

To be able to recognise a dim silhouette in dark, fog, or driving snow almost in a moment of time, to know intimately the response of the vessel to the wheel, the capacity to carry sail, the merits and demerits of harbours and anchorages and those watery sidetracks that would make progress possible when the recognised ship's run was untenable, their surroundings and directions – any or all of these might make the difference between progress and stagnation, success or failure, life or death. Hence, I never regarded it as truancy from more important work to take every opportunity of cruising, and in that autumn of 1912, between the closing of Indian Harbour for the winter and the time for getting into winter quarters according to plan, there was a great opportunity for an instructive trip. It almost summarily ended my career, but it stood me in good stead afterwards.[85]

Yale was to go south to Newfoundland for an overhaul before another season on the Labrador coast. The previous winter, she had been berthed at North West River and had incurred some damage to her steering gear in the spring ice. This was to be repaired and the seams of her hull recaulked and a thorough survey made for any possible damage from her grounding on Yale Rock. Fred Blake was not familiar with the route to be followed. He and Sam Pottle were to be landed at Mud Lake on her last mail trip, and those two, with Fred's elder brother, Captain John Blake, who owned a seven-ton schooner and was the best pilot for the upper waters of Hamilton Inlet, were to meet Dr and Mrs Wakefield and myself at Rigolet on my return north in an old yawl of something under twenty tons named *Roméo*, the property of Revillon Frères at North West River. A special pilot arrived from St Anthony, where Will Simms also belonged, to take her south, and a volunteer cook had been found in a student who was spending a winter north. These with myself made a crew of four. As soon as the hospital was closed, we left on our last mail trip.

While awaiting *Sagona* at Rigolet, snow was on the ground, and I made my acquaintance with the spruce partridge, a variety of grouse [ptarmigan] that relies on camouflage rather than flight. Any apparently dead stump sticking up out of the snow or a seeming bunch of drying spruce foliage may be a succulent meal if detected, but the experienced hunter will get a good bag when the novice will not even see a bird, and little Indian hunting dogs known as "crackies"[86] will find far more birds than the keenest-eyed hunter. During the berry season, the flavour is excellent, but on a diet of spruce the grouse is apt to taste somewhat strong for the uninitiated palate. Since it is usually impossible to put him to flight, the nearest attempt to sport (as well as the most economic method) is to shoot him through the head with a .22 bullet. When nature is in an abundant mood, these birds are almost as thick as flies. I have known 150 to be killed in the immediate vicinity of a trading post in a single morning. The prevalence of grouse and rabbits in Labrador follows a well-marked cycle in definite relation to the movements and abundance of predatory fur-bearing animals.

When *Sagona* arrived and we received our mail, a very different kind of trip up Lake Melville from that of the previous month awaited us. There was a sharp frost, the thermometer registering 14° F. There was also a wind, little less strong than on the other occasion and less fair in direction. As we foamed along with our lee gunwale deeply buried, our little tender was afloat on our deck, lashed fore and aft to the rigging. The boat was good for it, but the leash-line of the mainsail froze stiff and cracked like a dry stick, so we had to ease her. None the less, we made a fast run.

At Mud Lake, the nurse for the winter [Laura Coates] was already installed and was getting the makeshift hospital into some sort of shape for our prospective staff and patients. On our way out of the inlet, the most direct route would have been to go out of the bay on the south side, but we needed to take in more supplies from the closed hospital, and we also had left a cask of fuel oil to be shipped for the run south. When we regained Indian Harbour, the cask was gone. It had not been stolen but borrowed, under the impression that we should not be calling there again, and it was faithfully returned next summer. Meanwhile, it was a serious matter for us which almost led to disaster.

There were half a dozen late schooners anchored in the harbour. Another big breeze was brewing, which was to keep us inactive for the next two days. We managed to purchase twenty gallons of kerosene oil from one of these vessels, but this was really a drop in the bucket if we got baffling winds. It was October 21st when in the half-light of early morning we crept out of harbour and started to sail close-hauled across the wide mouth of the inlet. The wind was light then, but as the sun rose we picked up a spanking offshore breeze along the strand shore and had a splendid sail as far as Pack's Harbour, on the outskirts of Sandwich Bay. Then we kept away more southeasterly for Gready with the wind well on our quarter and bowled along in fine style. Turning nearly south again for another run of just about twenty miles to Indian Tickle, which is quite a separate place from Indian Harbour, [we found] the wind failed us, and we had to use some of our precious reserve of oil to make the harbour. We had put over eighty miles behind us according to the route that we had followed and over seventy as the crow flies, which was a very useful day's work.

Next day dawned dull and lowering. There was not enough wind to keep our sails out, and we should have done better to conserve our remaining oil, but the temptation to get ahead while the going was good was too much for our pilot, so we chugged along at barely four miles an hour from dawn till noon. Then the wind, which was northerly, freshened fast and snow began to fall. By five o'clock, there was a strong rising wind and sea, more snow, and a thoroughly dirty night in prospect. The few schooners going south more or less in company with us were making for Square Islands Harbour, and our pilot decided to run for the same haven. It was then that our troubles began.

Three narrow tickles lead into Square Islands Harbour, and in this wind the northernmost was the one to use. The entrance was very constricted, but there is no question that where those schooners went in, *Yale* could and should have followed. Our pilot was an old man and past his best. He is long since dead and I would not say any unkind word against him, for he was a most kindly old chap, but there is no denying that he erred and erred almost fatally. He was willing to go through the tickle under power but not under sail. Three times we bore up for the mouth of the tickle and three times sheered away. The third time we had emptied lanterns and every other container of kerosene into our almost-dry tank, but tossing about as she was, no steady flow of oil from tank to carburetter could be maintained, and for the last time the pilot sheered away and announced his intention of running for Battle Harbour.

That port was still over thirty miles away, and there was no prospect of getting there till far into the night, and such a night! We might well hit the rocks long before we saw a light from the lighthouse, even if we reached that neighbourhood unscathed. I did not know then as I know now that Occasional Harbour and Ship Harbour are but five and seven miles respectively from Square Islands Harbour, and either could have been reached before it was really dark. However, he had the say and on we went. We had picked up a passenger at North West River in the person of Monsieur Lescaudron, previously referred to as an ex-sailor of the French navy now in the employ of Revillon Frères, who desired to go to Battle Harbour or the nearest port that we touched at. He was now to prove a very valuable addition to our ship's company. Fiercer and fiercer blew the wind, thicker fell the snow, and the sea had become very heavy.

The first incident of note occurred just at dark. A wild cry of "Breakers!" and another of "Hard a-starboard!" The steersman whirled the wheel, the *Yale* sheered rapidly from her course, taking wind and sea more on her beam and rolling wildly. The boom of the foresail came over with a run and nearly took the pilot overboard, and we grazed past an iceberg by feet or yards, but not many of the latter. That was escape number one. Number two came two hours later, when we almost hit the rocks at the extremity of Cape Spear, nine miles from Battle Harbour. Even our pilot had now to admit that we were far more likely to find a watery grave than Battle Harbour if we kept on as we were going, so very reluctantly he put her SSE for ten miles out into Belle Isle straits. This was but a temporary palliative. The right thing to do would be to get clear and heave her to till daylight outside Belle Isle altogether, but he was never a deep water man and hated to go far from land. However, apart from another berg, it gave us some three hours of ease as regards any running ashore.

For a while it cleared, and we saw the eastern light on Belle Isle, but it soon shut down as thick as ever. Monsieur Lescaudron was at the wheel and I was on lookout for'ard, while the others were having a spell below and getting a "mug-up"[87] ready. Suddenly, a light stabbed the darkness almost over our masthead, as it seemed. The Frenchman shouted, "Here's a steamer on top of us," to which I replied, "No port or starboard lights." Once again we sheered away as the others rushed upon deck. Clearing a rocky promontory by what margin heaven only knows, we suddenly opened the western point on Belle Isle, on which is another lighthouse. There were now but sixteen miles between us and Cape Bauld, Newfoundland. Even under greatly reduced sail, we drove along uncomfortably fast with several hours of darkness yet to pass. The old pilot set a course calculated to take us clear of Cape Norman, on the western side of Sacred Bay, into the gulf, but either because of strong tides or because we made unusual leeway under shortened sail, dawn found us pretty well in the bottom of Sacred Bay, uncomfortably close to a bad lee shore. In the night, we had passed enough hidden dangers to have finished us two or three times over.

And now *Yale* had either to beat her way out of that bay or go to pieces, and fortunately for us she did the former. I still remember word for word the almost lyrical outburst of the old pilot when we finally rounded Cape Bauld and squared away along the French Shore. "I have been on many vessels," he declaimed, "but never on a better one than this. There's many a big schooner would have torn herself to pieces beating out of that bay this morning, and *Strathcona* (a little steamer of 110 feet on which he had often served) could not have looked at it." No doubt there was some poetic licence in this statement, excusable in a man who had been strained to breaking point, but there is no question that *Yale* had done a noteworthy performance for a vessel of her tonnage. She had sailed about 275 miles in just about forty hours of actual headway, much of it under shortened sail, and several hours just doing something under four knots on the engine, and her victory over Sacred Bay was a real triumph. The rest of the trip was uneventful, and a day or two later ss *Home* once more carried me in company with Monsieur Lescaudron across Belle Isle straits to Battle Harbour.

It was now October 26th, and it was already November when ss *Solway*,[88] which had replaced *Sagona* for this trip, arrived northward bound with Dr and Mrs Wakefield on board. I had known Wakefield in old days in England as a rugged athlete at swimming, football, and boxing, anything that promised a good scrap. One of the "bulldog breed," he was a man for whom, once his mind was made up, "sweet reason hath no charms,"[89] but none the less a man who had already proved himself in the Boer War and was to do so again in the Great War and also on two Everest expeditions. Some of his records in the Cumbrian Heights still stand today, I believe. His wife also proved to be an outdoor person with a musical talent that was no small asset in the sub-arctic before the days of radio. As already mentioned, Wakefield in his bachelor days had spent one winter at Cartwright, travelling from there northwards to Okak. It was owing to this, no doubt, that he had come so late to the coast on this occasion, for he had no difficulty in reaching Cartwright by the last steamer any more than we had now, Cartwright being but ten miles from the outside coast. But to delay arrival at Rigolet so late, with a hundred-mile voyage in a small sailing craft ahead, was quite another matter, as we were both to learn before we were much older.[90]

It was the afternoon of November 8th when we anchored off the company's post at Rigolet and found *Roméo* awaiting us. As it turned out, we had been within an ace of not finding her there at all. There had been a wedding at Rigolet and, leaving *Roméo* apparently securely anchored, the crew of three had gone ashore to share the festive occasion. Perhaps the romantic event stirred old memories in *Roméo* and sent him off seeking a Juliet. Anyhow, when the crew came out to go aboard for the night there was no *Roméo* to be seen. Pursuit in a small boat resulted in the capture of the truant, quite unhurt, after a stern chase of about ten miles.

It soon became evident that *Roméo* could not take all our freight. We were getting her on favourable terms with the two conditions that her owners' freight should receive priority of space and that if we lost her, $400 should be paid towards her successor. For the moment, the chief consideration was to get it all off the *Solway*, and what *Roméo* could not hold must go on the company's wharf by kind permission of the agent, Mr W.E. Swaffield.[91] The following day, which was still unfavourable for progress as there was a strong headwind with hard frost, we re-stowed her. We shipped the owners' freight first and then our own, in order of importance, leaving till last what we could best do without. The remainder was to be warehoused at Rigolet for the winter. Then we sat down to wait for a favourable wind.

We lodged at the government customs house, the summer resident having left on the *Solway* and permission having been obtained. November 9th and 10th came and went, and the 11th dawned without any shift of wind. About mid-day of the 11th, the westerly died out and a draught of wind came in from the east. We hastily closed the customs house and got aboard, but the wind was so light that when the tide turned against us we could not make headway and had to anchor only nine miles above Rigolet in a snug little salmon fishers' harbour at Snook's Cove. Of course, the summer houses were long since abandoned for the winter season.

On the morning of the 12th, before sun-up, we had just enough wind to stem the last of the down tide and got through the portal of the Narrows run between Eskimo Island and Caravalla Head. We hoped for a fine sailing breeze which would take us to North West

River before dark, but the wind was never more than light to moderate;
it turned snowy, and we were becalmed most of the night off Mulligan
Head, still over twenty miles out. We finally made North West River
next day, the 13th, where we landed what freight we had for Revillon
Frères. We were told that we might have trouble in getting through
Sandy Point run, and it was too late to risk anything with possible ice
in tortuous channels that night.

On the morning of the 14th, we left on our final effort to get into
winter quarters at Mud Lake by water. We had only about twenty-
five miles to go, and the favourable wind still held, or we should have
had no chance whatever. For the first twelve miles all went well. Then
we struck ice, a mere film at first but gradually getting thicker. Fred
Blake was slung in a bosun's chair from the jib-boom to break away
ice from the stem, while Wakefield and I, on either bow, smashed away
with oars or boat hook to protect the planks. Still it was cutting
steadily in, and still the fair wind thrust us ahead. Presently, we lost
headway, as the ice was now too thick, so the next expedient was to
take to the small boat and break a road for the yawl. Needless to say,
progress under these conditions was not rapid, and the short November day was slipping away. If we failed to get to Mud Lake, could we
get back to North West River? If we stuck, we had no supply of fuel
to last us until we could walk ashore perhaps. If we sprang a leak...?
There were about eleven hours of daylight, including morning and
evening twilight. It had taken us till about ten o'clock in the morning
to reach the ice, and it took us over eight hours to cover the next
ten miles. The final bar of ice just outside the river mouth was the
toughest obstacle of all. Wind and small boat both failed to get us
ahead. It was time for any remedy, however desperate.

Lashing ourselves with ropes which were secured to the mast, we
leaped, two or three together, on the ice till it foundered under us,
immersing us to varying depths. Then we scrambled out and leaped
again. It was touch and go now whether our planks would stand till
we got into the river. They did so, and in the twilight hour of evening
we passed Smokey Island with the last of the favouring breeze and then
pulled or towed old *Roméo* along the narrow channel into the Mud
Lake anchorage, rousing and startling the inhabitants with a stentorian
cheer as we dropped anchor. They had given up all expectation of
seeing us till ice travel began. Investigation next morning showed that
no less than five of *Roméo*'s planks were almost cut through, but we
had saved our freight and the $400 and, incidentally, had learned a
lesson never to be forgotten about the respect due to Hamilton Inlet
in the late autumn. It remained to ferry our load ashore, dismantle the
old yawl and see her securely moored for the winter's rest.

We now entered on a period of small village life in the sub-arctic early winter, of a kind completely new to all our party but Wakefield. First of all, there were a number of things to be seen to: the arrangement of our dispensary and stowing away of all our supplies, then the supply of firewood for three stoves. A middle-aged Eskimo, one of those who had been exhibited at Chicago,[92] had been engaged to cut and haul what firewood he could, but his efforts would not suffice. Fred and Sam had already lost some weeks of trapping time, but at least the pay on boats was sure, whereas trapping could either be far more profitable or far less so. Most of the able-bodied men were away trapping, and since medical work was not likely to be excessive, the best thing to do was to go out and cut some wood ourselves. A day in the woods with a four-pound axe is certainly a good appetiser, and other out-of-door pursuits were the hunting of spruce partridges and the beautiful white willow grouse and also white-coated rabbits. The latter were sometimes shot but more often snared. In the catering department, trout fishing through the ice sometimes proved a very profitable occupation. These practical household considerations being attended to, which included a good deal of sport and exercise, there was the problem of how best to use the six weeks or so before the long medical patrols began. Here were two doctors and a nurse in rather restricted surroundings from a professional viewpoint, and the small local population could not supply many ward cases.

There was a little surgery to start with. Wakefield and I each straightened one crooked leg of a delightful but rickety youngster who is now a hustling trapper and father of a family. There was a gynaecological case badly needing attention, and Wakefield ventured into the realm of the eye specialist in a worthy effort to restore sight to a blind veteran by an operation for cataract. This was only a qualified success through no fault of the surgeon. We also admitted a woman, wife and mother and still young, for consumption of the lungs. There were various reasons for admitting this case where there were so many that could not be accepted. The children were small and the father, who was a very successful trapper, could not get away to hunt unless his wife could be cared for elsewhere. Moreover, the children were all too likely to become victims of their mother's disease if she remained with them. The husband was only too glad to pay his wife's maintenance costs if he could get off and earn for his children. She was a very plucky and co-operative patient, but disease had gained too firm a hold and she did not survive the spring.

There were, of course, various minor ailments and accidents and one mental case, fortunately only temporary, which was a very awkward problem to handle in such surroundings. But apart from these few cases, there was still something to be done in the way of medical education of this little public. Weekly health talks were arranged, dealing as simply and directly as we could do with the main problems of health, as we saw them, in an attempt to stimulate the interest and secure the co-operation of those who should be most concerned in such matters. The doctrine of fresh air, of balanced diet in so far as it could be achieved, and of the disorders of digestion could be dealt with and particularly precautions against the spread of consumption. Prevention is proverbially better than cure, and there was room for a good deal of preventive medicine in any small community with few facilities hitherto available. Another thing to be aimed at was an improvement in local standards of midwifery as well as the care of the expectant mother and also the infant. Dental hygiene was another obvious line to work along. Finally, there was the social aspect of life, and it was a great interest to dip into local tradition and custom and to get beneath the surface with some of our neighbours. Of a few, long since dead, I can write freely.

It has already been mentioned that the little village fell into two divisions, lake shore settlers on the mainland and the residents on the island who had gathered around the now extinct milling venture. It was naturally the former who had the more developed and attractive homesteads. At the angle between the lake and the channel which circumvented the island was John Michelin's domicile. As the name suggests, he was of French-Canadian origin. He had two elder brothers: Peter, who lived twelve miles below North West River at Sebaskachu, and Joseph, who had a lovely homestead on Traverspine River, a small tributary of Grand River which joined the mother stream five miles from Mud Lake. John was then about fifty-eight or fifty-nine, of spare figure (fat men are almost unknown in Labrador, though women attain to ample proportions in some cases with their more sedentary lives). His wife was kindly and cleanly. The rest of the family still at home consisted of a grown-up son and daughter. A little wharf supplied landing facilities from the channel, and a neat wood walk led up to the house, past a well-tended garden patch on one side and a storehouse and small barn on the other. A small storm porch led into a spotless kitchen with a two-decker stove. Then came a cheery, light living room with two little ground floor bedrooms beyond. The upper floor provided further sleeping accommodation. To the east of the house were some beautiful trees, and behind was a fine hay meadow with a plantation of poplar varying the prevailing spruce and fir on the west side. Here was no illiterate wilderness inhabitant.

I still remember my gasp of astonishment when, on calling one day, John chattily remarked, "I see they have found the *Mona Lisa*." He

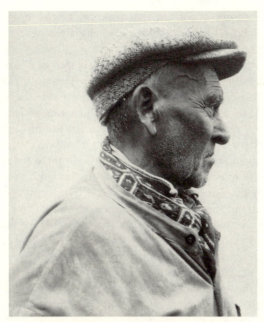

Uncle Joe Michelin (Fred C. Sears)

was an avid reader of the *Montreal Daily Star*. Truly, here was a pleasant, kindly, and prosperous sub-arctic homestead. To eke out trapping, John did a little branch business for the Hudson's Bay Company, which saved both local residents and nomad Indians many a weary mile between Mud Lake and North West River. He was trapping to within thirty hours of his death. Then, a sudden stroke and a quick, easy passing ended an honest and happy life at the comparatively early age of sixty-nine, for his brother Peter lived to see seventy-six, and Joseph, nearly nine-three, is now [1938] the grand old man of the inlet. Peter was a quiet old chap, reckoned an outstanding local carpenter as well as a cunning hand with the fiddle, but Joe was the most colourful of the trio, who shall later be met at his home.

Next to John Michelin's home was Captain John Blake's, a very similar kind of homestead except for the absence of barn and hayfield. John was a widower without children. He had a nephew, "Little" John Blake, who tended his fur-path.[93] [Captain] John was another quiet man but with a twinkle in his eye and a dry humour that often turned the laugh against a tormentor. He was shrewd and thrifty and had money salted away in Canadian securities. He was a man of the strictest integrity and as keen a reader as John Michelin and made quite a little addition to the proceeds of his fur-path with his little vessel. Later on,

John married again, and from that time on Uncle Johnnie and Aunt Sally were my host and hostess whenever I visited Mud Lake. He died at the age of seventy-five.

The third homestead on the lake shore was that of Mark Best, whose wife was a hustling Newfoundland woman [Susanna Lundrigan], an immaculate housekeeper, keen gardener, and capable manager. She also had a great love for domestic animals which has at least one rather comical sequel. A ewe with lamb having died, the old lady reared the lamb by bottle feeding. When, after her husband's death and with grown sons raising families of their own, the home went through some hard times, she felt compelled to part with the lamb to the Hudson's Bay Company's agent at North West River, who saw in it a desirable Christmas dinner. She stipulated that her one-time pet should at least be taken alive out of Mud Lake. So the week before Christmas, the agent sent his junior clerk with a team of husky dogs to transport the crated lamb. All went gaily enough across Goose Bay and through the portage between the basin and North West River Bight. As they came out on the latter sheet of ice in sight of home, but still over a mile away, the amateur teamster left the komatik to get a good warming run, but the dogs spurted too, and at the critical moment the man lost his footing. When he rose again the dogs were fairly off. Had the wind been from the lamb to the dogs, they would probably have run clear, ripped apart the crate, and killed and eaten the lamb before the clerk could intervene, but excited over their escape and thinking of the feed tubs at home, the rascals lost a chance which they would never get again. The astonished agent, who heard the din of the returning team, came out to see the lamb driving up in solitary state behind a big team which could have wolfed him in five minutes. Mark [Best] had two daughters, one of whom [Maggie], the possessor of a good alto voice, acted as choir mistress at the little church and the other [Esther] as schoolmistress of the village school. Both these young women had been to school in St John's.

Such were the three lake-shore homesteads and families in brief.

On the island, Blake and Pottle are already familiar names, to which can be added those of Broomfield, Goudie (more Scotch stock), and Hope. The latter was really an adopted name in place of a Scandinavian surname which it was hopeless to get local people to attempt to pronounce.[94] There were also two families of Whites, one on the island and one in Carcajou Cove, on the point of land between Grand River and the straight channel leading into Mud Lake. Baikie (Scotch again), Mesher, and Gear completed the selection of local names. There were in all sixteen families besides the hospital unit and a bachelor Methodist padre [Rev. W.S. Mercer].[95] The padre was a bold sailor who often cruised solo in his taut little *Glad Tidings* and was also a hardy winter traveller who drove his own team.

For social life, Mrs Wakefield initiated a young people's club for social evenings, and also we staged some sort of entertainment for the trappers and their families when the former came out of the woods for Christmas and the New Year season. Some of the men who went but a limited distance to their furring grounds or fur-paths came and went with some frequency, but the long-distance men emerged only once during the whole winter, for the festive season. And truly the northern Christmas had its charm, spent as it was among people so unsophisticated as to give full flavour to every aspect and incident. For decorations, needless to say, there was no difficulty over a perfect tree, and spruce and fir foliage made the best of wreaths and festoons. As a substitute for holly berries, those of the mountain ash, preserved in sawdust, made an adequate relief to the otherwise sombre green.[96]

For the New Year keeping, of which Donald Smith had made such an occasion, we all went to North West River. I was privileged to read the reminiscences of an old widow [Margaret Campbell Baikie] whose husband had originally come to the country as a young Scottish employee of the company and whose earliest memories went back to the days of Donald Smith. With almost feudal state, the postmaster [post manager] would receive his tenants. There would be a handshaking procession, following which the men would retire with him to drink a glass of wine while women and children received cakes and soft drinks elsewhere.[97] Then came sports, shooting for prizes, and wrestling. On the present occasion, our two ladies rode on a komatik while Wakefield and I walked with a group of trappers on snowshoes. The seventeen-mile tramp was but an appetiser for dinner and the subsequent sports. We were kindly entertained by Monsieur and Madame [Margarette] Thevenet at the "French post" (Revillon Frères) for the mid-day meal. Then came a football match on the shoal ice, Mud Lake *versus* The World, and a tug-of-war which was so protracted as to come very hard on unprotected hands frantically grasping a rope.

We went across to the Hudson's Bay Company's post for the night with Mr Heath[98] as our host. The shooting competition followed next day. Square dances were a feature of these celebrations at night. They took place usually in one of the warehouses of the company. On one occasion, the number and agility of the performers and spectators threatened a collapse of the floor. A group of men sallied forth and in a few minutes reduced stout firewood logs to the required length, jacked up the sagging floor, and it was a case of "on with the dance." One feature of the occasion has been omitted. At the passing of the old year, the company's big bell rang in the new year with an immediate accompaniment from the "Labrador band" of howling huskies. Then a salute of guns followed, and everyone shook hands with everyone else. There was little imported liquor in evidence, though "spruce beer" was brewed locally of very varying potency, and sprees were few and far between. Altogether, it was a very pleasant occasion.

On January 3rd, Dr and Mrs Wakefield and the nurse left for Mud Lake while I started out on a medical patrol of between seven hundred and eight hundred miles to Battle Harbour and back, as well as around the chief bays.

6

The Long Winter Trail

On January 3rd, 1913, stocky little Billy Murphy and I left North West River with ten husky dogs.[99] It was a strange kind of morning for January in Labrador. Within a few hours, thunder and lightening, rain, hail, snow, and then a quick shift of wind with a return of hard frost were experienced. Billy, who belonged to Battle Harbour, had driven for Dr Grieve for a term of winters and was familiar with a large part of the route to be covered by both Wakefield and myself. It was because Dr Grieve was out on furlough that he was available. He had arrived at Mud Lake shortly before Christmas, and the team had been useful in hauling home wood.

In those days it was customary for doctors to travel with two teams, one of seven or eight dogs to haul the doctor and one of nine or ten to haul the load. The latter consisted of grub-box and medicine chest, sleeping bags, tent, snowshoes and axe, and a reserve of dog-feed. This meant from sixteen to eighteen dogs and three men, which made rather a serious addition to the population of some one- or two-roomed cabin, especially if the whole party were hung up for two or three days by impassable blizzards. There were liable to be other travellers too to be accommodated, and in unfamiliar territory it was sometimes necessary to add a special pilot's team. While I naturally conformed to tradition for my first winter or two, a little experience and organisation soon enabled the second team to be dispensed with. The depositing of food supplies for ourselves at convenient points along the route during the open water season, together with careful arrangements about dog-feed and the hiring of a local team just to meet the emergency of a moment, all combined to make one good team do the work of two with little loss of speed and none of distance covered. The programme for this patrol was roughly as follows: first, to treat any cases that could be treated as we went along; secondly, to make a note of cases to be treated at hospital during the following summer; and thirdly, to become familiar with the people of the district covered, their mode of life, their problems, and their viewpoints. Fourthly, no better opportunity could be desired for the purpose of making a survey of manifest tuberculosis in a large district. It is true that the facilities of laboratory and x-ray plant must be missing, but what family history, signs, symptoms, and the stethoscope could reveal could be noted.

In the summer cruising, the considerations of weather and tides, of a safe anchorage during darkness and storms, also the relative importance of the institutional work during the brief open water season all combined to handicap any great progress in these directions. But while it was necessary to use all good opportunities of getting ahead on the winter travel, there were many long, dark evenings to be spent in solitary cabins or small hamlets as well as many days when travel would not be possible, and these afforded splendid scope for the work indicated above.

The intimate association of medical with social service has been stressed, and only house-to-house visitation could make this really effective. Also, it is by no means the most serious cases that always seek out a doctor, especially in a country with such limited communications, and it is by these personal visits that some of the most important patients are discovered and dealt with. This trip, then, really amounted to a culmination of the first year of survey by means of cottage hospital, cruising, and dog-team travel. The going was not very good to start with, and we had only one team. Apart from big teams kept at the trading posts, there were no extra dogs to recruit from amongst this essentially trapping population at the head of the inlet. It was in the Rigolet district that we hoped to get the nucleus of a second team, building up further as we coasted southwards. So the first day's travel was slow.

Five miles out was the first homestead, at a very picturesque spot known as Butter and Snow, probably named from the blending of late autumn foliage with an early snowfall on some remote occasion in the past.[100] Birches and larches would contribute to such an effect. Here, Fred Rich, hustling trapper, seal hunter, and trout fisher, who was also a keen and successful gardener, headed a household like a hive of busy bees. Skin boots were made, not only for the family but also for sale, and later on a little sawmill was to assist further the family budget. The report here was "All well, thanks," so we did not delay.

Eight miles ahead was the hamlet of Sebaskachu with three houses inhabited by old Peter Michelin and two married sons. We had been especially asked to call here to see a case. Sabaskachu lay in a deep bight where snow lay deep much longer than out in the main run of the bay. One or other of us was continually trotting to lighten the load and maintain as good speed as possible. Here we had our mid-day meal. It is almost an insult to go into a Labrador house when on travel and refuse a meal. If staying the night, tea and bread and floor space for the sleeping bag are a recognised minimum of Labrador hospitality. In the more prosperous houses, extras like butter and sugar and fresh trout or game meat are also gladly added. Apart from this, we supplied our own food. (In most households, it was usual for the men and boys to feed first, though family meals are on the increase nowadays.)

Leaving Sabaskachu, [we found] the next house lay five miles on, at North West Islands, where a patriarchal Scot was nearing the end of his earthly pilgrimage. It was the widow of old Tom Baikie who had an interesting story to tell, though we did not wait to hear it on this occasion. Her grandmother had been a Caravalla Eskimo in the Rigolet Narrows run. Some trouble at home had resulted in her wandering off up the north shore of Lake Melville alone with but a kettle and knife besides a little food. When she came to any stream too deep to wade, she would make a raft of windfall logs and long supple roots for lashings. One day, she was confronted by Mulligan River, the widest stream that she had met with. The smoke of her fire as she boiled her kettle while working at a raft attracted the attention of two Englishmen prospecting or trapping in the neighbourhood. They rowed over to investigate and took the woman back with them. She cooked and sewed for them, and later one of them married her. A daughter of this pair [Lydia and Daniel Campbell] married a Scotch immigrant in the next generation, and Margaret Campbell later became the wife of Tom Baikie. It was she who had kept a unique record of her life in the sub-arctic [*Labrador Memories*]. It was her account that I read of the New-Year keeping at North West River in the days of Donald Smith. Her reminiscences told, too, of the girlhood days when the family would move in a homemade little schooner from the winter home at Mulligan River out to the salmon fishing summer quarters at Moliuk, a few miles above Rigolet, and of the return voyages in the autumn, often stormy, when they would be held up for days together in island anchorages, berry picking and living a carefree picnic existence.

On one occasion, on reaching the winter home once more, [they discovered] a black bear had evidently fancied it for a summer residence. The sequence of events could be fairly accurately reconstructed. Having broken his way in, Bruin had evidently been considerably

annoyed to find another of his species ahead of him. He showed his
teeth, and the river bear did likewise. Believing that the first blow is
often the winning one, Bruin launched a terrific uppercut. The result
succeeded his utmost expectations. His rival simply vanished; his
paw was almost paralyzed, and a large mirror lay on the floor, smashed
to atoms.[101]

With womanhood came love's young dream to Margaret Campbell,
but the man of her choice sailed away, and later on she was married
to an honest, thrifty, diligent, but dour husband who realised little of
a woman's viewpoint. She was taken away to the head of Grand Lake,
forty miles from North West River, and during his long absences on
the fur-path she lived in dread of visitations from Indians, who were
persistent and arrogant beggars. She told of ways of hunting wild birds
and beast, of the raising of a large family, and of a life of mingled
romance, adventure, and drudgery.

From North West Islands, where there was nothing to delay us,
another three or four miles over ice took us to the mouth of Mulligan
portage, a short cut across the neck of land which separated the river
of that name from Lake Melville and which ends in Mulligan Head.
A mile or more through woods and marshlands and over a low hill
took us out on to Mulligan River. Just as we took the portage, we saw
a small covey of six willow grouse perched in a clump of willows. As
we needed any fresh meat that we could get, we halted the komatik
and unlashed my .22 rifle. It was a case of almost point-blank range,
with no excuse for missing, and I dropped three in quick succession
before handing the weapon to Billy. So long as they were cleanly killed,
the survivors were not alarmed, but somehow Billy contrived to miss
his first shot, merely scaring the living target, with the result that the
remainder took flight and soon vanished.

It was already twilight as we came out on the river and ran down
to its mouth, where was the two-house hamlet occupied by Hugh
Campbell and old Tom Blake, a remarkable veteran. Tom had travelled
quite extensively and read eagerly. At the age of seventy-five, he
celebrated his birthday by chopping seventy-five "turns" of firewood,
a turn being a log as big as a man can carry on his shoulder.[102] Not
long afterwards, he married his fourth wife, using the same wedding
suit that had done duty for his first matrimonial venture. He lived to
the age of ninety-three, active to the last in any way open to him,
though suffering from total deafness and a large degree of blindness.
When he could do nothing else, he would make shavings for the
household with a drawknife, largely by sense of touch.

Despite the lateness of the hour, we went on to Pearl River, three miles
further, as we had a forty-mile run in prospect for the following day

which we could not do unless we reached Pearl River the first day. It was my inexperience, being a novice, that had resulted in the loss of over half an hour's daylight that first morning, but it soon became clear to me that it was a cardinal sin to lose a minute of the precious daylight of those short winter days. Thenceforth, our routine was to rise an hour and a half before dawn and to be ready to set out as soon as we could see.

The memory of my first night's hospitality at a Labrador home is still a vivid one. The homestead at Pearl River was occupied by three Chaulk brothers, settlers from Newfoundland: Abner, Andrew, and Amon. (A fourth brother, Alexander, was dead.) Andrew was a widower with several surviving children, and Abner was skipper, his wife being a daughter of old Tom Blake of Mulligan River. We drove up in the dark, and friendly voices at once hailed me. "Go on in the house, doctor. You must be cold, sir. We'll see to your stuff." Passing through the usual storm porch into the main room, a combined kitchen and living room, I received a further kindly welcome from my hostess. "Haul off your things, sir." Off came a scarf, lashed around the waist of the dickey and then the dickey itself. This is a hooded short jacket without any opening in front except for the face. It can be made of native sealskin or deerskin, but I have always found these too hot. People who lacked warm underwear, however, might well be glad of them. Otherwise, the dickey can be made of canvas or cotton or any wind-proof textile. (The very best for wind as well as the lightest that I have used at all is Grenfell cloth, a textile named after Sir Wilfred.[103]) Then came the overalls. These again are often of sealskin, otherwise of ordinary canvas such as fishermen wear. It is only in mild weather, when wet snow is apt to penetrate canvas overalls and other clothing beneath them, that I have found skin-pants tolerable.

The extremities are another matter. They must be protected properly or trouble is certain. I was shortly to meet a young woman [Kirkina Jeffreys] who had been caught in a bad storm and had frozen her legs so severely that gangrene had set in. In the absence of a doctor, her father had performed a double amputation with his axe, which she had survived.[104] She had worn out one pair of false legs on the rough Labrador rocks and was shortly to start on a second. When these failed, she was reduced to waddling on her knees. This produced double "housemaid's knee," for which I was later to operate. No, no liberties can safely be taken with even sub-arctic frost. Deerskin moccasin with sealskin legs sewn on are much the warmest type of outside footgear, but whenever water is to be encountered, sealskin is to be preferred. Inside the boots or moccasins come two pairs of duffel "vamps," slippers of a blanket-like material which are worn over wool stockings or socks. The hands are protected by sealskin mitts with either duffel or knitted wool under-mitts. Even then, frequent exercise is necessary to maintain circulation in cold weather. The nose and chin are also vulnerable points with regard to which preventive chafing in good time is to be preferred to even moderate frostbite, though the latter is sometimes unavoidable. It is a relief to get rid of these cumbersome outer coverings at the end of the day's run.

The outer clothing doffed, "Would you like a wash before your tea, doctor?" Meanwhile, the load is being brought in. "We have feed all ready for the dogs, sir." But it is best to let the team cool off for an hour before feeding. Meanwhile, the armchair is brought close to the double-decked stove, the lower part a fire-box and the upper an oven. Billy goes through the same preliminaries as I while the table is laid. "Sit over and take your tea, sir. Make yourself at home, now." And the three brothers and Billy and I, together with another teamster bound east, gather round the festive board. A great dish of smoking venison is set before us with unlimited hot tea, bread and butter and cranberry jam, and some homemade cake. "Make your tea now, sir. Don't be afraid of it." Not that there is any need of such stimulus after the day's exercise and with that savoury venison inviting attention.

The meal ended, pipes were produced, and yarns were the order of the day. The talk turned on dogs and their sagacity, and one of the brothers told a tale of a new leader brought from another part of the country which, after a single journey across Mulligan portage and on across Lake Melville to the narrator's trapping grounds, re-crossed the bay over twelve or fourteen miles of ice in a blinding storm to end up right in the mouth of the four-foot path. "I knowed that if the dog could do that he could bring me on home," he ended.

I counted no less than twenty-seven firearms laid across the beams of the ceiling, varying from old-style muzzle-loaders to modern, hammerless ejector breech-loaders. Some of the older weapons could still shoot straight and hit hard. But a pleasant languor was stealing over me, born of fresh air and hard exercise, copious supper, and a comfortable warmth. "Stretch out when you wish, sir," perhaps a concession or perhaps a hint. Sleeping bags were produced and unrolled, and soon both family and travellers were stowed away for the night.

There was no loss of any daylight on the second day out. Sunrise found us well on our way. For ten miles, we followed the eastern shore of Mulligan Bight till, rounding Long Point, we squared away down Lake Melville on improving going, the snow and ice here being exposed to the full sweep of westerly winds. The mid-day pull-up was at Lowland Tilt, the property of Robert Baikie. (A tilt is a hunter's log hut in which he lives, or in a series of them, while at work on his furring grounds.) We now had to travel the windy area under the highlands for about fifteen miles.

At one point, the dogs seemed suddenly to go mad and started out in a wild gallop. "Traveller seal," shouted Billy, pointing to a shallow groove in the centre of the snow. A traveller seal is one which, having emerged from one of the regular breathing holes open all the winter, fails to regain it because of rapidly drifting snow and sets off in search of some other entry to the water. Gradually, the poor beast becomes exhausted, starved, and bewildered, and they have even been killed in woods or on hillsides. I have killed three in one afternoon, hardly having to go out of my way to do so, but needless to say such good fortune is by no means common. The pace was kept up, and presently a black dot appeared on the ice ahead. The dogs strained yet harder, and we bore rapidly down on the unfortunate seal, which had winded us and was making a clumsy but futile effort to increase its ungainly progress. As we neared the creature, Billy dropped a dog drag over each runner, dashed out ahead with the whip as the komatik slowed down, and succeeded in holding back the team while I shot the seal. Here was a good supper for the dogs, at any rate, so we added the carcase to our load and pushed on towards Valley Bight, where was the home of Bill Shepperd.

Bill was a character. It is no insult to his memory to say that in a community with a limited vocabulary, Bill was known as the biggest liar in Labrador. This did not at all reflect on his dealings with his fellow men but was rather a tribute to his prowess in the sphere of extemporised fiction with no intent to deceive. Possibly, frequent repetition did make some of his tall yarns true to himself, but it did no one any harm if he thought himself a champion in the noble art of self-defence or if he whiled away many otherwise dull hours with flights of romance. The only objection was that Bill, when wound up, often showed no signs of running dry when others wanted to go to sleep. Experience soon proved that the only way to adjust this difficulty was to take the wind out of Bill's sails with a yarn that left him gasping. Thereafter, concoction of these fictitious bombs occupied many an hour of chilly travel towards Valley Bight, either from east or west. Even if he had a long tongue, Bill was neither fool nor laggard as trapper and salmon fisher or as opportunist in various other sideshows, including agriculture. His homestead, widely isolated as it was in every direction, was a natural pull-up for travellers. At any hour of the night, as well as by day, cold and weary and hungry men were sure of the same welcome and good cheer. There was always dog-feed and human

feed too in abundance, and since he died, the sad transformation that
has come over Valley Bight has caused him to be missed greatly by
those who remember the good old days.

I was allotted a clean little room to myself with the added luxury
of a hot tub, also an excellent supper and then the night's programme.
Two songs he sang, each of something under a hundred verses. One
was about a pirate named Manning, a most unpleasant person.[105] Just
as the unfortunate lover had been made to walk the plank and the
innocent maiden was being butchered in the cabin, Bill added to the
vividness of the scene with a wild step dance. The effort ended
with the richly deserved execution of Manning and a tag of "Rule
Britannia."[106] The second song, also an affair of blood and thunder,
found me nodding at what should have been the moment of the highest
dramatic effect, but besides these poetic numbers there were many
items of prose, relevant to local life and events, which were both
entertaining and informing. When Bill ventured into "high" English,
he sometimes achieved startling effects, as when he tried to discuss
denominations and called them "abominations." In suitable doses, Bill
was a sure cure for depression.

The following morning, refreshed by their supper of fresh seal meat
and encouraged by the best of winter going, the snow being wind-
beaten to the hardness and flatness of a floor, the dogs romped gaily
over the fifteen miles to Caravalla Head, at the entrance to Rigolet
Narrows run. The run itself is a poor place for komatik travel. The
rapid tideway is seldom if ever frozen across, though a few of the
larger coves afford safe ice, but the ten miles by boat is increased to
nearer fifteen by dog-team through having to follow an irregular
shoreline. This has to be done by way of "ballicatters,"[107] a corruption
of *barricades*, indicating shore rocks covered with ice and snow and
also by short portage paths over miniature cliffs or points where the
ballicatters are impassable. In all but the coldest weather, there is
seepage from the bog-land between the run and the hills, and water
overruns the ballicatters, producing "quores," a term the derivation of
which I never have been able to make out.[108] These are areas of ice
with water flowing over them, often forming an inclined plane sloping
towards the water. Needless to say, they are dangerous if not impassable, and there are portages cut inside the worst spots. There are a
series of dwellings belonging to Eskimos or half-breeds in this run in
winter, as well as the deserted dwellings of salmon fishers from the
head of the inlet, so our progress was deliberate.

One scene always remains in my mind with regard to this part of
the route. In one wretched hovel, a single room, were gathered no less
than sixteen people. On a rude wood bunk lay an old man coughing

away his life in the last stages of consumption. A middle-aged woman, reposing on the floor, was in little better condition. A young woman crouched dog-like beside the stove, her clothing rather obviously limited to a single porous dress. There was an atmosphere difficult to breathe in, with no ventilation at all, and the air must clearly have been laden with bacteria. Close by was an empty shack, but they preferred to aggregate in one. Perhaps there was no stove or other equipment available for a second household. Naturally, eating and drinking vessels were shared by diseased and healthy, if anyone there could be healthy. It was a depressing household and a depressing district, and what could be done about it?

At Rigolet, Mr and Mrs Swaffield gave me a most kindly welcome at the Hudson's Bay Company's post, and Mr Swaffield very helpfully offered to send his team for a day with me dog-hunting while my team rested. We set out the following morning for Ticoralak, where dwelt two brothers, Jerry and Austen Flowers, each of whom sold me a good dog. I had also secured a second teamster, Peter Oliver, a man who badly needed work and who also possessed two well grown pups, rather young for such a trip but not to be rejected when dogs were scarce. This raised our total to fourteen. Sometimes the bay is fast outside Rigolet, enabling the traveller to cross on ice and greatly shortening the run to Cartwright, but such was not the case this year, and we must needs go back up the Narrows run, cross the bay from Caravalla Head across the head of the long cul-de-sac of Back Bay, previously referred to as the original estuary of the Grand River and Naskaupi River systems, and so on to the two-house hamlet of Pease Cove, where dwelt two Wolfrey brothers, Jim and Willie: Jim with his married son Sam and Willie with his son-in-law, Peter Pottle.

Back Bay is an evil locality. In the first place, it is a region of rapid tide-rips and bad ice, and secondly it is the worst place for drift that I know of on the whole coast from Battle Harbour to Nain. It is right in line with the seventy-mile basin of Lake Melville and is a narrow funnel between high hills. Into this is swept all the accumulated drift snow of the lake above. After any bad blizzard, which almost invariably comes with an easterly wind, when the wind chops round to the west, down comes the light snow, swept by a following gale, and whirls and roars down Back Bay, sometimes for many days in succession. There used to be an interval of over twenty-five miles between next-door neighbours in this bay, and it was a cruel journey from house to house.

The very next year to this, a travelling fur-buyer who was after live silver foxes for breeding purposes almost lost his life, together with his teamster, on the shores of Back Bay. Leaving Pease Cove against the advice of the local dwellers and relying on the speed of an exceptionally fine team credited with covering ten miles in the hour on more than one occasion, they expected to cover the distance within three hours by the simple expedient of following the south shore. But this was by no means so simple as it sounded since the shore in question was considerably indented and very rough. In crossing big bights, they were all too apt to keep either too far in, in which case they landed on a lee shore and had a punishing ordeal to work out again round the next point, or if they kept too far out they were apt to get onto the north shore, where the houses were not to be found. And this is what they did.

Just where a long point runs out from the south shore, the whole axis of the bay inclines a bit more to the southward, and they crossed to the north shore, where the very worst of the storm was to be met with. Had they turned the point referred to, they would have been in comparative shelter for some miles and would have found no difficulty in reaching their objective. Now their only chance to reach the houses was to re-cross the bay with the wind abeam, or nearly so. If it was bad before the wind, it was far worse across it and utterly impossible to stem it at all. The dogs were demoralised too. All that they could do was to dig into a snowbank amongst a few scattered dead trees, which would at least supply fuel, and make the best shelter that they could with the komatik bridging over the imperfect roof. The furious wind eddied the snow into their poor shelter, making it difficult to keep a fire going at all and filling their eyes with smoke. Tent they had none or kettle. A preserved milk tin was the best substitute available for a kettle. The storm lasted unabated for two nights and part of three days. When the lull came, the teamster was almost completely blinded with snow and the trader not much better off. But they had at least acquired a healthy respect for Back Bay.

We had to portage inside Pease Cove head to reach the hamlet and unharnessed our dogs at Jim Wolfrey's. Jim would not equal Bill as a raconteur, but he had a bear story to tell. Many years before, he and another man had been hauling home firewood on a stormy day with very heavy drift flying. Much of the road was in a well sheltered wood-path, but there was a stretch of open marsh and ice to be crossed on the way home. One team included eight dogs and the other seven. Suddenly, the dogs became wildly excited and despite their heavy loads fairly bolted. Then there began a wild uproar, and the men found that they had run foul of three polar bears. Curiously enough, husky dogs, which usually are afraid of wolves, never hesitate to attack the far more formidable King of the North. By the time the men had secured their guns, there were five dogs left out of the fifteen. Unencumbered by traces, the dogs can usually keep clear of a single baited bear, but the number of the enemy and the hampering traces had been too much for them.

The next morning, fortunately for us, Back Bay was on its good behaviour, and we ran down it with little difficulty. Our teams were still on the light side, especially since two out of fourteen were puppies, and we had to nurse them carefully, so we contented ourselves with reaching the Back Bay hamlet of two houses for that day, where we put up at Joe Pottle's. There was a marked change, however, in the type of homestead since we left Valley Bight. At Pearl River and at Bill Shepperd's, there had been such an atmosphere of comfort and confidence and independence. These were now missing, and sadly missing. There was still kindness and hospitality to the limit of capacity, but there were also uneasiness and the pinch of poverty and a noticeable change in physique.

At Pease Cove, I purchased the most beloved animal that I have ever owned and, I think, as fine a female husky as I have ever seen. Ribble, for such her name seemed to be, was a beautiful black and white animal whose offspring were to be the mainstay of my teams for many years to come. From the day I bought her, she was devoted to me, and woe betide any other dog that sought caresses from me in her presence. She was a wonderful mother, and to see her with her puppies was a delight. Quite early in their lives, she would start school, preparing them to make their contribution to the Labrador band. Seated on her haunches with the little class lined up before her, she would throw back her head and utter a series of long-drawn, wolf-like howls which were characteristic of her race. The youngsters would respond with their ridiculous falsetto squeaks with a comical effect. Again, when they were first put into harness, she loved to run ahead of them as they frantically paddled their short limbs in an effort to keep up with her long, easy stride. Soon they would collapse, and she would look round with a friendly grin of encouragement. But legs and wind soon lengthened, and they would become mature members of the team. They were always good workers and never once vicious, towards human beings at least.

Poor Ribble. It was her maternal devotion that was to end her life. Having produced a litter of puppies at Indian Harbour one early summer or late spring, she was kept with them for six weeks, but just before she was to be separated, she fell from grace and made off in the night and killed some hens belonging to a fisherman's wife. She was promptly banished to the island two miles away, where the rest of the team were spending the summer. But the next time that the dogs were visited, Ribble was missing and was never seen again. Evidently, she had tried to swim back to her beloved puppies and had been carried away by a strong tide.

"If you never saw poverty before, doctor, you will see it today," said Billy the morning that we left Back Bay for Flatwater Brook hamlet, and he spoke the truth. But again, why? Flatwater and West Bay, the next hamlet which was on the strand shore, were simply abounding in natural resources: salmon early in the summer and cod all the season, when there was any; and trout in the brooks and ponds and the finest smelts that I have seen anywhere to be caught through the ice for much of the winter and spring; and eider ducks haunting the coast there whenever there was an open water, all through the winter, as well as the migratory ducks in their season; and deer to be found on the peninsula, sometimes in every year; and numbers of ptarmigan and other grouse as well as many rabbits; and then the fur-bearing animals and endless berries. Why, they ought all to be living like fighting cocks. One year when I went there, three families had killed over one hundred each of the great snowy owls, which they eat with much relish.

There was one definite difficulty that these people had to contend with, as I presently learned, but only one of a material nature, and that was their borderline position between two trading districts. They lived over thirty miles from Cartwright and a bit more from Rigolet, and it was genuinely difficult to get salt for their fish and also to get their fish to market. There was one other difficulty, and that lay in themselves – lack of initiative. Had these people been under a capable leader to tell them what to do and to see that they did it, I believe they might have been at least self-supporting, if not prosperous. As it was, the few who were inclined to succeed despite difficulties were kept down by parasitic neighbours who sponged on them. In the midst of abundance, they were economic and physical tragedies.

I have always been convinced (and still am) that a capable district commissioner of the type that has done such admirable service in other parts of the Empire, with a reasonably free hand and a quite modest budget, could have had Labrador running on oiled wheels despite race difficulties and any others within five years, if not within three. That this great country, teeming with natural resources, should fail to support a permanent population of under five thousand, for the summer fishermen really affected the question very little, seemed and still seems absurd and disgraceful. The community had no representation and no administration worthy of the name, and a race of professional paupers was growing up unchecked.

"We prefer to pay $10,000 a year and hear no more about Labrador" was a perfectly authentic politician's utterance about this time. It represented a definite policy of laissez-faire, and its effects have been growing – on a relief bill that finally became an emergency at a time when the colony was least prepared to face it and also the production of an unemployable section of the community from the point of view of Big Business. The dole, flung out either for no returns at all or else for returns quite unmarketable, which the dole parasite produced on a semi-starvation diet, might at least have been reduced in cost by sawmills turning out marketable timber, which again would have tended to produce able-bodied and reasonably skilled woodsmen. Philanthropy, which has certainly made its mistakes and had its faults in Labrador, as elsewhere, has nevertheless been blamed for failing to handle, without the necessary authority, problems that those responsible made no attempt whatever to handle themselves, while recommending those who did try to provide a palliative to mind their own business. Granted, it must be that many of the older generation were past praying for in their armour of ignorance, tradition and prejudice, But there was a younger generation, many of whom were redeemable, and many of their elders need never have sunk to their present level. Of that I have what is to me irrefutable evidence.

Leaving West Bay, we ran on to Woody Point and the North River and so into Cartwright, eight days out from North West River, three days having been consumed in a detour to Rigolet and Ticoralak. There I was the guest of Mr Peter Smith[109] of the Hudson's Bay Company, who again very kindly rested my teams while I went to Paradise – not in a chariot of fire[110] but to the village of that name by dog-team. I was taken up the bay by a young Labradorman named Jim Pottle, who was later on to drive for me no less than seven winters. At Paradise were a score of families, which meant quite a clinic, of course, and I spent twenty-four hours there, booking several patients for Indian Harbour the following summer.

On leaving there, our first day's run took us via Goose Cove and Roach's Brook Bay to Sandy Hills, where lived old Solomon Burdett with a heart of gold and a tongue like a summer squall. A mission padre told me a few years later that he had never been quite so nonplussed in his life as under old Sol's hospitable roof. His offer to conduct Divine Service was welcomed, but when this was in progress the dogs outside started a free-for-all fight. Up bounced Sol from his knees and fairly shot to the window, whence he anathematised the combatants for a good five minutes while the padre stood stunned. The forces of evil effectually quelled, Sol devotedly subsided onto his knees again. His intentions were excellent though execution was undoubtedly faulty.

A forced march of some forty-five miles took us from here to Long Pond, where was another winter settlement of a number of families. We were now traversing another very depressed and depressing district, soon to become the worst of the whole Labrador coast for the dole, with an almost continuous processing of relief applicants parading between Table Bay, the next south of Sandwich Bay, and Battle Harbour, some northward bound to Cartwright and more southward bound to Battle Harbour. It was a manifest stronghold of tuberculosis, and any protest against unhygienic habits was liable to be resented. And when one turned from the difficult older generation to the younger, of whom so much was to be hoped, the desired relationship was none too easy to establish. "Now, then, if you ain't a good child I'll send you to hospital and the doctor will cut your head off" would be the exclamation of some harassed parent anxious to secure quiet for the guest, and my prospective allies would shrink away in horror from this bloodthirsty monster.[111] So another thing became evident. The one hope for many of these children was to get them away from home, sad as such a conclusion was and great as were the responsibilities that it carried with it.

Another sidelight on the economic problem of the individual was afforded by a little detour to the whaling factory at Hawke Harbour. The last whale of the season had been left as a benefice to the local people for dog-feed. Any man could come and chop a load from the great carcase and carry it off, but according to the sacred law of Labrador hospitality, every teamster who came must be offered a meal by the local caretaker of the premises. Up to date, and it was still but mid-January, the unfortunate manager had fed 153 teamsters.

The last stages of the journey to Battle Harbour provided the most acute surgical case of the trip thus far. At George's Cove, a hamlet of seven households, was a young man with a face like a football and a large discharging abscess in his neck who could not separate his jaws enough [for me] to examine the teeth thoroughly. By exercising almost intolerable leverage, I managed to extract one from the centre of another abscess inside the mouth, but I strongly suspected that this was not the only guilty one. However, it was the best that was mechanically possible for the moment, and having issued dressings and an antiseptic mouthwash, I promised to call again on my way north.

The next day, after twelve days of travel ahead, during which we made over three hundred miles, and five more days occupied in detours around Rigolet and Cartwright, we ran into Battle Harbour, having to go some distance up St Lewis Sound to find good enough ice to cross on. We drove up to Billy's home, where I received a very kindly welcome from his parents. Old Billy Murphy, his father, was mailman from Battle Harbour to Long Pond, where he transferred mail to a courier from Cartwright, and he was a noted pilot and hardy traveller.

7

The Same, Concluded

While our weary teams rested at Battle Harbour, Billy and I, after one day spent there in seeing cases, started off on a tour of St Lewis Bay with a fresh team. Billy wisely made for the more remote hamlets and houses while the weather was fine and, when change threatened, brought off a characteristic example of the opportunism which goes so far towards making a success of komatik travel. We had cleaned up on the south side of the bay as regards the more distant units and had crossed to the north side, intending to spend the night at an isolated home there, but as the sun sank there was an unsettled look about the sky, and when the moon rose there was a big ring around it. We had no wish to be caught and detained by a long storm at this point. About twenty miles away was the Lodge,[112] the biggest winter village in the bay. If we could get there before the storm broke, we could spend a day or more to some purpose. So after a few hours in which to digest their suppers, the uncomplaining huskies were harnessed, and we set out for a night ride.

Hours before daylight, snow began to fall, but we had then got over the worst part of the road, across the wide stretch of open ice, and into a well-marked approach to the Lodge. A little later, we roused the head man of the village from his beauty sleep, and there was still time for a nap in our own sleeping bags before a new day dawned. The storm was a severe one and kept us there till late on the second day, but we were able to get a house-to-house visitation done, let the storm rage as it would, instead of kicking our heels in a lone cabin away up the bay. After two days' rest for ourselves at Billy's home,

we were ready for the return trip. I had promised to be back as near
as possible to February 16th to allow time for Wakefield's northern
trip. Coming south, the prevailing winds had been in our favour, but
now, homeward bound, it was to be one bitter storm after another,
together with the hardest frost that I have ever experienced.

We hoped to travel with Old Billy as far as Long Pond, as he was
due for another mail trip. We left together on the last day of January.
We were across St Lewis Sound before the wind had reached its height,
and crossing the neck of land between St Lewis Sound and Alexis Bay
we had some shelter. When we came out on the shores of Alexis Bay,
the music had to be faced. A mad whirl of drift was coming down the
bay before a gale of bitter northwesterly wind. It was only a four-mile
crossing, but that was enough. The dogs declined to face it, and it was
then that Old Billy showed his mettle and his skill as a pilot. Running
out ahead of his team, he induced his leader to follow him, the other
dogs falling into line. Hugging the back of his komatik came Billy's
team, with Peter's in close attendance behind. Often, it was quite
impossible to see the next komatik ahead or behind, but the dogs kept
touch with the komatik ahead, and Old Billy ran steadily on. He was
aiming for a single house on the north shore of the bay, and just as
we struck the land he found his dogs and their traces all tangled up
with the feed-stage [scaffold][113] of our prospective host. (The feed-stage
is a structure of rough logs, raised sufficiently high from the ground
to keep such luxuries as seal meat and fat from the reach of canine
raiders.) It was certainly good shooting on Old Billy's part to have
scored a bullseye on so small a mark, running blind across a four-mile
stretch of ice in a whirlwind of drift.

After the conventional mug-up, we pushed on to George's Cove,
where was my dental patient. The abscess on his neck was almost
healed and his jaws were far more movable, but there was still considerable swelling of the gum from which just the top of the crown of
another offending molar peeped coyly forth. This must evidently come
out. It was so exquisitely tender and the patient so nervous that a
general anaesthetic seemed to be indicated. I cleared the deck for action
by expelling all but a travelling fur-buyer, who kindly consented to act
as my assistant. When the patient was well under, I started on a job
which I expected would take but a minute or two, but time after time
the forceps slipped off, and it was only after some blunt dissection with
my fingers that I could expose the tooth enough to see that instead of
sitting at the conventional right angle to the jaw it was set [impacted]
at an angle of 45 degrees. No wonder that the forceps had slipped. At
this point, I made a further discovery to the effect that I had an interested audience. A whisper made me look round, and there was the
entire adult population of George's Cove, with children struggling for

points of vantage between their seniors' legs. I charged them with brandished forceps, threatening wholesale extraction for anyone who ventured back till I was through and then completed my task.

I was then assured that there was a very similar case at a lonely home eight miles to the westward, entailing a detour and the loss of Old Billy's company. I was told that the husband and father had begged that I would on no account go north without calling there and that he had stated his intention of delaying a trapping trip to await my coming. In the face of such a statement, there was only one thing to be done. So next morning, when Old Billy headed away north, Young Billy and I started on a hard westerly punch of two hours or more. When we arrived, it was to find that the whole thing was a delusion and a snare. The man was away in the woods, and a damsel who had had toothache some time ago was better and had no desire for any extraction, thank you. Homicide and arson being excluded from our procedure, there was nothing [for us] to do but to accept a mug-up and get back on to Old Billy's trail. There was no hope of making Long Pond that night, but Billy told me that his father kept a tent [tilt] standing on the shores of Cape Bluff Pond, really a considerable lake over twenty-five miles in length, for use when he could not reach between George's Cove and Long Pond in one day, so we decided to spend the night there.

We made Long Pond the following forenoon, arriving just as another severe storm began. The next morning our host, Harry Hopkins, advised us not to leave. Snow fell thickly, and a strong northeaster drove it as it fell. It was a poor day for crossing the barren lands between Long Pond and the shore. Billy felt confident that he could reach the shore, in which case we could follow it to Porcupine, another settlement of some little size as Labrador settlements go. So we started and got through all right, but that very day a shocking tragedy occurred within a few miles of us. Just as we reached Porcupine, the wind swung from northeast to northwest, and a comparatively mild temperature gave way to hard frost. It was such a change as this that Harry Hopkins had feared for us, and it was to prove fatal to another traveller.

A lad of about sixteen left a house on an island to drive to some friends on the mainland with a nice free wind. His leader was a good one and was well used to this run, but the boy carried no compass, and the shift of wind caught him out on the open ice, steering by the wind on his face. When the dog, who knew his road, wind or no wind, went right on for the house, bringing the wind more ahead, of course the lad thought the dog was going astray. The whole melancholy story could be reconstructed from the telltale tracks which persisted afterwards. At first, he would naturally try to turn the animal with a word, "ouk, ouk, ouk" for "right" and "rah, rah, rah" or "urrah" for "left."

These, together with an "a-a-ah" for "stop" and almost anything for "get on" are all that a husky hears, or should hear, from a driver while under way. The more talk, the less ready obedience and understanding of the driver's wishes. (A crack of the twenty-five-foot lash will wake up a sleepy team to a more lively gait, and an occasional cut for a chronic shirker or other kind of offender completes the discipline.) Evidently the leader, sure of himself, had been reluctant to obey his young master's order. In a team, the hindmost dog must be some fathoms from the driver or he will be run over on any steep down-grade. The leader in a team of any size will be from fifty to sixty feet from the driver, often out of his sight in drifty weather.

When the leader would not turn from what he knew to be the right line, the driver had run out alongside the team and forced him to turn off with the whip. Once again, the intelligent beast had sheered back to his right line, and if only the boy had let him go, he would soon have sighted the shore and familiar marks and would have realised the situation and trusted to his dog to find the house. But a second time he had run out and cracked the whip till the dog turned off, and that sealed his doom. Further and further from their objective they drove, and if the lad realised his error, it now meant a bitter stem right into the teeth of the wind, which he simply could not face. In despair, he turned the komatik on its side as some protection against the wind and lay down under its shelter, never to rise again. And for six days and nights, the "savage brutes" lay starving near the boy's body without molesting it. He was then found by searchers whose previous efforts had been foiled by the persistent wind and drift.

We were able to keep going but not with full day marches. Our smallest pup was found dead one morning. He must have found something salt to eat, Billy thought. Salt will simply kill a working dog outright very often. The other dogs were looking the worse for wear too. By the time that we regained Cartwright, another had given out and had to be left behind. This time, I was to visit the north shore settlements of this bay [Sandwich Bay]: Dove Brook, Separation Point and White Bear River. As I went up the bay, the local thermometers were registering −60° and −62° F. I do not think that they were accurate, as cold is largely a matter of altitude and remoteness from salt water, and at Mud Lake at the time (which is 150 miles from the shore, whereas Sandwich Bay is less than thirty miles in depth) the lowest temperature recorded on a really reliable thermometer was −55° F. Still, it was cold enough. From White Bear River, I booked a patient for Indian Harbour for the summer for an operation that saved one prospective victim of consumption from premature death to a long life of normal activity. At Separation Point, I stayed at the house of Fred

Brown, the leading gardener of Sandwich Bay, who made his garden a real asset to health and economics. At Dove Brook, I stayed at the home of two perfectly charming old brothers, Silas and Tom Painter. Salmon fishing and carpentry were their chief means of livelihood. The home always had a delightful atmosphere. In their long lives, they were closely and happily united, and it might almost be added that "in death they were not divided,"[114] as Tom did not long survive Silas' death. Their honesty, industry, and kindliness made them highly respected as well as beloved members of their little community.

We left Cartwright late one afternoon, running across to North River for the night so as to get a better jump off for tomorrow's run, when we hoped to make Flatwater. Stopping at a lonely house a little way off the direct line, where we had been asked to call, I saw an old man with advanced cancer of the liver. Before I could speak, he read his sentence. Quite unafraid, he asked to know the whole truth. "Thank you, doctor. I had a mistrust it might be something like that." And that was my first and my last meeting with old Will Learning. At North River, there were three houses on the south bank and a single one at which we planned to stay the night, rather hidden away in the woods lining the north bank. I was detained on the south side until after dark seeing some cases, and as it was still blowing and drifting one of the men offered to walk across with me, a distance of nearly a mile.

We set out and were well out on the river ice when I happened to glance back and saw what appeared to be a husky dog following us. Thinking it might be one of my companion's dogs pursuing him, I called his attention to it. We halted and the animal did the same. We called, but whereas a dog would have run to us, this animal halted, irresolute. "Why, I'm blessed if that isn't the wolf!" exclaimed my companion. On my way south, the victim of a dog fight had been hung up in a tree until there was some better way to dispose of the carcass, but a long-legged, agile wolf had come and managed to dislodge the dog's body, which it had devoured at leisure. Ever since then, the beast had haunted this neighbourhood.

It was extremely improbable that the wolf would attack two men. Careful enquiries had failed to elicit a single instance of actual attack on mankind by Labrador wolves, except for the single case of a wolf, supposedly mad, which ran amok and attacked four men. There are several instances of wolves stalking men with possible sinister intent. One man who was stalking deer happened to glance backward to find himself being followed by a pack of wolves running into double figures, but they immediately took to flight on his turning on them and opening fire. Others have had somewhat similar experiences, but no one so far as I can learn has been killed or even bitten by a wolf. It is strange

that the dogs, of wolf descent themselves, will usually cower before a
single wolf, even when in a pack themselves, yet will always attack a
polar bear. I believe that the Labrador dog is a mixture of wolf and
Mongolian chow originally, though this is conjecture, admittedly.

Obscure as is the full genealogical table of the Eskimo, as is made
clear by Birket-Smith, there has clearly been a free communication at
some time across the Arctic belt from Kamchatka [in far eastern
Russia] to Greenland, and it seems at least possible that Mongolian
dogs should have found their way across.[115] Certainly, a red husky dog
can look very like a chow at times, though the latter is not so big. On
the present occasion, we saw no more of the wolf before we parted at
the house of my host for the night, but my pilot did prefer to borrow
a weapon before he started back alone.

The following day, we made Flatwater all right and, egged on by
the irrepressible Billy, I made good one omission of the southward trip
by extracting from Israel Williams his famous adventure with a great
horned owl. One spring day, Israel had gone off hunting with some
companions. The nights were short and not cold, and they did not
bother with a stove in the tent but preferred an open fire outside. In
the grey of morning, Israel crept out to rake together the still smoul-
dering coals of last night's fire, preparatory to boiling the kettle for
breakfast. In the half light and also the red glow which developed as
he blew on the coals, Israel's shock head looked convincingly like a
plump spruce partridge to a marauding horned owl. Silently, the owl
swooped, and the long talons seared Israel's scalp without getting a
firm hold. The owl slipped right onto the coals, and doubtless a smell
of sulphur was added to an atmosphere already more than sufficiently
charged. Then, on the morning stillness arose the despairing wail of a
lost soul. Convinced that he was about to pay the penalty for all the
sins of his harmless life, Israel beat all his previous sprinting records
in a dash for freedom to the west, while the owl, equally convinced
of unholy agencies at work, flew eastward with a velocity exceeding
that of Israel.

From Flatwater, instead of reversing our outward route via Back
Bay, we struck off across the old delta to Tinker Harbour, on the south
shore of the eastern basin of Hamilton Inlet, outside Rigolet. There
was a little series of hamlets on this shore, but with the bay still not
fast within five miles of Rigolet and the Narrows run, we should have
to come all the way back to the foot of Back Bay unless we could get
a pilot across an old portage route that led from the south shore to
the head of Back Bay.

Any regrets that I may have felt about a possible wild goose chase
were soon to vanish. Coming to the little hamlet of Turner Bight,

I entered a house, to be confronted by a scene not easily forgotten. On a bed lay a young mother, raving in puerperal insanity,[116] a dead infant close by. Another child, or what had been a child for nearly two years, lay awaiting burial when the paralysis of grief and bewilderment should pass off enough to permit a grave being dug in the frozen ground. Where quiet and order were essential, there was crowding, noisy grief, and chaos. The house was quickly cleared of all except those who were really needed, and never surely did a hypodermic of morphia do much better service. Fortunately, the condition was largely toxic, associated with convulsions in childbirth, but there was nothing except dry bread and tea in the house, so that our reserve of extras, carried for just such cases as this, was a perfect godsend. Before we left, the mother was rational, the simple funeral rites completed, and the relief over the first had considerably softened the other blows.

On arrival at John's Point, we eagerly asked old William Mugford about the old portage route. He was not encouraging. It had been unused for twenty-seven years, he declared, and he was the only man who knew it. He was too old to take us, and we might as well return on our tracks, but this did not carry conviction. Turning to his son and son-in-law, who stood by, I asked if they, with all their knowledge of the neighbourhood, could not find a way across the neck after consultation with the old man. They were perfectly willing to try, and as it turned out the next day they were never at fault for twenty minutes together, and long before sundown we were lodged at Pease Cove once more. Half a day's march or less took us to Valley Bight, where we were hung up for two and a half days by another heavy storm, with plenty of time to listen to Bill's yarns. A fellow guest under Bill's hospitable roof was Monsieur Lescaudron, who had shared with us the somewhat venturesome cruise in *Yale* the previous autumn. He was eastward bound, but so bad was the storm that he was as helpless as we, even though the wind had changed round to the westward, making it a fair wind for him and a headwind for us.

Meanwhile, time was passing. Until this storm came to handicap the final stages of our journey, we had been well within our schedule when we reached Bill Sheppard's on February 11th, but it was the morning of the 14th when we left, and then not because it was fit to leave. In all these years, I have never taken such a buffeting from wind and drift as we took during those next two days between Valley Bight and North West River. The first day, it took us eleven hours and a half of gruelling work to make forty-two miles, on going which was not very bad if only it were not for the pitiless wind and drift snow. We had to keep off from the shore a bit because whenever the dogs sighted land they bolted for the nearest shelter. Frequently, we had to stop and comb the frozen drift from the eyelids of the poor beasts, who were almost blinded. The worst punishment was for about two or three hours before noon and for about two hours after noon. After that, the drift would pitch down gradually, and we improved our speed with less punishment coming to us. And the second day of this great stem was worse since between Mulligan River (where we sampled Hugh Campbell's hospitality this time) for most of the way to North West River we were in those deep bights where the snow was slowest in packing and the going was vile. It actually took us from seven in the morning till half past eight at night to make twenty-four or twenty-five miles.

On February 16th, true to schedule, we crossed Goose Bay to make Mud Lake, a local team of two dogs which were hauling a two-hundred-pound load easily keeping pace with our exhausted teams. One pup had perished, one dog had been left behind, and now another had to be shot, and several more were in pretty poor shape. It took ten days' rest to get back into travelling order. For these casualties, I partly blame my own inexperience, looking back over a span of years. I was on my mettle as a greenhorn. Cross-country running at Repton and Oxford had given me endurance, and I was honestly inclined to believe that if I could keep going, husky dogs could too, but the dog needs understanding. He is wonderfully tough and willing, but he has a skin and feet as well as a stomach to be carefully tended, and it does pay to give him fairly frequent days off.

The salty, cheesy mixture that forms on the surface of salt water ice, without a sufficient covering of snow, will take the pads clean off a husky dog's feet if too long exposed to such conditions underfoot. Also, some dogs have far more trouble than others with balls of hard snow forming in the fissures between their toes in rather mild weather. These cause abrasion and then ulceration if careful attention is not given to removing them before trouble occurs. Worst of all for dogs' feet is the shell which forms like plate glass on the surface of deep snow when a partial thaw is followed by a rapid frost. Breaking through the shell into deep snow, the leg is simply shaved clean of hair as with a razor and then the skin lacerated, and the worst of it is that if caught by such conditions in a bad region for dog-feed or human supplies or in medical emergencies, it may be unavoidable to drive through shell. I have started off a long trip by breaking shell solidly for three and a half days ahead of my team on snowshoes. If we waited till conditions improved, we might sacrifice the greater part of the travelling season, and once when caught north by a sudden rainstorm, which was immediately followed by hard frost for eleven successive days, we averaged ten miles a day, breaking shell ahead of our discouraged and bleeding dogs the whole time. That is what takes the spice out of komatik travel far more than a frozen nose or chin.

As regards his skin, the hard-working husky generates a good deal of heat even in the coldest weather. He always works with a long tongue hanging out, which is continually warmed by his breath. Also, the harness gets so much warmer that rime [frost], and then ice forms on it. The harness must be religiously thawed and dried every night when in this condition or the poor beast's skin will suffer, as do the feet in shell, and he will be severely chafed and frost-burnt under the shoulders. In spring, when the melting of the snow erodes the surface of the ice by day and then night frosts produce cutting knobs and edges, it is customary to boot the dogs with home-made sealskin boots, but the sealskin is often irresistible as a canine mug-up. In winter, it is too cold to boot the dogs, as the lashings of the boots would strangulate circulation in the feet.

As already mentioned, the husky is peculiarly intolerant of salt when working in winter. In summer, he can swim and wade in the sea and catch flounders and sculpins and other fishy creatures, but salt is poison in winter. Unfortunately, much of his unsavoury food must be preserved in salt and then washed out before use, and sometimes there is still too much salt left in carelessly soaked feed, or salt scraps are left exposed with dire results. Sometimes the rascals raid a store, to their own undoing. Apart from this, the husky is fed but once a day and lacks table manners entirely. Supper is a strictly competitive event, and the husky needs plenty of time to digest his meal before being driven again. All these things cannot be realised off-hand, and whatever blame was due to me, the first conditions were almost unprecedented and have never since been equalled in my experience. At least lessons were learned which bore fruit, and I have never since known such a tale of casualties in any team under my control, except when an epidemic of rabies fell like a thunderbolt upon us and our dogs.

Leaving Mud Lake in the last days of February, with the longer March and early April days ahead of him, Wakefield made good headway on his trip to Nain and back. It was certainly not that he had chosen a softer job for himself. He was the last man to do that. He had definite reasons for preferring the northern trip that year, and he could not possibly have foreseen what was coming to Billy and me any more than we could. Mrs Wakefield may well have had some misgivings during his absence, knowing of his previous narrow escape on the Big Neck on that same route (of which more anon) and his reckless nature; but on this occasion, he had no very strenuous experience and came back early in April in the pink of condition.

There are two or three memories of that spring still interesting to me. The first of these was the beginning of acquaintance with the Montagnais Indians, unfortunately not of a happy nature. Their chief of those days, Michel Ashini, came to see Wakefield and myself with a suspicious hoarseness, coupled with other evidences of tubercular activity. Larynx and lungs were both attacked, and he was a doomed man with but a few weeks to live. However, it was a beginning of relations between the *toganish*, or doctor, and the second of the native races. Another memory is of my first visit to old Joseph Michelin's homestead near the mouth of Traverspine River, a tributary of Grand River. It was a beautiful spot with a remarkable settler. At seventy-two, Joe could trot across Goose Bay without turning a hair, still less boiling a kettle. At eighty-three, he was still going off trapping for three weeks at a time with no companion. I ran into him at ninety-one, returning home with a fine cross-fox, just taken from one of this traps. Now at ninety-three, while his trapping activities are about over, he still finds sufficient interest in life to speak hopefully at times of passing the century.

Fishing through the ice, here as in other places, at once provided sport for young and old and also a valuable contribution to the larder. One day when only the children were out fishing on new ice, one boy [John Michelin, Joe's grandson] suddenly went through and was soon being carried along by the current under the clear ice surrounding the hole. Without a moment's hesitation, one of the boy's sisters seized the little axe used for chopping fish holes, dashed ahead of the drowning boy, chopped a large hole in a twinkling, and fished out by far the biggest catch of that eventful day.

Nor was this the only adventure that the younger generation at Traverspine could tell of. One day, some of its members were badly scared by a strange, barely human face peering at them through some willows. In alarm they rushed home and told the news. Joe being away, his wife seized a gun and, dimly seeing a figure through the bushes, fired both barrels, knowing that it was neither neighbour nor Indian. Thereafter, the creature avoided the place by day but haunted it by night. Tracks were found of which patterns were preserved. Watch was kept from places of concealment at night, but without result. The lumbermen had started work at Mud Lake at this time, and some of them joined in the hunt, but with no success. The creature evidently had a mate, as double tracks were seen, and also sounds of domestic strife were heard, with loud lamentations from the weaker member. No capture or killing was ever effected, and the affair remained a mystery. That there were gorillas or even chimpanzees in sub-arctic Labrador seems impossible. Only lately, I received from an English relation who had visited here and heard the story a newspaper cutting regarding "snowmen" [the Abominable Snowman] whose tracks were reported by Himalayan explorers. Possibly there may be a clue here to the mystery of Traverspine, Labrador.[117]

There remains one final feature of that winter's programme to be recorded. Wakefield, who as already mentioned had served in the Boer War, was an officer in the Legion of Frontiersmen. This was the creation of Lieutenant-Colonel Driscoll, himself a veteran of the Boer War.[118] The enterprise was planned to have every possible able-bodied man of the British dominions ready to serve the Empire in time of need, not only as a soldier but in the special capacity for which his normal career had fitted him. Pilots were to be available for uncharted waters, guides for little-known tracts of land, engineers, artisans, cooks, clerks, etc. The misplacing of bad soldiers who might be good in some other capacity, needing much weeding out and loss of time, money and effort, had impressed itself deeply on the mind of this thoughtful officer. It was unfortunate for him, as well as for many others, perhaps, that the legion was still very young with a total membership of about twelve thousand when the Great War broke out, and so much had to be gone through which Colonel Driscoll had planned to prevent. Wakefield had enlisted some members on the Labrador coast, and at Mud Lake we used to have Frontiersmen's evenings, with boxing, single-stick, and elementary drill. When the Great War came, Wakefield's work was not without its fruit, and a small but effective group of natural snipers found their way to Flanders from Britain's least known and unrepresented dependency.

While Dr and Mrs Wakefield were to remain at Mud Lake till open water, I still had to get out to Indian Harbour on the last of the ice to begin the projected extension of accommodation there. Billy Murphy had left for Battle Harbour as soon as possible after returning with Dr Wakefield from Nain, but I now had some dogs of my own, and in the last week of April we set out. With me went Fred Blake and Sam Pottle, who were again to join *Yale* for the summer, and also Peter Oliver as teamster. We were to pick up one or two others outside. We had a terribly sloppy journey with little frost. Marshes were bare of snow often, but the ice was often under a layer of water and slush almost knee-deep. At other times, following big cracks which had formed between the shoal and deep water ice, we careered gaily along in almost effortless progress.

The finish over treacherous sea ice was a bit risky, but we got through on May 1st and were marooned by drift ice and water for the next six weeks, with the result that the one-time chapel had been converted into quarters for all male in-patients as well as all out-patients before our new season opened. By then, eight months had passed with no news from the outside except that brought by three letter mails. To send a telegram would require a 650-mile round trip between Mud Lake and Battle Harbour. None the less, the winter had been full of human interest and not without professional opportunities. Every home on a large section of the coast had been visited and its problems at least partly realised. The dog-team travel too had had the charm of novelty as well as a most healthy physical effect. For me, both country and community had a very real interest and charm. There were definite problems to work on and at least something to start work with along some lines.

8

Second Summer at Indian Harbour and Back to Mud Lake for the Freeze-Up

We had our little difficulties during that May month on Indian Harbour island. We were not a skilled construction gang by any means. Fred and Sam were tolerably handy with ordinary tools, but neither was by any means a finished carpenter, and the rest of us were not in the same class with them. Peter as well as John Rich, the first Labradorman to greet us when we landed in 1912, were more used to rough-hewn logs than to lumber, and I was regretting my preference for athletics over the carpenter's shop in school days. There had been no weatherproof place in which to store our lumber, which was saturated; by the way of economy, rough lumber had been sent, and it was our task to plane it and tongue and plough it with hand planes. As a preliminary, we had first to dry it, a dozen boards at a time, in the kitchen. Progress, therefore, was slow if sure.

The hour of sunrise and also of sunset would usually find some of the party out on the western point of the island, waiting for a shot at flying ducks, as we depended on our guns for any fresh meat. Sam, by virtue of his office on *Yale*, was elected cook, which of course reduced his hours of carpentry considerably. The frame had also to be made for the partitions. Gradually things took shape as partitions rose and rooms were "ceiled"; and as the end of our job began to be in sight, we took more interest in maintaining a lookout for the first signs of an icebreaker working her way north through the great ice-field that ever formed a large fraction of our view from the summit of the island.

It was on June 8th that we saw a smoke and then the vessel, which turned out to be not our old friend *Sagona* but the new and powerful

Kyle,[119] of more than twice *Sagona*'s registered tonnage, a vessel with graceful lines. She brought no passengers for Indian Harbour hospital, but we heard that we were actually to have a second Labrador mailboat for that summer, the *Invermore*,[120] which was no boat for ice. She was said to be on her way north, incidentally with the person that I most wished to see on board [Mina Gilchrist]; but as it turned out, *Invermore* got jammed into some harbour by ice and had to stay there, and it was not till *Kyle* had been back to St John's and caught up with her again that her passengers were able to resume their journey north.

Just as *Kyle* had left us, a schooner was seen coming out of the inlet from the direction of Rigolet, and it turned out to be John Groves'[121] vessel from Goose Bay, near Mud Lake. When I had visited Goose Bay hamlet the previous spring, I had seen a rosy-cheeked youngster [Wilfred Groves] who was to have an outstanding career for a Labrador boy. I little thought then that this child, fifteen years later, would have completed a brilliant career at a technical training school in Canada and a college in New York State and would be on the staff of an American technical college instructing young Americans, many of whom had started with so much that he had lacked.

When John's schooner came to anchor, who should appear but Dr and Mrs Wakefield, who had hoped to embark on the steamer which had just left. So they must now possess their souls in patience[122] at Indian Harbour. However, navigation had opened early this year as compared to many years, and it was not very long before *Kyle* reappeared, bringing my fiancée and a second nurse [Helen M. Smith]. Furthermore, a real medical student assistant was to arrive on the following boat. When he came, Sandy proved to be a real acquisition, well up in his work after studying in Germany as well as the United States.[123] He was fond of laboratory work, which had never been a strong point of mine. Naturally, he lacked practical surgical experience, but he had plenty of ambition to get such experience. Particularly anxious was Sandy to extract a tooth. Of course, I had to be careful as to what I passed on to an unqualified man, and Sandy's patience was sorely tried.

One day, I was summoned to see a case a few miles off by motorboat. During my absence, a fisherman arrived with an offending tooth which Sandy felt sure was just made for beginners, so he got to work. I made an unexpectedly quick trip, and on my return I heard a weird noise proceeding from the out-patient room. Reconnoitring carefully through a window, I beheld the following tableau. The central feature was a pair of dental forceps, at either end of which pirouetted Sandy and the patient respectively, the patient attached to the forceps by a molar which, too late, he had decided he would rather keep. Sandy's hair was a rich red, but his face surpassed his hair on this occasion. A nurse, helpless with hysterical laughter, leaned precariously in a corner. At that moment something happened, and the patient suddenly abandoned his tooth, which remained triumphantly brandished in Sandy's forceps. Then the patient reacted nobly and showered blessings on Sandy's head, and the incident was ended. None the less, although we persecuted Sandy about his first extraction, he did yeoman service that summer and has made his mark since, especially in regard to some problems connected with influenza.

We settled down to a busy and happy summer. The new accommodation proved to be no mere luxury. Our in-patients increased by 50 per cent, as did our operative work. The generous gift of a new operating table, which rejoiced our eyes, was especially opportune, as the museum specimen which I had found there on arrival in 1912 had shown a most disquieting tendency to collapse under the patients at extremely inconvenient moments. Now we could at least be sure where the patient was to be found during an operation. The same generous donor had sent a complete lining of white sanitas for the bare walls of our new ward and operating room. Some new instruments also made a valuable addition to our equipment.[124] My winter itinerary also bore fruit in the marked increase in the proportion of Labrador patients as compared to those from the Newfoundland fishing community.

One early case of this season illustrated the need of child-welfare work in this region. *Yale* brought in a rickety two-year mite of a girl, still bottle-fed, who weighed exactly the same as an eight-month infant in the same ward and who seemed considerably less intelligent. For lack of anything to chew on, the whole of the first dentition had decayed, producing a condition of the mouth which alone condemned the unfortunate child to chronic blood poisoning. There was simply nothing for it but wholesale extraction, a shocking state of affairs. As a finishing touch, the grandmother, an old dame of the managing type who was responsible for much of the damage, had come to show our nurses how to look after the child. To dismiss the grandmother involved a short but painful scene, followed by a violently abusive epistle from her husband. I was not yet a justice of peace (though that was to come within a few weeks), but I felt sure that there must be something in Newfoundland law to cover such cases, and I therefore ignored all demands that the child be returned home. We kept her the whole summer, and cod-oil, sunlight, and a balanced diet, as well as some discipline, started the work of rehabilitation. When she went home in the autumn, it was with some very pointed instructions and with an ultimatum that unless these were carried out they would have to hand over the child for good. She is now the mother of a small family.

Besides Sandy, I had another medical student in his first year of study
who had come mainly for outside work on the reservoir, etc., but when
Yale arrived from a mail trip with thirteen people on board for the
hospital, only two of whom had been summoned by me and including
only one other real patient, I decided that a little censorship was needed
on board. Thereafter, either Sandy or his junior travelled on *Yale* and
controlled this traffic, at least to the extent of rejecting obvious pleasure trippers. The junior medical student referred to developed many
years later into a specialist in brain surgery, though at his first introduction to operation room procedure, as we did an appendix, he was
not much attracted.[125] We had nearly fifty cases under general anaesthesia that summer, as against twenty-five in 1912.

The case of all others that lingers in my mind from that summer of
1913 was that of a widow from Makkovik district [Anna Christina
(Andersen) Perrault] who had left two girls in their early teens behind
her when she came to hospital. She was suffering from a disease that
was considered quite incurable and which was also painful and disfiguring. But while we could not cure, we could at least relieve for a time,
so she remained. Just to be nursed, to have food that she had not had
to think about and of greater variety and delicacy than she had known,
and to have no household duties to supervise – these things alone were
enough to make her feel so much less miserable that she began to hope
for recovery, and it was a hard task to disillusion her. When it came
to a choice of going home at the time when Indian Harbour hospital
must once more be dismantled or of coming up to Mud Lake to end
her days in comparative ease, she chose the former, and as I said good-
bye to her on the *Kyle*, I fully expected not to see her alive again. The
sequel may as well be told here.

When I reached Makkovik on my dog-team travel the following
winter, I heard that she was still alive and made a special detour to
visit her. The home was a little single-roomed cabin in a solitary spot
on the shores of a long fiord with the nearest neighbour normally seven
miles away, which is a long gap in a winter storm. But now another
similar cabin, quite nearby, was occupied. It belonged to a settler from
Newfoundland named Abraham Morgan. As a rule, he used this cabin
only for seal hunting for a few weeks in each autumn, as it was close
to a rapid tidal rattle which kept open long after the neighbouring
waters were frozen over. His real winter home was about fifteen miles
away, where all his winter firewood was already collected in convenient
nearness to his trapping ground. Last autumn, when it came to a
matter of leaving that helpless trio to themselves, Abraham Morgan
and his wife [Ellen][126] could not do it. So they had sacrificed their
comfortable home and were wintering in the comfortless cabin. The

one man must now cut, haul, and split firewood for both households and also hunt for both; and the devoted couple had shared the night vigil by the dying and suffering woman's bedside. This service had been going on since October (and it was now February) without repining or relaxing. It made one feel very small. Abraham Morgan could not preach a sermon and he knew no theology, but it seemed to me that he had more of the essentials of religion about him than many who were more eloquent and occupied more exalted positions.

Another patient from the same region was "Long Tom" Broomfield, who arrived at Indian Harbour in a truly shocking state, leaving a wife and several small children behind him. An abscess almost the size of a melon overlay and also burrowed under the pectoral muscles on the right side of his chest. An area of skin the size of the palm of my hand had sloughed right away, leaving a raw surface through which protruded part of two ribs. Very shortly before, that man had been forcing himself to fish. How he had done so almost passes comprehension. The abscess could be and was dealt with forthwith. But what lay underneath those carious looking ribs? I removed them, as they could not possibly recover and were only doing harm; but this little operation only confirmed my worst fears of a deeper abscess in the pleural cavity. Dr Little was his only chance now, and to Dr Little he went as soon as he was fit to be transferred. He lived till spring and then succumbed. So there was another family of young orphans to be provided for, and in Labrador there is never any delay in making such provision, though all too often the burden must be borne by people who already have as much or more than they can really undertake. Can it be wondered at if we declared something of a crusade against tuberculosis?

The outside work on the reservoir was exasperatingly held up for a time by a difficulty over land titles that came like a thunderbolt. Happily, it was adjusted in time but cost valuable weeks and postponed our running water facilities for an extra year.[127] Still, substantial progress was made that summer. At the valley head was a series of two pools in a narrow ravine. It was necessary only to throw a concrete wall across the ravine, reaching down to bedrock, to prevent any overflow down the eastern slope and then to dig out the marshy soil and loose rocks around the pools and throw another concrete dam across the ravine to the westward. The lower pool then made the main reservoir, with the upper pool as a reserve, and 180 yards of piping conducted the water down the valley to the hospital.

One little venture into auxiliary social economic service marked this first period of work at Indian Harbour. It was noticeable that the local Labradormen fished at a great relative disadvantage as compared with the Newfoundlanders, owing to the scantiness and poorness of their

gear. Inferior boats and no traps left just hook and line fishing open
to them, and that only in fair weather. Of course, this meant that
commercially they were not regarded as worth fitting out with expensive gear. But was such pessimism really justified? And were there not
some better men, also lacking gear, who might be brought in to stiffen
up the poorer prospects?

With the help of a generous friend, an experiment was carried out.
Two crews were formed, one to fish at Indian Harbour, where I could
at least show some interest in their activities, and another at Bluff
Head, between ten and fifteen miles up the inlet. Each crew was
provided with a good outfit, trap and trapboat, dory, an outfit of
provisions, hooks, lines, grapnels, etc. If they could make good and
redeem the gear for their own, then the refunded money was to be
used to offer the same facilities to another crew. If they failed, they
would at least have had a chance. For the crew at Indian Harbour,
I had to hire a room and stage from Mr Jerrett. He at once concluded
that I was trying a flutter [speculating] for myself and strongly dis-
suaded me. I doubt if he ever quite believed my explanation, but provided
any fish caught was sold to him and that there was no competition
with his business, he shrugged his shoulders over my obstinacy, merely
prophesying the loss of the capital.

For skipper, I secured a man of whom I heard good reports as a
fisherman and whom I meant to employ as my own teamster for the
following winter, George Pottle. With him were two of his brothers
who were making a poor living in the Rigolet district and John Rich.
It was rather a proud moment for me when, after a single summer's
fishing, Mr Jerrett said to me, "Doctor, I have watched those men of
yours, and they are fine men. They can put away a load of fish just
as fast as my own men. If you can get together some more crews like
them, I'll be glad to hire them rooms and stages." And for a time, an
increasing number of Labradormen did mix with or fish alongside
Newfoundland crews in this harbour. The Indian Harbour crew did
redeem their gear, but the Bluff Head crew, with less supervision and
poorer leadership, were frankly not a success. They lost time coming
after salt, and they often lacked bait when the crews at Indian Harbour
had it, and they needed hustling a bit.

Winter plans had also to be thought of ahead. (Dr and Mrs Wakefield
had found another field for their energies.) On October 1st, the
Rev. Hubert Kirby[128] arrived from Cartwright, and my fiancée and
I managed to find time to attend our wedding ceremony. After our
marriage, my wife and I were to return for another winter to Mud
Lake, and the other nurse was to accompany us. Dr Grieve was to be

back at Battle Harbour and would patrol the coast to Cartwright while I took from Cartwright to Nain, as Dr Grieve had a further stretch to cover southward and westward from Battle Harbour.

Schooners were once more speeding south, and fish was daily spread on the bawn or was being shipped. And then came Sabrina, who was a young pig. Her Newfoundland owners had brought her north in the spring to fatten and then sell. As fresh pork was an unwonted luxury in Labrador, we had agreed to take her, expecting to be able to keep her alive until we could freeze what we could not eat within a reasonable time of slaughter. One afternoon, I heard a din recalling somewhat that which accompanied Sandy's first venture in tooth extraction, but this was outside the hospital. Investigation revealed Sabrina holding the centre of the stage under strong protest. Tugging at her ears was the white-moustached old veteran who owned her, while his son, who was almost helpless with laughter, shoved astern. The veteran was almost breathless, but the pig seemed to have plenty to spare for vocal purposes. When she was finally secured on the new premises, she went on a hunger strike worthy of any of the early militant suffragettes, which was finally ended by an irresistible offering of smoked salmon.

Sabrina had, seemingly, been something of a family pet and made no bones about inviting herself to dinner in the staff dining room. She was also found one morning snugly ensconced in the bed of a patient in the fresh air shack, who had rashly left the door open. I do not for one moment insinuate that she had been allowed these liberties at her former home, but if you gave Sabrina one inch she would take several ells. She also seemed to consider it her special duty to chaperone newlyweds wherever they went. She could climb like a goat, and rocks were as futile as insults to discourage her. Altogether, she proved such an impossible pig that it was decided that her presence alive on *Yale* simply could not be faced. So when *Yale* returned from the inlet after taking up the nurse and a maid to get ready the building while my wife and I had a honeymoon on a deserted island, Sabrina figured forthwith on the casualty list, and it was to be a long time before we attempted any more traffic in pigs.

The hospital finally closed, we left for Rigolet, where we had to await *Kyle* for mail and also to ship Will Simms back to Newfoundland. *Yale* was to winter at Mud Lake. At Rigolet, just as *Kyle* came, a tremendous electric storm burst over us. The temperature shot up to 67° F. in the last week of October, and a heavy gale of westerly wind followed with a tropical downpour of rain. On the first of the breeze, *Yale* sped back ten miles to Ticoralak, partly for shelter and partly to pick up a young woman who was coming up the inlet for domestic service with us that winter. Even the *Kyle* followed us there for refuge, for this was no common storm.

Before it really broke, my wife and I had gone ashore to see about the maid and also to see the people, of whom there were three families. The approach to the shore was across a shoal hundreds of yards in width, with great boulders sticking up everywhere. We were just rowing off again to go aboard and had almost reached the deep water where *Yale* rode at anchor when the first real squall came with a deluge of rain. We were simply blown backwards, bumping from rock to rock and being drenched to the skin before we could land. We were fortunate indeed in finding so cosy and clean a refuge as Jerry Flowers' hospitable roof. The house was spotless, the quarters simple but comfortable, and the food abundant and palatable. An element of comedy was afforded in the attempt to fit us out with dry clothing. My wife, long and slim, made a strange figure in the Sunday best of short, plump Mrs Flowers, and it was the overalls of the long, cadaverous Jerry that would accommodate my lower limbs, though a guernsey proved more stretchable further aloft. All that night and most of next day, it blew with little abatement. When morning came and we saw *Yale* riding to two anchors and diving bows under, we realised how lucky we were. It was nearly two o'clock in the afternoon before *Kyle* could leave before the wind, and it was not for yet another twenty-four hours that it was worth our while to put out to beat against it. At last, on the morning of October 29th, we put out, intending to run on all night if conditions were favourable.

As we passed Rigolet, the schooner of that name was loading at the company's wharf. A laughing wager was flung at us that they would be in North West River before us. Running on all night with a free wind, we reached that point early next morning, but it was three weeks before *Rigolet*[129] arrived there, and she was frozen out of her intended winter anchorage at Mud Lake altogether. As she had a large fraction of our winter supplies on board, which she was to have brought right to our winter quarters, this was a matter of considerable concern to us. Before October ended, we were once more ensconced, though hardly snugly, in the old lumbermen's shacks at Mud Lake, which were far from weatherproof. We had a recruit to our party in the person of a young southerner from South Carolina, Flinn by name,[130] who came prepared to make himself generally useful and did so.

In November, there came one of those long Indian summers that occasionally occur. Every trace of frost, snow, and ice disappeared. We could picnic in the woods in ordinary summer costume with comfort. George Pottle was a fine axeman, and he, Flinn, and I did much outside work while awaiting *Rigolet* and a return of the frost. But always there were either baffling winds for the schooner or dead calm. She was a flat-bottomed old tub and therefore very poor at beating to windward. Before the middle of the month it turned cold once again.

On November 14th, we had become so uneasy about the *Rigolet* and our supplies that we felt we must try to do something. Possibly, we thought, the vessel might have reached North West River and been detained there for lack of a pilot for Sandy Point run. So George Pottle, Fred Blake, and I, with faithful Sam, rowed across Goose Bay and walked over the portage into North West River, only to find that there was no sign of the missing schooner. There was nothing to do but to get back with all speed after arranging with Monsieur Thevenet to warehouse our freight on his side of the river, handier for the dog-team transport, which would not be impossible if the schooner reached North West River at all.

We ourselves had a hard time in getting back to Mud Lake. A strong and frosty westerly wind had sprung up and blew right down Goose Bay. We could not possibly row across wind and tide on a straight course for Rabbit Island without foundering but had to dodge and sidle our way across by keeping the wind and waves on our starboard bow. This meant our being continually showered with spray, which froze as it pitched on us and also necessitated frequent bailing. It was long after dark when we landed on Rabbit Island, drenched through and half frozen. Happily, the island is thickly wooded, and we got into good shelter, made an extra windbreak of spruce and fir brush, built a roaring fire, boiled a kettle, and stripped off most of our wet clothing. Then we tried to snatch what sleep we could until about two in the morning, when the wind began to drop, and we were soon able to get afloat again and complete our journey.

Two days later, a rowboat got through from North West River, bringing news that *Rigolet* had reached that place the day after we left and would now winter there, which meant that we must haul seventy-five cases of supplies averaging over seventy-five pounds each across Goose Bay on ice. I was particularly concerned about a new travelling medicine chest which had been ordered, ready filled for the winter's travel, but could get no news of it. We learned that the *Rigolet* had been wind-bound at St John Island until the crew ran out of food supplies and that they had been compelled to return to Rigolet for more. It took her altogether from October 28th till November 15th to make the eighty miles or so between Rigolet and North West River. Remembering *Roméo*'s ordeal in Sandy Point run in mid-November of the previous year, they had decided to be satisfied with North West River as a winter haven, although the running ice in spring over there was apt to constitute a serious risk to the vessel that took the chance. However, that seemed to be the lesser of two evils.

As soon as the ice formed across Goose Bay thick enough, it was believed, for safe dog-team travel, we started out on our task of transport. Making up two teams from my own and some borrowed dogs, we set off in great style. George Pottle and another man went on one komatik, and I made my debut as teamster on the other with Flinn as passenger. There were about two inches of light snow on the smooth ice. All went well until we were abreast of Rabbit Island, when suddenly four of my dogs went through the ice. Shouting to Flinn to throw himself off, I did the same, landing on ice still sound enough to bear us. Seeing what had happened to us, George stopped his team just in time, as a long fissure thinly covered with unsafe ice, concealed by the snow, ran off from the point of the island. Where we were, this fissure was eight or ten feet across, but it narrowed down to two or three where the other komatik was, so we made a bridge of George's komatik and all walked safely across.

Meanwhile, my dogs, feeling cold after scrambling out, had bolted. If they had only gone in the right direction, I would not have blamed them, but the scoundrels went off at a tangent and gave me a six-mile marathon before they lay down for a nap in an alder bed, having hit the shore about three miles from the portage. On my side, diplomatic relations were liable to be broken off when I got within speaking distance, but they grinned and wagged their tails so ingratiatingly that there was nothing to do but to beg them not to mention it and assure them that I was fond of exercise. Just in sight, away across the ice, a black dot represented the faithful George, faint yet pursuing. Flinn, who was no distance runner, had joined the other komatik and driven on.

While I could not fairly be blamed for losing my team under such circumstances, professional pride demanded that I should get them started, and that in the right direction, before George arrived, though I really should look foolish if they ran off around Sandy Point. It was pretty slippery going on the thinly covered ice, and I did not want to lose them again. Happily, all went well this time. I picked up George, and we joined the others in the portage. We had hoped to get back with a load that night but had lost too much time now. One of George's dogs, which had strained a muscle on the slippery ice and had been turned loose to make his way back to Mud Lake, managed to arrive wet and caused wild rumours to circulate which almost persuaded my bride of six weeks that she was a widow. But on the following morning, as we were making more sedate progress across Goose Bay with big loads, a scout appeared on skates and sped back with reassuring news. Unfortunately, a heavy fall of snow soon spoiled this good going. High tides caused water to overflow the ice under the snow, causing deep slush which made hauling a very tedious process. However, all was eventually transported, but the one thing of which no trace could be found was my travelling medicine chest.

We then settled down to a period of life very similar to that described in regard to the previous early winter. We had brought a little boy from far north [Stewart Dickers], who suffered from a tuberculous hip, into winter quarters with us. Fresh air being an important part of his treatment, all through the Indian summer mentioned above and again in the warm spring days, we used to put him up on a low roof out of reach of the dogs. (Unfortunately, the disease had too firm a hold for recovery to occur.) Christmas came and went again, and we attended the New Year's keeping once more at North West River. As there was no Dr Wakefield to share the use of my teams this time, I delayed my start till some days later than the previous January. This time I was to go into Eskimo territory, from which the little sub-tribe around Rigolet had become widely separated.

Among the short trips which I made locally before setting out on the main itinerary was one to Kenemich, where I visited the home of old Malcolm McLean, a remarkable settler. Malcolm had already been almost fifty years in Labrador at this time. He had originally come out as a servant to the Hudson's Bay Company at North West River but had later struck out as an independent salmon fisher and trapper. In addition to these main activities, this industrious and resourceful Scot had tried about everything that the country offered. He had cultivated the soil with some success. He had kept cows and churned his own butter as well as produced milk. He had imported sheep and made his own spinning wheel and spun his own yarn. He had also worked for two or three lumber adventurers, and because of his honesty and ability he had become local manager for each in turn. With the help of two successive partners [wives], he had increased the population of Labrador by no less than twenty-two inhabitants, yet he had always maintained economic independence. At the age of over seventy, sensing the overcrowding of the furring grounds, which was bound to mean distress unless wage-paid labour came, and wishing to prepare at least some of his sons for such labour, he collected some abandoned machinery and set up a sawmill, which added many hundreds of dollars to the family income over a term of years. In his eighty-ninth summer of life, he and his second wife were tending the salmon nets so that his unmarried sons would be free for the sawmill work. He was ninety or ninety-one, I believe, when he died. He was indeed a settler of the kind that Labrador needed and that would ever get the best out of the country. But for his huge family he might have been a very prosperous man.

9

Northward by Dog-Team into Eskimo Territory

On January 21st, 1914, we went away on a trip which covered between twelve hundred and thirteen hundred miles. The first hundred of these was over ground already made familiar. From Rigolet, where Mr Heath had been transferred from North West River in the company's service and acted as host this year, we were able to take a direct route to Cartwright, as the bay was fast, which was a great cutoff. I was again disappointed at Rigolet in my quest after the missing medicine chest, and Cartwright was now my last hope. I had brought what could be spared from Mud Lake, but I could not denude that station too drastically. Two more days' run took us to Cartwright, whither Mr and Mrs Swaffield had gone from Rigolet post, and there I finally had to abandon hope of the medicine chest for this winter's travel. All that I could do now was to make a detour to Indian Harbour on my way north and fit out there for the remainder of the trip. I had hoped to connect with Dr Grieve at Cartwright, but he had not yet arrived, and there seemed to be no idea when to expect him.

The day that we were ready to leave Cartwright was ushered in by a hard northeasterly wind with a blizzard of snow. Mr Swaffield tried to dissuade us from leaving, but George seemed confident, and it was only nine miles across to North River, whence we should have a shoreline to follow. It might be called George's native heath hereabouts, so we made a start. I was forthwith to get a salutary lesson in the importance of safety tactics in komatik travel. I had a compass with me but did not get it out, as George seemed so sure of himself.

Two hours at most should see us in sight of the north shore. There were islands to the west of our course and Huntingdon Island to the east. But much may happen in two hours.

We struck off from the base of Flagstaff Hill, just outside Cartwright settlement. All that we had to do, as it seemed, was to punch away to windward, as the course was northwest from Cartwright to North River. The first inkling that we had of anything wrong was that the ice we were driving over was new and not too thick. In a little lull between squalls, we also saw a little "flat" close to us. George was then able to put two and two together. The wind had shifted four points within an hour of our leaving Flagstaff Hill, and we had gone away up the bay instead of diagonally across it and had almost got into Main Tickle tidal rattle, where seals were sometimes shot and retrieved with the flat. This was a practical demonstration of the fact that it never pays to take chances when you have the means to make certain. If I had been checking our course by the compass instead of letting George steer by the wind, we could not possibly have got onto bad ice, which might easily have cost us a ducking and then a very severe exposure, if nothing worse. I have already quoted one fatal tragedy through steering by the wind, and it is not the only one that has prematurely ended a young life. This time we had got off easily, and having realised our position we could now set a course for North River, where we arrived without further misadventure.

North River always has a humorous significance for me, not because of the little encounter with the wolf but owing to the fact that once, when trying to cross it on glassy new ice in a strong wind, I simply blew away standing upright and was carried a long distance out of my way. I was in company with another man who had got ahead of me, and, being taller and broader than he and holding more wind, I drove down on him and sent him flying and then sped on till I finally hit a snowbank. Fortunately, there was no open water at hand. The same season, however, a Sandwich Bay man from Dove Brook was driving along the north shoal of the bay on a similar surface, and he did blow away, dogs and komatik and man, till he went off the edge of the ice into deep water. Fortunately for him, his dogs, once their feet were wet, secured enough hold on the ice to scramble out. Hitching the traces under his arms, he received some support, clinging to the edge of the ice also with his arms, the sleeves freezing on. Still, without help he must have perished, but another teamster was driving along behind him and witnessed his plight. To be too hasty in attempting rescue was but to share his impending fate. The rescuer had to cut footholds in the ice all the way across the entire belt before he could draw the victim out of the water. With his clothes a sheet of ice and freezing water between clothes and skin, he was hurried to the nearest house. Most fortunately, he escaped any sequels such as pneumonia.

Continuing our way north, we crossed the bay outside Rigolet to Ticoralak and then turned eastward for a while. At Rocky Cove, seventeen miles east of Ticoralak, lived another real character, old Arthur Rich, one of the few stout men I have ever met in Labrador, but he was old. The first time that I met him was on the way out to Indian Harbour in the late spring of 1913, when I arrived at his door before four in the morning, roused him from slumber, and asked him to pilot me across the nine-mile neck to Rocky Cove, which none of my party knew. He invited me to come in and wait for a frost, to which I retorted that we had waited for one for two weeks but had kept moving, and unless we did keep moving we might never reach our destination. Finally, he declared that he would come as far as the dogs could haul him, but if they came to a standstill from that point he would turn back home. As he was clearly a man who knew his mind, there was nothing to do but to accept his condition. To my great relief, the komatik never did lose way altogether until we reached the shore of Pottle's Bay, though it was touch and go at times. From Rocky Cove we went on to old Steve Newell's. He was the mailman between Rigolet and Makkovik, a very difficult sector of coast, and Steve was a noted traveller and pilot like old Billy Murphy.

Poor old Steve. I always felt that he received a very raw deal. He did mail service for almost thirty years, and for twenty-eight of these he received remuneration at the rate of $20 a trip for service, which was subsequently valued at $75 a trip. Had he been paid at the latter rate, he might have laid by a little for his blind and declining years. For his blindness he had himself to thank, alas. Years before I met him, he had had the misfortune to suffer from an ulcer in one eye, which had destroyed the sight of that eye, and as infection can readily travel from one to the other I several times tried to persuade him to part with the almost useless member to safeguard the remaining one, but he was timid and always put it off, and put it off till too late. One winter when I was on furlough, the disaster occurred against which I had warned him. A severe inflammatory light-up in the old ulcerated area spread infection to the good eye, with much suffering and total destruction of sight. For the rest of his life, poor old Steve rocked in darkness and remorse, crouching on a low bench day after day. The Labrador rocks are no safe road for a blind man.

From Alliuk Bight, we had to make the detour to Indian Harbour for drugs. This occupied a whole day of circuitous travel amid doubtful areas of ice, but we returned adequately equipped for the rest of the itinerary. To get from Hamilton Inlet to Makkovik involved crossing the intervening peninsula at one of two points, either the Big Neck already referred to, between Ticoralak and Tuchialic, or across the Pottle's Bay barrens, which was our route for this occasion. It was Dr Wakefield, with his own drivers and a special pilot, who had almost perished on the Big Neck a few years previously. It is a crossing of between twenty-five and thirty miles as the crow flies and a good thirty-five by the route that has to be followed.

Coming south, as they [Wakefield's party] were, the traveller begins with an ascent of three miles up the course of a mountain brook, emerging onto Tuchialic Pond. Crossing this diagonally, a further ascent is made [by the traveller] up a shoulder of hill, whence in clear weather can be seen Mount Gnat on the south shore of Hamilton Inlet. Then the route crosses undulating mossy uplands for about twelve miles with a sudden descent to a small river. Swinging to the left up this stream for three quarters of a mile, the invisible path enters a wood-skirt to lead to Wilson's tilt, where a former Hudson's Bay agent of Rigolet post [James Wilson][131] used to maintain a log hut for occasions when he could not cross the neck in one day. Then a gradual ascent to the crest of Half-Way Hill, from which at last a wide panorama of the western basin of Hamilton Inlet comes into view. Then a gradual descent through scattered woods to a well marked knobby little hill, at which point the route swings away west through wood-skirts, marshes, and ponds till another sharp descent leads on to Fox Cove Brook, which is followed for seven miles to the shore. It is a most picturesque route and a fine shortcut if things go right, but in a blizzard of snow or whirl of drift, those upland, trackless barrens are very inhospitable, and it is essentially a tract of land to be crossed with no needless delay, if crossed at all.

Wakefield's hunting instincts were almost his undoing. Coming across fresh caribou tracks when right in the middle of the neck in threatening weather, the temptation to follow the tracks proved [for him] irresistible. It was always a case of "Just another half hour. We must be close to them." Then the storm broke, and it was a case of a race to regain the komatiks and the one sixteen-year-old lad left with them. The party actually got so near the komatiks that when they fired guns, the answering howls of the dogs were audible. But a difference of opinion arose as to whence the sound proceeded, for echoes play strange tricks in those gulches, and the wrong counsel prevailed. So they wandered away from supplies and comparative safety, as they had food and could have camped till the weather cleared if the storm did not last too long. For two days and nights they wandered or crouched in the best available shelter around a fire. They had but a small tobacco tin in which to melt snow for a drink, and they were reduced to chewing at sealskin mitts to ease the gnawing pangs of hunger. On the third day, they staggered out to a house on the north shore of the inlet, just about all in. A relief expedition had promptly to be despatched after the boy. He was found at his post, where he had been left. He spent one uneasy night snatching a nap on the komatik in a sleeping bag. The dogs, without attempting to molest him, did try to tear a dog-skin mat from under him, so he felt it was best to drive back to Tuchialic for dog-feed, as he could not trust hungry dogs for another night. He felt confident that the leader could take him there despite the storm, and his faith in the animal was justified. But having replenished supplies, he drove right back again to the rendez-vous and remained there till the relief party found him.

After that, there seemed to be a superstition against piloting doctors across the Big Neck which it took years to live down. I have crossed several times since, but it was five years before I took my first trip across. The Pottle's Bay barrens afford a much shorter crossing of the peninsula, not far from its eastern point. It is only about twelve miles from shore to shore, but it is very difficult country in rough weather. A single stunted tree or a rock of peculiar shape are the landmarks, the finding and identifying of which make the difference between reaching shelter and safety or having a comfortless and perilous night out in some cases. Of course, it is possible to travel from shore to shore by compass, but to do so would land the traveller into every kind of obstacle and difficulty. It was only by following the little leads by way of small marshes, ponds, and gullies that the old hand would cross with ease where the novice would have a ghastly time. We were to find out all about that later on. For the time being, the barrens were on their good behaviour, as if offering a civil welcome to strangers.

We even met a team coming the other way which left a fresh trail for us to follow if required, a trail that a storm would none the less obliterate in less than an hour. I noticed that our pilot's leader simply disregarded the new trail, crossing and re-crossing it in the most independent fashion, and I remarked on this to the driver. "Yes, doctor, that dog has only been across here once in his life, but he is going the same side of every stick and rock as he went the first time, and he will go that way every time," was the reply. And here was further food for thought. A good leader, the brains of the team, is almost beyond price.[132] Some dogs are born foolish and get more foolish every day they live, and these will fail at a pinch. Some will go ahead at all only if they have a track to follow. Some go ahead but don't care where. Others will follow a shoreline slavishly, however crooked, instead of cutting across the coves. The dog that will take his own line, run straight or carry a photographic record of every crook and turn in his canine brain: this is the one to trust in emergency.

Our first stop was at the shack of an Eskimo widow, Lydia Tooktishina. This was a home of tragedy. During my first summer at Indian Harbour, I had received an application for copious disinfectants for funeral preparations at the home of an Eskimo family that had presumably had ptomaine poisoning of which the father and two children had died, leaving the widow with one other child. The death had occurred in the early spring, and the bodies had remained frozen till recently. It was just questionable if burial were possible or if a funeral pyre would have to be made of house and bodies. And here were the survivors of that gruesome tragedy. The widow was chopping wood, hunting and fishing, and doing all a man's usual work.

Fifteen miles further on, at Bob's Brook, we found shelter with an old friend in new quarters. Willie Wolfrey had migrated from Pease Cove hither with his son-in-law and daughter, hoping to make a better living. The next day we ran on to Tilt Cove, nine miles ahead, and then Tuchialic nine miles further on again, lying under the shadow of mountains up to three thousand feet in height. From there, a five-mile run took us to Pomiadluk, where dwelt John Cove, the pilot of Dr Wakefield on the occasion of the trip across the Big Neck referred to above. While he had escaped on that occasion, John Cove was not fated to die in his bed. He, together with several members of his family, was drowned by the foundering of a motorboat but a little distance from the home.[133]

Another twelve or fourteen miles took us to Seal Cove, where we spent the night after a good day's work. It was of course all strange terrain to us. Between Tilt Cove and Seal Cove, the shore is very exposed, for the most part, to easterly and northeasterly winds and seas, and the ice there is apt either to be very rough or to break up altogether, leaving the traveller a choice between cliff climbing or at least one very wild neck inside the outer hills. This again was to be revealed to me fully later on. On the present trip, the going was splendid. But we had had our share of fine weather for a while. We had hoped to reach Makkovik before another storm, but the following day we could make a run of only seven miles and chose a detour from the direct path.

From Adlavik, where lived Jim and Harry Andersen, had come an appeal for a medical call with promise of ample dog-feed from Jim. So we went out there and arrived just ahead of a storm which kept us there for two nights. The Andersens, of whom there was quite a clan in the Makkovik district, were of Scandinavian stock. At Jim's I ran into the first of the members of the Moravian Mission that I had met, the Reverend Mr Lenz.[134] On a coast where gossip is rife, I never heard other than good of this little German padre. The Moravian work on the Labrador coast was already about 150 years old, their pioneers having come at a time when death was not an unlikely reward for their zeal. Although well on into middle age, this wiry little Moravian was as active as a cat and possessed of a high physical as well as moral courage, as I was to learn for myself. A most deplorable incident occurred during this visit. There were four teams of dogs around the homestead that night. Usually, the odoriferous seal meat, with other over-ripe feed for dogs, is kept on an elevated stage, well out of reach, but some people prefer little store-shacks, as was the case here at Adlavik. A canine raid was carried out the second night, and dogs burst their way into the store and not only raided the supplies of seal meat but tore up a valuable silver fox pelt worth perhaps $250. It was not possible to lay the responsibility at anyone's door.

When we were able to make a start from Adlavik, I had to make another detour to visit an Eskimo patient, but Mr Lenz, who was taking Jim along to Makkovik with him, promised to await me at Big Bight, the last hamlet before Makkovik, which was inhabited by two Broomfield families, so that we could go together for the last eight miles over Kill-a-Man Neck. This pleasant sounding locality consisted of a small mountain pass, ascended chiefly beside a brook full of cascades whose waters were forever bursting their icy bonds and turning the snow into a freezing mixture of ice and water. The last part of the ascent was almost a chimney, down which after a snow-storm such as we had had the wind would be driving the light snow in a whirl of blinding drift. It was to be no picnic on Kill-a-Man Neck that day.

After the conventional mug-up at Big Bight, where I booked quite an important case for operation at Indian Harbour the following summer, we set out to tackle the neck. We pushed our dogs from foothold to foothold on the cascades, floundering after them. The intervals were better till we came to the chimney – that was blinding, stifling. But for Jim, we could not have got through. The pilot who had come with me before I met Mr Lenz curled up completely and wished to retreat. However, though bad indeed, it did not last very long. Once we reached the crest, a more or less level half mile took us to a gradual descent, though abrupt at times, which became more and more sheltered as we came down into wooded land, then across a pond and some marshland to another brook, which we followed out to its mouth in the bottom of Makkovik Harbour, or Flounder Bight. Here were the Moravian mission-house and church and a hamlet of four comfortable cottages inhabited by Andersens and Mitchells as well as the home of George Jacques (pronounced *jock*), who was in the employ of the Mission. Here I was kindly welcomed and most comfortably and hospitably entertained by Mrs Lenz. The luxury of a little privacy in a comfortable room, tastefully served food, and a hot bath were creature comforts not to be despised after the past days. I was already three weeks out from home and was to be away another six weeks, and interludes of this kind amid the wear and tear of the tripping were certainly refreshing.[135] A weekend afforded excuse for prolonging the visit beyond a single night, and I had no quarrel with the delay.

Greatly refreshed, we left Makkovik for Hopedale. Seven miles out from Makkovik, we stopped at the house of an old Welsh settler, Tom Evans, who had a self-appointed mission to help out doctors travelling in this region. This was a delightful spirit to meet. Before I had left Makkovik, I was told, "If you come to help us like this, doctor, you shall never want for dog-feed or a pilot and team to take you anywhere around." And in a quarter of a century, that undertaking has never been violated. Tom's contribution was free pilotage to Hopedale as well as to any other points in the vicinity. Tom, like old Solomon Burdett, had at once a golden heart and a tongue that brought him trouble. The former was evidenced by the fact that he had given a home to one of "Long Tom" Broomfield's children [Stanley]. He and his wife, having no children of their own, were never without one or more little waifs to whom they gave a good home and some useful training. From a surgical viewpoint, Aunt Harriett was a notable case in which a complete cure of advanced cancer of the breast, both breasts being involved, had been achieved by Dr Wakefield by an extensive operation done some years previously. It left some limitation of move-ment and frequently discomfort after work, but to the end of her life she had no recurrence of the dread disease, and she always lived an active and useful life.

After a detour up Kaipokok Bay to see the dying widow referred to in the last chapter, we set out northward with Tom. Again we had to diverge from the direct route to go up Island Harbour Bay in answer to another medical call. We stayed for the first night at a little hamlet at the entrance to the bay. It was here that a young trapper and salmon fisher of Scotch ancestry [Ted McNeill] had approached Dr Grenfell, when the doctor appeared on one of his extensive summer cruises, with an unusual proposition. "Doctor," he said, "if you will take me back to St Anthony and give me one hour's schooling a day, I will work for you ten hours a day." The youngster was not kept to the latter of the bargain, but a few years later this young man went to a first-rate technical training college for just over a year. Thereafter, he

returned to St Anthony and became master carpenter and then con-
tractor in reinforced concrete construction and has erected buildings
worth hundreds of thousands of dollars. I met his old parents and his
brother on this occasion.[136] The other inhabitants of this hamlet were
Lyalls, also of Scottish descent.

The following day was devoted to the ascent and descent of Island
Harbour Bay to see [Samuel] a brother of Jim Andersen, who lived at
the head of it. When we reached the house, I was greeted by a man
who from his manner almost might have been a courtier, though he
lacked a courtier's vocabulary. None the less, he was very far from
illiterate, being a great reader and deeply versed both in the botany
and ornithology of Labrador. But by contrast, he was sadly disfigured
as to his limbs with very extensive eczema. It was probably of largely
dietetic origin, as it was a condition prevalent in the family clan and
seasonal in its onset. Inadequate treatment had enabled it to spread to
a shocking extent, and there was not much that could be achieved in
his present surroundings. I had to have old Sam for two long sessions
at Indian Harbour both to cure and to give instruction in prevention
or early treatment. Thereafter, he never got into such a state again.
This dietetic eczema was to become widely realised in the Great War.
I have seen much of it since out here, and I have certainly seen some
cases clear up under treatment of cod-oil in addition to local application, which resisted the latter alone. This looks as if a lack of animal
fat was a provocative condition, and this is often experienced in the
spring months.

From Island Harbour, we made a run of thirty-five miles to Hopedale,
where was another Moravian Mission station presided over by the
Reverend and Mrs Hettasch.[137] Here the kindly welcome and hospitality of Makkovik was repeated. My first welcome from an Eskimo
community like that of Hopedale was a thing to remember. The whole
population swarmed out onto the harbour ice. As many as possible
crowded onto our komatiks till the teams were almost brought to a
standstill, and the usual final dash to the house faded away to nothing.
The women wore their gayest dickeys, and the fashionable white-
bottomed Sunday boots were much in evidence. The air resounded
with greetings of "*aksunai.*" (In Labrador, I have always understood
that this meant "be strong," but according to Freuchen, in Greenland
the greeting is "*sunak sunai,*" meaning "How glad you are to be
here."[138]) Handshaking was universal. The Hopedale Eskimos were
evidently determined that a visiting doctor's time should not be wasted,
and they were prepared to provide a clinic of indefinite length, but
Mr Hettasch, who acted as interpreter and knew the patients, was a
great help in sorting wheat from chaff with reasonable speed.

For an unqualified practitioner, Mr Hettasch had done some truly heroic surgery. In emergency, this level-headed clergyman had amputated an arm at the shoulder for gunshot wound and another at the wrist, not only doing the surgery but also giving part of his attention to a very amateur anaesthetist at the same time. The one qualified doctor of this mission, Dr Hutton,[139] who was a veteran of seventeen years of service, had recently retired. His hospital had been at Okak, some sixty miles north of Nain and the capital of Eskimo land in Labrador, perhaps, though much about the same size as Nain in population. So Mr Hettasch occupied a very responsible position in the Eskimo community, while a goodly proportion of the surgical cases, apart from such emergencies as those mentioned, were naturally sent to hospitals, where there were greater facilities. Of these, Indian Harbour was now the nearest, so this link now being formed had a very real value towards future co-operation and mutual understanding. Mr Hettasch proved to be an expert photographer and a keen naturalist, a man who was also blest with a keen sense of humour, without which no one should stay long in Labrador. Little did he or I realise, as we talked together in the spring of 1914, the death blow which was to fall on that little community within five years in the shape of that terrible aftermath of the Great War, the Spanish Flu.

I noticed that both in Makkovik and Hopedale, as was also evidenced in Nain, a reserve of wooded land had been established in close relation to the settlements to prevent improvident vandals from cutting out the last of the trees for firewood. Moreover, the Mission stations set a good example in opportunist small-scale agriculture even this far north, though the Eskimos were not imitative in this line.

One feature of Hopedale in time past, which was no longer to be seen, was the annual appearance of the great migrating herd of caribou, which used to come right across the harbour and would take a day and a half to pass. Whether the deer moss became eaten out on this route, which is apt to happen, or excessive depredations made Hopedale to be considered an unhealthy place for caribou by those most concerned, I cannot say. There are stories of wholesale slaughter, with dogs scavenging on mouldering carcases of animals recklessly slaughtered, but these may be exaggerated.

Naturally, the Moravians felt the impending fate of their Eskimo friends very keenly. They frankly admitted that their own pioneers had erred, with the best intentions and quite pardonably, at a time when no one realised the relative susceptibility of these aboriginals to white man's diseases, by encouraging centralisation for purposes of physical, educational, and medical service; and they deplore the fact that now, in a generation when these dangers were realised, the Eskimos had become too sophisticated for decentralisation and a resumption of their natural nomadic existence. But for the export of natives for exhibition outside, they naturally had nothing to censure.

After a most interesting little visit, we pushed on northward once more. The stretch of coast leading from Hopedale to Big Bay bears an evil reputation owing to another komatik tragedy which had occurred a few winters previously. A whole family [Lane] left their home in Passion Week to attend the Easter festival at Hopedale. They were overtaken by a furious blizzard on the way, and once again a shift of wind bewildered unskilled navigators. Travelling round in almost a complete circle, they actually re-entered their own bay, passed their home, and went on into the bottom of the bay. Forced to camp without any stove, they froze or starved to death before the prolonged storm abated.

At Big Bay, we were the guests of old Samuel Broomfield. He and Tom Evans were great rivals. Sam secured a long lead in fame by sending a sealskin tobacco pouch as a birthday gift to His Majesty, King George V, and received an acknowledgment. Tom later made up some leeway by receiving an invitation to a White House wedding in Washington when Mr Francis Sayre,[140] who had visited the Labrador coast and had met old Tom, was being married to a daughter of the late President Wilson. To witness one of their verbal clashes was no bad entertainment. Sam proved to be the soul of hospitality and made me a very handsome offer as his contribution to the itinerant medical service. The family, besides doing well with fish and fur, often killed seals by the hundred in the autumn. The value was, of course, largely in the hides and partly in the fat, but it meant that they had unlimited dog-feed. He offered to put up my travel-worn teams for a good rest while I finished my journey to Nain with a fresh team. His neighbour, Jim Lane, would take me to Nain. Needless to say, this offer, which included hospitality for my teamster, was altogether too good to refuse.

The following day, Jim Lane drove up with only six dogs to take him and his fifteen-year-old boy and me and our load for a sixty-five-mile run to Nain and a similar distance back. When I expressed a doubt over the smallness of the team, Jim said he thought they could do it, and he was right. Sam Broomfield had at that time the finest team of huskies I think that I have ever seen: a mother dog for leader, still young and lively, and two litters of her male pups born only six months apart, great upstanding animals of about two years and eighteen months in age. There was perfect harmony and united action, a magnificent team. (Jim Lane had another litter of the same breed.) We were travelling in company with another team of seventeen dogs from Hopedale to Nain, a mob rather than a team, and any time that Jim called on his six they would romp away from the seventeen.

Fifteen miles out from Big Bay, we ran into the Davis Inlet post of the Hudson's Bay Company. The agent, a young Englishman of the name of Handford,[141] who was then unmarried and, with no companion but a spaniel, greeted me like a long-lost brother and openly gloated when another fierce storm descended on us and penned me there for no less than four days, being about the worst storm of that winter. In the servant's house alongside the agent's lived the mother of little Stewart Dickers, the tubercular hip case that was spending the winter with us at Mud Lake, and I was sorry to have to give a very guarded report on the boy. When at last we got away, the going was so much spoiled that we had no chance of doing the fifty remaining miles to Nain in a day. We spent the night at the house of an Eskimo named Anton. Here I ate seal meat (not raw) for the first time. If the seal is young and shot rather than drowned in a net, there is really nothing objectionable about the meat, provided the fat be removed. The livers, hearts, and tongues might well be those of pigs or cattle, so far as flavour is concerned.

I had been travelling in company with a young Englishman who was accountant to the Moravian organisation, and he and his wife entertained me very kindly at Nain. The missionary in charge, the Reverend Mr Townley,[142] also English, was very co-operative and conducted me on a medical round of the village of three hundred, interpreting for me as Mr Hettasch had kindly done at Hopedale. I remember that he took me to see one unfortunate heart case with the second slowest pulse rate that I have ever counted. His heart beat only thirty times per minute. (Once in London, in my training days, there was a similar case in the wards with a pulse of twelve per minute.) Needless to say, the poor fellow had not long to live. When we were ready to leave for Nain, Jim Lane came to me in great trouble because one of his beloved dogs had been set upon by a pack of Nain dogs and severely mauled. He would live but could not possibly work at present. So the crippled beast had to be left behind, to come south with the mailman on his next trip, and we had but five dogs to take us back to Big Bay. Those five splendid animals hauled two men and a boy and our load almost fifty miles that day to a lone house to the westward of Davis Inlet, where I was summoned by a medical call to see a sick child.

I was struck by two or three differences between methods of komatik travel away north as compared with those in vogue further south. The northern komatiks were far longer, averaging from sixteen to eighteen or more feet, where the southern komatiks averaged from ten to fourteen feet. There was a reason for this. Where there is more timber, there are more narrow portage paths, and long komatiks are not practicable. In the Rigolet Narrows run, it would be simply impossible to work with a long komatik on the ballicatters and short, steep portages connecting with the shoreline at awkward angles. The long stretches of open ice, with barren land where there is land to be crossed at all, is far better suited to long komatiks. These, of course, bear up far better than shorter ones on snow that is not hard packed or on a weak crust that tends to founder under a shorter komatik, as the weight can be better distributed.

Another northern custom which saves dogs much labour and men much time is to water the runners before leaving for a run. An icy coat forms immediately and this will last as long as it hits no rocks or bare ground or hummocks of ice. If it gets knocked off, it needs renewing all over, as alternating patches of ice and iron prevent smooth progress. Finally, the northerner changes the "shoeing" of his runners more often than the southerner to suit the snow and ice conditions. On salty going, where scanty snow on salt water ice forms a sort of mixture of ice cream and cheese, iron drags more terribly hard where whalebone meets with little resistance. All these points are of very practical value to the traveller.

The second day out from Nain, we reached Davis Inlet early, with plenty of time left to go on to Big Bay, but it almost cost a physical struggle with the lonely and hospitable Handford to do so. He had rounded up several patients from scattered homes in the neighbourhood to meet me there, but there was nothing to hold us up long, and we had a duty to old Sam Broomfield, who had entertained my teamsters and dogs for nine days instead of the expected three or four. When we reached Big Bay, the dogs were so fat that it looked as if rolling would be their best mode of locomotion, and the two teamsters were in much the same condition. However, with a three-hundred-mile journey back to North West River ahead, there would be ample opportunity for slimming again. As if they had not done enough already, two of the Broomfields came with us as far as Hopedale, so I saw that splendid team in action and rode behind them.

From Hopedale, I was asked for another detour up into Adlatuk Bay to the home of Willie Mitchell, brother of Robert Mitchell of Makkovik. Here was a very comfortable and prosperous home. Willie acted as chieftain for a little colony of three or four families. It was a wonderful region for fur-bearing animals, with a fine salmon river and a tidal rattle that afforded good fishing through the ice in its neighbourhood for rock cod. It was also a place where grouse abounded. In the summer, they moved out to Hopedale for cod fishing. They were also good seal hunters. The home was clean and comfortable, and among its equipment was a small organ on which Willie performed creditably. There was but one thing to regret at the time, and that was the presence of tuberculosis. One of the daughters had a diseased bone in one foot. I have followed this case for twenty-five years. The foot eventually healed after a summer at Indian Harbour and some months in plaster of Paris. Then the disease appeared in the breastbone, where it also healed. Then came a term of healthy years and she married. (Fortunately, perhaps, there were no children.) About three years ago, signs of kidney trouble began. She had two periods of hospital treatment, but both sides are affected, and it is only a matter of time now. At least the disease had spared her lungs all these years, and she has had a comfortable and by no means useless life.

We reached Makkovik without further delays, and from there we ran for Seal Cove. Here I heard that I was needed in a judicial capacity at an Eskimo home on an island seven miles away. When we reached the house, it turned out that the woman was bringing an action against her husband for assault. As the plaintiff could speak no English and I could speak no Eskimo, the husband who was defendant had to act as interpreter for his wife. One could not help feeling that it was a great chance for a free translation, but I believe that he honestly did his best while he rather mixed up the case for the defence with that for the prosecution. He admitted that his wife was not at all bad as women went, but she did suffer from delayed cerebration when it came to carrying out his commands with the speed and dexterity to which he felt himself entitled. What could any self-respecting husband do but try to stimulate the cerebral cortex? And what more handy implement could be found for such a purpose than a billet of firewood all ready to hand in the box by the stove? Such was the gist of his discourse.

I explained that however degenerate the times and regrettable the change, the best husbands did not treat their wives in this fashion nowadays. He had been guilty of bad form as well as of assault. Since there was no prison handy and he had no means of paying the fine, he would be bound over to keep the peace for six months, and to stimulate his own memory he would cut one thousand turns of wood for the over-lofty and cold church at Makkovik, which was the only public institution in the neighbourhood. This the defendant promised to do, suppressing his candid opinion of justice, I suspect. It was a year before I saw the defendant again, and then he came forward and greeted me effusively. He was no man to harbour malice. Moreover, he had seen light amid the darkness, reason in justice, method in her madness. He had cut the turns, and his wife had carried them on her shoulder from the woods to the shipping point on the landwash.

Disappointed in our hope of crossing the Big Neck, we went on to Lydia Tooktishina's the next day and re-crossed the Pottle's Bay neck into Hamilton Inlet. We were now in the home stretch, though we still had to ascend the long cul-de-sac known as Double Mer, which opens into the main bay a few miles outside Rigolet. Here dwelt nine widely scattered families. We called at Rigolet for mail before making this detour, and just as we were leaving a team came in, hauling a young Church of England schoolteacher who was stretched out in his sleeping bag and racked with rheumatism. These travelling teachers would go from house to house and hamlet to hamlet, spending anything from a few days to a few weeks at a time and living with and like the people whose children they taught. Needless to say, accommodation and food varied greatly and seldom on the side of luxury, and facilities for teaching were not convincing since the teacher and pupil met under conditions unsuitable for both. I admired the devotion shown by some but could not see in this system a justifiable use of youthful talent, enthusiasm, and health. This was the first of several itinerant teachers whom I was to meet as patients. Having covered Double Mer, we crossed to Lake Melville by the portage leading to Bill Shepperd's but did not spend a night there this time, so any new fictional effort of Bill's had to be postponed. It was the sixty-second day of our absence when we finally crossed Goose Bay and regained Mud Lake.

That spring, I visited Kenemich again, where another company was just starting on a small scale what was to prove to be yet another premature and abortive timber venture. This again had but a short and unhappy career. I found that old Malcolm McLean had recently had a narrow escape. The Reverend W.S. Mercer had been bound to Kenemich by dog-team on a pastoral visit when he saw what looked at first like a seal on the ice ahead. The dogs saw it too and promptly bolted. As he drew nearer, the padre saw that it was no seal but the head and shoulders of a man in deadly peril. Malcolm had got onto bad ice, which foundered under him. He was holding grimly on to the last, with no hope of getting out unaided. Stopping his dogs with difficulty, the padre took his long whip and crawled cautiously towards the hole. Too much haste might easily end in a double tragedy. Presently, he was near enough to shoot out the last of his whip so that the end was within reach of the drowning man, who seized it and wound it repeatedly around his wrist. Then, taking a further grip with both hands, he was slowly drawn out of the hole to safety. Then, wrapped for the moment in the dogskin mat to be found on most komatiks, he was rushed home and laid in warm blankets and dosed with hot tea, and the tough old veteran was soon none the worse.

One night that same spring, I was roused from sleep by an urgent knocking below to find Monsieur Lescaudron arrived with a team from North West River. It was a case of childbirth, and things were not looking too good. In a few minutes, we were off on a wild night ride to the wildness of which a hard snowstorm added to the darkness not a little, while the finishing touch came from some runaway puppies, offspring of our leading dog [Ribble], which had chased the team across the bay and were lightheartedly playing with their fond parent and distracting her from her job. The result was that we went astray and took a long time to find ourselves again and pick up the portage. However, all ended well. Yet another night summons for a ten-mile walk on snowshoes by moonlight sounded so dubious that I sent the applicant back with some tincture of ginger and promised to walk over in the morning. By then, the ginger had done its work, and the aftermath of an overdose of pancakes was a thing of the past.

The remainder of March and the month of April soon sped by, and in the last week of April it was time to go out for another period of marooning on Indian Harbour Island to complete our task of the previous spring.

10

Third Summer at Indian Harbour: Outbreak of War, Back to England and ...?

We had just such a trip down Hamilton Inlet to Indian Harbour in the spring of 1914 as that experienced the previous year: warm days, wet snow or bare ground on the land, and water and slush on the ice, with intervals of slipping when following big cracks. Ribble's puppies were now in harness, proud team members, and worked with a will. With me was Flinn, also Fred and Sam, George and Peter. At Valley Bight, Bill Shepperd joined up, having generously offered to come and work "just for my grub, doctor." Fred's eldest son, Judson, a boy of fifteen, came along as cook so that Sam could act as full-time workman. The members of the Indian Harbour fish crew also appeared as we went along the outer basin, so that we numbered fourteen in all when we reached Indian Harbour. When we reached the hospital, there was no need to put a ladder up to the roof to uncover the chimneys and work from above at lowering shutters as there was a convenient snowdrift leading right up to it.

Ducks abounded, and with such a gang work was going ahead gaily when a thunderbolt fell upon us. One morning, an immense flight of ducks was sighted in the eastern basin of the harbour. A hunting party was told off, consisting of Flinn and Bill Shepperd and one other who went off to where a small flat was kept for such purposes, ready for launching off the edge of the ice. Soon after they had disappeared, we were surprised to hear a single shot. We supposed that they must have seen a seal and decided that one shot would not disturb the ducks. But in a minute more, a man appeared running.

"Mr Flinn is shot," he gasped.

"Not dead?"

"No, not dead."

Without waiting for more, we seized the komatik and ran it down to the scene of the tragedy.

It was an old, old story. The loaded gun carelessly laid in the boat before launching, a slip and clatter, a loud report, and the charge tore through the planks of the little flat and still at point-blank range, though with diminished velocity, brought up on Flinn's right leg. He was laid on the komatik and hurried to hospital, where I examined the limb. The kneecap might be called the bullseye of the target. As we cut away the clothing, numbers of loose shot rattled onto the floor. Several others were half embedded in the skin around the knee. Only in two places were there wounds right through the skin. I could feel that the margin of the kneecap was fractured, but that need not mean that the intricate joint was pierced, which meant a grave risk to the limb if not to the life. One bad sign was to be noted right away, though. On the trip down the inlet, Flinn had acquired a moderate degree of water on the knee, and clear watery fluid was unquestionably seeping through one of the wounds. It was still possible that the joint had escaped infection, though no longer probable.

The skin was carefully disinfected with iodine and alcohol, sterile dressings applied, and the limb put up on a splint for complete rest. Labrador being considered free from tetanus, there was nothing more to be done but watch and wait. Within forty-eight hours, it was clear that there was going to be trouble, and a nice pickle we were in: nurse and nearly all instruments 150 miles away at Mud Lake, no anaesthetist apart from the surgeon, no proper cook, laundry, or invalid diet. I did a drainage operation on the joint, finding no loose shot there or any visible sign of shot having entered the thighbone. But a single pellet, which would leave no visible entry wound in the cartilage, would be enough to cause endless mischief. I washed the joint out frequently with mild disinfectants, and for the next three or four days things seemed to be going well. Temperature and pulse fell to normal, and the patient was comfortable. On the sixth day, there was a sharp rise of temperature and on the seventh high fever with rapid pulse.

We were in for it now with a vengeance. An infected thighbone, an amputation, necessarily high up, with an infected joint on the table to threaten the amputation wound, and only rawest of raw amateur assistants. I had to put the case to Flinn, who reacted heroically. I spent half the night sterilising equipment and trying to get some ideas of asepsis into my chosen assistants and of the dangers and other elements of anaesthesia into Fred Blake. It was too cold for ether to volatise well, and I was no expert at spinal anaesthesia, so it had to be chloroform. For a saw for the bone, I had my choice between a carpenter's cross-cut saw or a small surgical instrument meant for finger bones and such like or axe. I wished afterwards I had chosen either the cross-cut or an axe, but I chose the smaller instrument because it was more readily sterilised. This was an error, as speed was important and tardiness as big a risk as an incompletely sterilised tool in an operation where sterility was practically impossible to maintain. Another difficulty was added by the lack of a tourniquet. Rubber goods are readily rotted by frost, so we had taken everything of rubber away into winter quarters, where we could protect them. Bandages were a poor substitute for a tourniquet. But I engaged a special assistant to compress the femoral artery higher up. Even at that, the operation was bound to be far from bloodless.

[I] having made the best preparations that I could, we started off. At one stage of proceedings, the amateur anaesthetist overdid the chloroform, and I had to drop everything in a hurry and do artificial respiration. Fortunately, the patient soon reacted to this. The operation was then completed without further misadventure but with almost a certainty of wound infections, which duly occurred. For more than a week, I feared that destruction of tissue would necessitate re-amputation later if the patient survived. For nineteen days, I was day and night nurse, and it was a continuous nightmare; and if it was a tense time for me, what about the patient? Gradually, infection subsided, the wound cleaned, and first the life and then the remains of the limb could be declared safe.

Flinn, who was heroic throughout, began to talk of a man of his acquaintance who had also had an amputation through the thigh, who could dance and "skate like a streak." This optimistic mood was to be painfully clouded, not by any fresh setback to his own progress but because the first steamer brought news of the death of his widowed mother. I am glad to say that once that shock passed off to some extent, his own progress was well sustained, and he, like his friend referred to above, was able to lead an active and happy life.

Navigation opened late that season. It was July 1st when the first steamer arrived, and fishermen northward bound in schooners told us that they had been indulging in dog-team drives as they coasted along the Labrador. Dog-team on Lake Melville was actually prolonged into June, an altogether unwonted state of affairs and one that I have never known to be repeated since. It was a matter of considerable concern to me, as *Yale* did not arrive with my wife until July 1st, and our first son [William Anthony Paddon] was born on the 10th. It was again to be a record summer, with eighty-four in-patients and over eight hundred out-patients. Great fields of ice came driving south, and repeated in-winds packed the ice on the shore, penning northward-bound schooners into harbours and seriously hampering steamer traffic. Old *Invermore* met her doom within a few miles of Indian Harbour, being forced off her usual course by ice and running ashore to become a total wreck. We were overcrowded with refugees from her, awaiting a relief vessel, but even the powerful *Kyle* was herself jammed in for a week near the scene of *Invermore*'s disaster.

The wreck brought us one patient, at least. After *Invermore* was abandoned, raiders crowded aboard to loot her. One party discovered some liquor, and under its influence one man undertook to explode a signal rocket with a sledgehammer. He arrived at hospital with his face in a shocking state, and it seemed to be almost a miracle that the sight of both eyes should be unimpaired. Eventually, the amorphous mass, which resembled a pumpkin rather than a face, took on definite features once more, and ultimate disfigurement was amazingly slight, considering what the condition had been. Despite the tragedy of Flinn's leg, the work had gone on to completion, and the extra accommodation was certainly welcome. Running water was now available, though the full plumbing system was not completed till 1915.

And then, into this whirl of activity came the declaration of war in Europe. Wakefield, who was then at Battle Harbour, was off like a shot. He had at least a qualified assistant to whom he could hand over his patients. I had Frank [Babbott] back with me as student assistant this summer, but while he was as conscientious as ever and progressing well with his medical studies, it was impossible to saddle him with the responsibilities of the place. Wakefield having gone to St John's, beyond which point even his ardent enthusiasm could not get him for a long time, I advised local Labrador frontiersmen to await any instructions from headquarters, either of the Legion of Frontiersmen or the newly forming Newfoundland Regiment, before leaving the coast. The government had all that they could contend with in Newfoundland and did not want untrained men crowding in at present. I was due for furlough after this season closed, and my own problem could be settled then. Meantime, my hands were more than full. We had two nurses again that summer, and they were by no means idle. Fifty-nine cases were operated on under general anaesthesia, and two successive Sunday mornings found us operating on acute appendix cases landed from schooners. A little outbreak of typhoid at no great distance brought us four cases of that exacting disease. Of course, the war was to affect profoundly both fish and fur markets. While the importance of food supplies was immediately enhanced and fish gradually rose to a figure hitherto unprecedented and never since equalled, fur was at first a luxury, and the bottom fell out of the market. Yet within eighteen months, a totally new class of buyer had arisen, and the demand soared as did the prices. For the third time, we closed down the little hospital after a spell of work, the figures of which almost doubled those of two years ago.

On a stormy, rainy black night, after we had gone to bed in happy assurance of being undisturbed, *Sagona*, which had replaced *Kyle*, crept into harbour and blew an imperious summons, and we had to make a hurried toilet and exit. Icebreakers were in great demand, and Newfoundland had sold part of her fleet to the Russian government. *Kyle* had replaced s s *Lintrose*,[143] the successor to *Bruce* on the Cabot Strait route. At St John's, we transferred to the old *Mongolian*,[144] of about five thousand tons. (I believe she was the first trans-Atlantic vessel to alter her course in response to orders to abandon the north of Ireland route to Glasgow and Liverpool owing to submarine activities.) And so we came to the England of 1914.

Immediate personal affairs attended to, I waited on Colonel Driscoll of the Legion of Frontiersmen, offering to resign my present position and join up if he thought I ought to do so. After hearing the facts, he had no hesitation. "You must go back to Labrador. Your duty lies there," he declared, and although a colonel's son myself and despite the fact that it was not pleasant to be "one of those who did not go," I felt convinced that he was right. That question settled, I took a postgraduate course in operative surgery and visited old haunts at St Thomas's Hospital. And now, at last, there was time and opportunity to summarise the impressions and conclusions of two and a quarter years of Survey, which had included three periods of cottage hospital work at Indian Harbour and over 2,500 miles of dog-team travel besides a considerable amount of small-boat cruising. The results were as follows.

With the country itself, I was both charmed and intrigued. The beauty of the fiords inside the grim coastline fascinated me, and my imagination was caught by the evidence of great natural resources which, in my belief, would one day make of this little-known and thinly populated country a productive and prosperous region. The immense latent waterpower, the great timber reserves, and the almost certain mineral wealth, as well as the vast tundras of reindeer moss, all offered great hopes for the future, whenever the time should come. The salmon and trout streams held great attractions for sportsmen, and artists could also find boundless scope for exercise of their talents. Moreover, even the fisheries were as yet almost undeveloped, alike in regard to variety and modern improvements. As to the people, the plight of the Eskimo and Indian survivors called forth a sense of compunction and a feeling of responsibility which extended to the mixed stock. Also, I had found in many of these frontier dwellers a very real interest and charm. The boat and dog-team travel interested and attracted me greatly as well as the human factors. In regard to work, it was clear that it must be to some extent a bridging of the interval between chaos and cosmos, the primitive and the developed.

Exploitation of a new country for industrial purposes always constitutes a real menace, in many ways, to pioneer settlers and settler stock. To try to prepare the present population for the inevitable change was a worthwhile quest. To produce a good standard of public health with such evils as tuberculosis and nutritional disease reduced to a minimum; to produce employable citizens fitted not only physically but mentally to play a worthy part in their country's history and development; to build up a corporate feeling and co-operative effort; and also to aim at economic improvements so closely associated with health problems – here was a programme replete with interest and big enough to afford full-time interest and activity. But in order to carry out any worthwhile part of such a programme, pills and potions and surgical instruments and small wards were not enough. Education must be the first ally of medicine, while the importance of the rising generation and of getting handicapped children out of handicapping homes have already been emphasized. The significance of agriculture in this programme was hardly realised as yet, though it came to loom very large later on. The value of small auxiliary industries was also noted.

With regard to institutional work, the scarcity of communications was a strong objection to any one centre. The Labrador community fell into well-marked sub-communities determined largely by geographical considerations. Each main bay was like a little world of its own. Battle Harbour, Cartwright, Rigolet, North West River, Makkovik, Hopedale, and Nain were all natural little capitals, and the trading stores also contributed to the demarcation of districts. To develop one sub-community at the expense of others was a thing to be deplored. The Moravians were already at work among the Eskimo community, while they were not completely self-dependent for medical service. In regard to the mixed stock, cottage institutions in each of the chief sub-communities seemed to offer a far better prospect than any one bigger central plant.

The people must, early in the campaign, be taught to recognise the value and use of natural resources all ready to their hands. Crude cod-oil, edible berries, and plants, the latter including many edible fungi with a high nutritive value if sensibly and conscientiously used, could alone give a powerful setback to disease due to undernourishment, and elementary hygiene as part of a rational education could do the same with regard to the deadly tuberculosis. A child welfare campaign, including boarding schools and orphanages which could be combined under one roof, was of vital importance to the success of the whole enterprise. Under the Children's Act,[145] a justice could remove any child from a home where, on moral or economic grounds, the youngster's welfare was threatened, and this could be and has been a powerful lever with refractory parents. Such a plan would also afford opportunity for routine care of juvenile throats and teeth, and so many of the evils that flesh is heir to[146] have their origin in diseased tonsils, redundant adenoids, and carious teeth. Domestic science could be inculcated in a way that would transform cooking, clothing, and general home nursing, first aid to the injured, and care of infants. Such cottage institutions could be real model homes for the homemakers of the future, with little that they could not copy in homes of their own.

It was my firm conviction, too, that there were just as bright brains in Labrador as elsewhere if only they received opportunity for self-expression and vindication. It produced a strong inward protest to hear one supposedly responsible for education of that time in one district declare that "the fourth reader is enough education for any child in Labrador." Why should not Labrador produce its own nurses, schoolteachers (both of which have since materialised), and doctors and clergy? Again, the standards of native midwifery were depressingly low, but there was no reason why the more intelligent and cleanly of the local women should not receive some instruction, not only in delivery but also in prenatal care of the mother and also postnatal care of mother and infant.

The lack of administration in this unrepresented community has already been touched on. All that we saw were minor officials during the summer season with no real authority to do anything and no real opportunity to form a first-hand opinion of the problems involved. And what was true of the state was largely true of the church, though not equally true. The ecclesiastical powers that be, like the political, found plenty to occupy them in Newfoundland. Education was denominational, subsidised by government.

Then there was trade, which profoundly affected individual economics. Naturally, the viewpoint of traders must clash with mine at times, but I have no wish to conduct a one-sided argument. I have eaten the salt [been a guest] of many traders out here and have received not only neighbourly kindness and friendship but also much co-operation and generous support for my work. While outside his office the trader may be the most philanthropic of men, inside it he is there to make money for his company. Trade and charity obviously can hardly run in double harness in the same office. Labrador was not and is not ready for co-operative methods, and there is no scope for the profit-sharing schemes of big firms which are to be found in some places outside. I have always been an outspoken opponent of unopposed trading, being a disciple of Adam Smith[147] through studies in political economy at college and having seen nothing since to upset my early convictions. That is my position, in brief. But I have seen first hand the trader's side of the case as well as the customer's. Nor do I forget that it has been trenchantly said that in the ideal revolution, while politicians and business captains might meet with some violence, the biggest contribution to the crimson tide would or should be made by the blood of the philanthropists![148]

Such were the data then to hand for formulating a plan of campaign. How long would be the time available for working at it? Whence would come the sinews of war?[149] How far would it prove practicable to transmute theory into practice?

PART TWO

Foundations

11

Back to Labrador: Founding of North West River Cottage Hospital

It was early in June 1915 that SS *Carthaginian*[150] cautiously nosed her way through a loose field of pan-ice into St John's harbour. Among her passengers was a young Anglican priest whom I will call Father Henry.[151] He was a type of the Church Militant[152] that is always a refreshment to meet: deep without being ponderous, tolerant without being lax; always human, cheerful, and kindly and blessed with a saving sense of humour as well as with eloquence; and, finally, deeply interested in the material as well as the spiritual welfare of his parishioners. The one thing that Father Henry lacked for prolonged successful work in Labrador was the degree of self-interest required to pay due regard to his health. It was this, combined with other causes to some extent, that was to limit his service to a single decade of effective work in Labrador. He came to replace the Reverend Hubert Kirby, a man by no means without vision but who had been sadly handicapped by lack of funds to transmute vision into accomplished fact.

A padre's lot in Labrador is a strenuous one[153] if he is worth his salt. A fearless and competent sailor, Father Henry none the less almost ended his career at its outset one wild night in the wide mouth of Hamilton Inlet, and within his first year in Labrador he was to have an experience well worthy of record. Starting out in the spring, as soon as there was open water, to visit some outlying parishioners in an outboard motorboat, [he found] a shift of wind brought in the ice again and drove him ashore on a tiny islet off the end of the long promontory known as Cape Porcupine. Being alone and quite unarmed, it was a little disturbing [for him] to find the small rocky refuge already occupied by a very able-bodied polar bear. They were hardly a stone's throw from the cape, so near and yet so far, but neither man nor beast cared to trust to the drift ice in the narrow tickle, which was of the small, pounded-up grade. For the rest of the long spring day and for a good part of the short night, which seemed perhaps longer than the day, padre and bear kept the circulation moving by pedestrian exercise. Once, inadvertently, they approached each other closely enough to have shaken hands, but although there was no breach of diplomatic relations, they avoided contact. At last, while it was still dark, a change of wind occurred which was welcome at least to one of the pair, and Bruin, without even the courtesy of "after you," plunged into the tickle as soon as the ice opened up enough to make the passage possible and disappeared on the mainland. If ever a sociable soul was grateful for solitude, Father Henry was on that occasion.

Ice conditions, which were again very bad, delayed our departure for Indian Harbour, but there were very substantial compensations. The makeshift winter hospital at Mud Lake was to be a thing of the past, and a permanent cottage hospital, at first for winter service but later to become an all-year little institution, was to take its place. It was to be erected at North West River, which with its two trading posts was always alive with comers and goers and was also far more accessible and central than Mud Lake, especially with regard to late autumn navigation, as we already knew somewhat to our cost. The building was to be the gift of a generous individual [Mrs J.S. Lockwood] as a memorial to her mother and was to be called the Emily Beaver Chamberlin Memorial [Hospital]. Also, whereas I had so far worked at Indian Harbour with unqualified assistants, a young doctor was to be there for the season about to begin. This arrangement would enable me to keep an occasional eye on progress at North West River.

Yale too was to play a definite part in the enterprise, her contribution being to carry all the cement required for the basement from Rigolet up to North West River, where it would be landed by the mail steamer. (Her mail service, which had always tied her up rather unduly, was being discontinued.) This transport would involve at least six trips and would serve to bring the whole inlet into closer touch with Indian Harbour during the summer. As the mail service of *Yale* was discontinued, the old crew had been dropped. I now ran the boat with one young lad to look after the engine and one young volunteer cook-sailor. It is an old saying that "Providence takes care of fools." I still had all too little experience of these very poorly charted waters, and we had to go day and night to do our transport work with the cement in time to have the basement ready for the arrival of the schooner. We

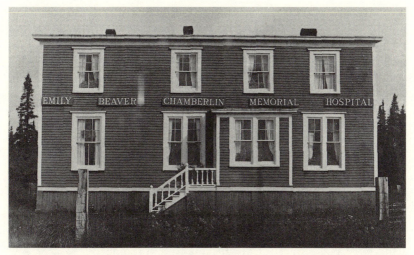

Emily Beaver Chamberlin Memorial Hospital, North West River, 1920 (Faculty
of Medicine Founders' Archive, Memorial University)

cruised over 2,500 miles that summer without either boat or men being
the worse.[154]

Dr Thomas[155] proved to be 6 feet 4 inches in height. We had a
tedious voyage north with frequent fog, and it was already July when
we reached Indian Harbour. A real plumber and a skilled carpenter
arrived to put finishing touches to our work of the last two seasons,
so that hot baths were at last added to the list of attractions at Indian
Harbour. As soon as I could manage it, I left in *Yale* for a trip to North
West River to choose the site for the new cottage hospital and to
engage local workmen who were to construct a concrete basement
under the supervision of one experienced workman from outside. The
superstructure, with a team of carpenters and a mason, was to follow
later on a schooner chartered by the contracting firm.

I soon found other things to think about besides the building enterprise which, incidentally, was to prove a perfect godsend to the local
people at a time when fur was almost worthless. I purchased for a
friend in England three beautiful cross-fox pelts for a pathetically low
figure, even though I gave 33 per cent above the current price with
the full consent of the person mentioned. Twelve months later, those
skins would have been worth four or five times as much, though of
course we had no idea of this at the time.

Tragedy had overtaken an old friend during my long absence. Fred
Blake, while away alone on his fur-path, had had the misfortune to
wound one of his knees with an axe. The joint had become infected,

a very serious condition, and it was a wonder that he had survived to tell the story. He had been found before he starved or froze, and with the freemasonry that prevails among these long-distance trappers he was hauled back home to Mud Lake. This year there was no doctor or nurse or hospital such as had been available for the two preceding winters. A round trip of about two hundred miles was made on his behalf to try to connect with Dr Grieve, who was known to be travelling the outside coast, and divert him to Mud Lake, but in vain. Still, his tough constitution held out, though it was a sorry wreck of a man that arrived at Indian Harbour hospital. The limb eventually healed, but Fred's trapping days were over. Nor was poor Fred Blake the only victim of misfortune. Will Goudie, a fine-looking, upstanding trapper in the prime of life, exhibited to me a swollen and discoloured wrist which caused a very sick feeling to come over me. Here was a family man whose children were still of tender years and whose right hand must be sacrificed if his life was to be prolonged.[156]

We had another passenger awaiting us too for the run out to Indian Harbour en route for St John's and then for Flanders fields. The first little local detachment of the Legion of Frontiersmen was going to join up: a Hudson's Bay Company clerk, Mr Peter Smith; Fred Goudie, a brother of Will; Robert Michelin, one of old Joe's sons; "Young" Johnnie Blake, nephew of old Captain John Blake; and a very smart young Eskimo, John Shiwak, humorously known as "The Duke of Mud Lake." The last two were looking their last on their native land, though they knew it not. And others were not to be far behind them. There were Dan Groves, Charlie Mesher and Billy MacKenzie, all of whom were to find a soldier's grave; Heath and Learmonth,[157] clerks of the Hudson's Bay Company, as was Blackhall[158] also, who was to experience a German prison camp. From Sandwich Bay too went other volunteers. Five memorial tablets deck the walls of the little church at North West River today. Murdoch McLean[159] too went and returned unscathed. Robert Michelin, wounded and returned as a cripple for life, is still a hustling trapper today.[160] A brother of Robert's, "Job,"[161] who was in St John's when the trouble broke out and joined up there, became an instructor in machine gunnery with the rank of sergeant. The Eskimo lad John Shiwak achieved a modest notoriety as a sniper.[162]

It was blowing a strong headwind as we left North West River, and some of the gallant defenders of King and Country were sorely discomfited. With her new 22 HP engine aiding her sails, *Yale* thrashed her way to windward gallantly, but with many a wild caper. When we reached Rigolet, what should I find but another case almost exactly like Will Goudie's. This time, it was the right wrist of John Blake III,[163] an employee of the Hudson's Bay Company at Rigolet. And so another

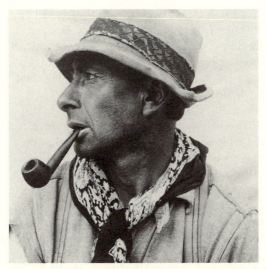

Murdoch McLean (National Archives of Canada
PA 148588)

young family man must be mutilated. Altogether, the return voyage
was rather a subdued performance in regard to merriment.

Fortunately, the ordeal for the two victims of tuberculosis was not
without its compensations. John Blake is still very much alive twenty-
four years later [1939], and he has simply refused to be handicapped
by the loss of his right hand. Disdaining an artificial limb, he has
wielded an axe, driven dog-teams and tended traps as well as steered
the company's successive sailing boats or motor craft attached to the
Rigolet post. Will Goudie showed the same indomitable spirit, though
he was to have but eight years of full activity before the disease struck
again and secured a death hold. However, this did give time for his
children to mature considerably. The eldest, alas, was to follow his
father to the grave, a victim of the same scourge, but a younger son
and daughter have grown up to share the care of the courageous
widow. Within two years of his amputation, Willie actually went three
hundred miles away into the heart of the country to take up new
furring grounds in a determined effort to maintain his independence,
his heroic partner going with him. When the disease recurred and he
knew that he was doomed, Will maintained to the end an unembittered
cheerfulness that gained him the respect of all who knew him. It was
my sad task as well as my privilege to find a market for his last fox,
a pure black pelt except for the tip of the tail, that a few years earlier
would have been worth some hundreds of dollars but could then fetch

only $50 in local markets. However, with the cordial approval of three interested fur traders, I secured double that amount by private sale, making a little nest-egg for the survivors to carry on with. With these and other surgical cases, as well as medical patients in the wards and plenty of out-patients, Dr Thomas and I did not find time hanging heavily on our hands when we were together.[164]

Our most dramatic case of the summer was that of a young Newfoundland fisherman who arrived on his schooner from far to the northward in a truly shocking condition. His right arm and hand were one vast abscess from fingers to shoulder. No less than fifteen incisions were required to open up its many recesses and eleven drainage tubes to afford egress to the pus. And as if that were not enough, he also proved to have a rather acute attack of appendicitis. This put us in a dilemma. If the appendix ruptured, he would probably die, but he was in very poor condition for an operation, the dangers of which would be gravely increased by the proximity of that awful right arm to the necessary abdominal wound on the right side of the body. The only thing to do was to chance a rupture and hope the attack would subside, which fortunately it did. The arm took a month to heal, after which the patient had a further fortnight of convalescence. Then we removed an appendix nearly ten inches in length and showing very severe inflammation. How it had failed to rupture was a mystery. After more than two months in hospital, Stephen sailed away south without a cent for his summer but alive to fish another season.

It never rains but it pours. That same summer, yet a third case of tuberculosis of the right hand or wrist came to me at Indian Harbour. This time it was the hand that was involved, and there seemed a good chance that the disease was limited to the tendons of the back of the hand, so I sent him to Dr Little for X-ray photography and any surgery that might be deemed necessary. I heard afterwards that a conservative operation was done in an attempt to save the hand, but amputation had to be performed later.

In the intervals of surgical work, I would run off in *Yale* and take yet another load of cement from Rigolet to North West River. Despite her fine seagoing qualities, *Yale* was ill-adapted for this work. The cement was in barrels which weighed three hundredweight each. On deck it made her top heavy, while to stow ten or eleven barrels down in the saloon meant clewing up the sleeping bunks, sacrificing the dining table, and eliminating every shred of comfort that *Yale* possessed. However, it was not for long at a time, and it was a light price to pay for the facilities and comforts of the new little institution. Our usual load was ten barrels, but when an SOS came for a rush cargo, as inexperienced work had caused a threatened collapse and the schooner was imminent, we crammed the last sixteen barrels into her somehow, which left her badly out of trim and down by the head, and hoped for a fair wind. If we had met a strong headwind, we should have had to jettison cargo or founder, but after being becalmed most of the night we did pick up a northeaster at dawn, which was the wind we would have chosen of all winds, and triumphantly delivered the cargo a few hours later.

Another interesting contact that summer was with the Montagnais Indians at North West River. I received notice from the customs officer at Rigolet that an Indian who had been christened Sebastien and had come to be known as Pasteen[165] had unlawfully captured a live fox in summertime and had the animal in captivity at North West River. It was my duty to see that the animal was liberated. At first, the captor demurred strongly and stipulated that if the fox must be liberated, he and his family must be fed for the entire summer. To point out that he could neither legally sell the fox nor live on it for the period named did not seem to be an argument that appealed, but the fox was finally freed. I fear I was not popular with the late owner of the animal, and it was a real satisfaction when the opportunity came not very long after to render the victim of my judicial procedure some service as a doctor. His old squaw, who must have weighed something near 250 pounds, had the misfortune to sprain her knee, and I was asked to call at Pasteen's camp. It was a simple enough case to treat, though it gained me kudos with the Indians (especially with the stout lady's husband) far beyond my deserts. And a second visit in the dead of winter, when he was encamped in a remote corner of Sandwich Bay, put the *toganish* (doctor) "next to the Great Spirit" with this grateful Indian.

Such gratitude can be embarrassing at times. Years later, on the occasion of a visit of His Excellency the Governor of Newfoundland to North West River, I had to share with the local representative of the Hudson's Bay Company and Father O'Brien,[166] the Roman Catholic priest who annually visited these remote parishioners, the entertainment arrangements. The final item was a visit to the Indian camp. When we reached the tents, the picturesque figure of Pasteen appeared. To him, through an interpreter, Father O'Brien explained who the distinguished visitor was and whom he represented, to all of which the Indian vouchsafed an indifferent grunt, and when he spoke he merely remarked, "I want to see Dr Paddon." Fortunately, His Excellency enjoyed the joke.

The cruising was of the greatest interest to me. Any lover of the late Erskine Childers' *Riddle of the Sands*, a book with a purpose that attracted much attention in Germany as well as in England shortly before the Great War, would find some resemblance at least between the cruises of *Dulcibella* and *Yale*.[167] True, *Yale* was twice the size of *Dulcibella*, and I could not begin to compare with Davis as a sailor, but just as he ferreted out uncharted channels amid the Frisian Islands, so I cultivated the byways of the Labrador fiords with the view to being able to find sheltered waters and to make progress when the main ship's run would be untenable or would mean hard punching with small results. And just as Davis was forever running ashore and "kedging off,"[168] all as part of the game, so we too developed the habit of carrying empty oil drums to haul down under *Yale*'s bilge, as had been done with such success when she lay on Yale Rock, in order to help float her as the water rose. In comparatively sheltered waters, we knew we could not do her much harm, and we never did. After seventeen seasons of rough and tumble work, she was still able to be sold and has since been sold twice more and is still in commission at the age of twenty-nine. This practically acquired knowledge of these uncharted runs did repeatedly stand us in good stead, and she came unscathed through gales and high seas, dark nights, thick fog, and blinding blizzards repeatedly, and few better sea-boats have ever floated. No doubt it might have been much better done, but it was done and with a definite object.

The schooner duly arrived, and the superstructure rose rapidly on the basement. After the lapse of time and the disappearance of the original building, it is perhaps permissible to say that both the contractors and ourselves had much to learn about sub-arctic construction, and in our case at least the lesson was to be learned by experience, the best though sternest of teachers. In the first place, to economise in material and space, presumably, the building was nearly flat-roofed, which meant that snow would lie thickly upon it, and as the snow melted the roof was sure to leak. Secondly, the rooms were far too lofty, which meant that our drinking water would freeze on the table when a person on a ladder would find more than enough heat around head and shoulders. Thirdly, there was far too much cold passage space, which should always be reduced to a minimum except in buildings of heavy construction with a big central heating plant. Again, with a range preferred to one of the cookstoves in common use in the country, the servants would have to wear overcoats in the kitchen until about eleven o'clock in the morning in really cold weather. There was a hot-air central heating plant, as it was too risky to use a water plant, but the walls were not sufficiently substantial to keep out the cold effectively at −40° F. In the building which succeeded the first one, all these defects were to be corrected. Meanwhile, it was only during the dead of winter that most of the defects were of any significance, and when compared to our quarters of the last two winters, these were palatial.

There was a three-roomed family apartment and a nurse's room, with a common dining room. As the institution could not be run without a staff, the patients' facilities had to be in accord with the funds available. The whole enterprise was experimental, and it had been impossible to foretell the final cost, so that expenses had had to be conservative. To begin with, we had a single small ward besides out-patients facilities. Of course, the service was to be largely itinerant, but a second ward was obviously needed for sex separation. When the donor [Mrs J.S. Lockwood] heard of the difficulty, she at once put a further sum towards the necessary addition, and an oblong building was converted into one of t-shape, which gave not only the extra ward but also a much needed room for social service purposes. These will be discussed later.

Our closing of Indian Harbour and the move into the new winter quarters was to be little less memorable than our first experience of autumn cruising in 1912. The schooner fleet had gone south, and Indian Harbour was abandoned by the summer quota from Newfoundland, so that only the hospital remained. But a series of hard westerly gales delayed our departure for nearly two weeks after *Sagona* had taken the last of our patients south. Day after day it blew. Engine trouble had robbed us of our power when we most needed it. We were only a very light crew, though we had an altogether excessive allowance both of passengers and freight. Two trips had been planned to North West River, but the endless headwinds, coupled with the loss of our engine, forced us to make a single trip do. At last there came an improvement more apparent than real, since a momentary lull only served to introduce a fresh and violent storm. We felt that we could not afford to miss any chance, as we had to reach Rigolet before *Sagona* somehow. The engineer, Albert Elson, and our volunteer cook-sailor, Layard Hughes, had to go south on the mailboat, and we had to pick up two more hands to help me to take the *Yale* on up Lake Melville. To make a start meant having to beat our way out through the narrow western tickle, which was no easy task even for a highly skilled crew. However, up came our anchor, and we got under way.

With our engine, we could have run out of the tickle in a few minutes with perfect ease and safety, and if it then proved to be rough outside, we could have run back for shelter again. We hoped to be able to reach the landlocked run on the north side of the bay with which I had now become pretty familiar. Just as we were going about in the narrowest part of the channel, a foul eddying gust caught us and put us ashore in a twinkling. We were now in an awkward plight, as no help was available and another prolonged gale was upon us. The first thing to be done was to get the women and our little son ashore and to open up part of the shuttered building again. We had started out with the proverbially unlucky number of thirteen aboard, and while I am not superstitious and would contentedly sail on Friday the 13th with thirteen people on a boat of thirteen tons whenever asked to do so, this was not the first time that the old proverb had been justified by events. We were on the far side of the harbour from the hospital, which made everything just a little more difficult. We had to unload *Yale* to lighten her as much as possible, and as it was too rough to ferry the freight across to the south shore, it had to be landed on the rocks near to the wreck without any shelter available.

Our main anchor was set out right over *Yale*'s stern, as the wind had backed several points and was driving a nasty short lop right into the little cove where we lay aground. The kedge was set out from the bow in such a manner as to tend to pull her head round into the channel any time that she floated. Unfortunately, the water had been just about high when she struck, and the strong westerly wind prevented any high tide, though the unloading had lightened her considerably. She actually did float from about three-quarter flood tide till high water and then to one-quarter ebb, but so hard did it blow that we simply did not dare to attempt to get her off for fear of dragging our anchor and getting harder aground. The high tides were about noon and midnight, and if the mid-day efforts were cold, the midnight struggles were bitter. Snow lay on *Yale*'s decks. Day followed day. If *Sagona* beat us to Rigolet, we were in an awkward fix, in any case; moreover, with no one left at Indian Harbour, *Sagona* was not likely to come within miles of the place, at any rate, to anchor.

At last, on the third afternoon, the wind showed signs of dropping out, and on the night tide we got her off. Next morning, there was a hurried loading, embarkation, and departure, and at last with a free wind we made Ticoralak about dark that evening and anchored for tide for a few hours. Long before dawn, sooner than risk missing the steamer, we started towing *Yale*, in the absence of wind, on the morning up-tide to Rigolet, which place we reached before *Sagona*. So that difficulty was surmounted. For the run up Lake Melville, we had secured the services of John Shiwak, Sr., and his son Will, the father and brother of the Eskimo sniper mentioned above, whom they were never to see again. We could not have wished for a quieter, more civil, willing and efficient crew. With their help, we reached North West River without any further misadventure.

12

Systematising the Service: Further Insight into the Problem of Poverty

With the opening of the North West River cottage hospital, we entered on a new stage of our work. While there was still plenty to be learned about the country and the people, the stage of Survey might fairly be said to have given way to the stage of Foundations, of which the new little institution was the first but by no means the last. It is the house not built with hands that outlasts any structure of timber or even of concrete,[169] and we now had a centre both for local development and also wide radiation of ways and means of building up public health and welfare. There was abundant scope not only for the activities of doctor and nurse but also for exponents of every branch of domestic and social science: cooking, needlework, laundry, child welfare, vegetable and flower gardening, home canning of natural resources, poultry yard, and barn – anything and everything that could help a family budget or add to the comfort, efficiency, and attractiveness as well as to the health of Labrador homes. Here my wife was in her element, while she still found occasion for many a comeback as nurse and anaesthetist.

Example ever speaks louder than precept. Enquiries had already come from a distance of 150 miles to ask if we really treated our small son as we had advised others to treat theirs. When it proved that the child did sleep out of doors by day, even in the dead of winter, under the lee of the house in sunshine; that his window was open at night; and that he was fed only at regular hours; and that as he grew older he was put to bed regularly at an hour that gave him long nights of good sleep; that he was allowed to eat what was considered good for him and not what older people had or what he cried for; and that despite all these restrictions or exposures he weighed twenty-six pounds at six months and over thirty at a year! – well, these were facts that could not be gainsaid, and they did have an influence on the conduct of other homes as time went on. And when he and his small brother[170] went careering along behind a team of small puppies in a coachbox on their own little komatik, other miniature komatiks soon appeared. Young mothers who had suffered from too much indoor life began to exercise themselves as well as their children, with real benefit to their health. While many housewives already made beautiful bread and cooked to perfection the fish and game meats that the country afforded, there was still much to be imparted to those who were interested to add to the variety and economy of their kitchen produce. Much, naturally, had been learned about dietetics since the original settlers came to this region. I remember seeing in one home in Sandwich Bay a bad case of beri-beri where there was actually everything in the house that was needed to keep the disease at bay. There were potatoes, rolled oats, dried peas, and beans, and a patient partly paralysed because he would eat only bread and butter.

Another vivid memory is of a half-witted mother arriving at Indian Harbour with an infant just about ready for weaning. In any case, the mother was in no condition to feed the child herself. It was about noon when they arrived, and the ward maid brought a plate of baked beans for the woman and a bottle of milk for the infant. When the nurse happened to come in, the woman was quaffing the last of the milk with much relish, and the baby was munching contentedly at the beans. No wonder I heard tales of infantile convulsions till I began to wonder if there could be such a thing as epidemic epilepsy, but investigation repeatedly proved that the heavy meal of the day was administered shortly before the child went to sleep or that a fond father or uncle had emerged from the woods, sold his fur and conferred a generous dole of candy on a receptive member of the younger generation. Our own domestic servants afforded a starting point for the campaign, and a number of these during the long term of years have carried into homes their own recipes and regulations which commended themselves by practical experience.[171]

Again, instruction is often made more acceptable if combined with a little entertainment, so my wife inaugurated the Young People's Club at North West River, at which an hour and a half of work would be followed by a social hour. This little institution became the dynamic for any public-spirited effort required in the community interest, with occasional wider application. During the Great War, the proceeds of the sale of work produced on club nights went to swell Red Cross funds in 1916 and to support a North West River cot in the British military hospital at Étaples in 1917.[172] Since 1918, the proceeds of these spring fairs have constituted the bulk of the local support to the cottage hospital and the auxiliary services which were added later. Thus, the club became a sewing class, open to all women and girls over fifteen, and later on a little furniture factory employed men as profitably as the women. When education and agriculture as well as livestock farming were added to the medical service, the effect on community health and economics was much enhanced.

That year marked the emergence of a small village from the tiny hamlet at North West River. In the same year as the hospital service started, the first little day-school was inaugurated by our nurse, as her medical duties did not take her full time; and the same summer that saw the hospital come into being also witnessed the erection of the first church. This was under the supervision of the Methodist Church of Newfoundland, though the headquarters of this missionary enterprise was still at Mud Lake, North West River receiving only occasional pastoral visits. Meanwhile, the doctor here, as at Indian Harbour, carried on as "parish priest."

Settlers began to come in, attracted by the threefold facilities offered by village life, but at the same time it behoved the breadwinner and housewife to think twice, carefully weighing the advantages of isolation against those of settlement life. In the first place, the solitary dweller had his own woodskirt, water supply, and trout stream at his door, whereas the bigger the settlement grew, the less fish and meat there would be per family and the more accessible firewood would soon be cut out, involving greater expense of time and strength to bring the winter's fuel to the home. On the other hand, until a boarding school materialised, this isolation must mean the dependence of the children on their elders or on occasional itinerant teachers for education. Moreover, in a settlement there is always apt to be work to bolster up bad furring winters and fishing summers. Such were some of the earlier problems to be faced by ourselves and our neighbours. It was also possible now to systematise to some extent the itinerant service radiating from North West River.

Usually, it was possible before November was out to visit the settlements to the south and southwest by dog-team – Goose Bay, Mud Lake, Traverspine – involving a round of between fifty and sixty miles. Early in December, the suburbs to the east and northeast became accessible – Butter and Snow, Sebaskachu, North West Island, Mulligan River, and Pearl River – a round slightly more extensive than the first. Apart from emergency calls, this was the extent of travel before the new year. In the rest of the time available, teamster and dogs would be employed in hauling home firewood.

Then there were the outings after trout, caught through the ice, and the hunting of spruce partridges and willow grouse and rabbits, all of which combined healthy exercise with variety of food and also economy. The local people made quite a combined business and pleasure expedition after berries in the autumn before the snow came, whole families camping out in likely spots and picking a whole winter's supply. "Red berries" or "cranberries"[173] were simply allowed to freeze till required, as were bakeapples, unless (as often happened later on) they were canned. Raspberries and [red] "currants" [*Ribes glandulosum*] would often be preserved too.

Another valuable auxiliary food supply was afforded by great shoals of smelts which infested the river mouth just about the time of the freeze-up and could be caught by the hundred in nets or later through the young ice. There was beauty too in abundance, the changing foliage of autumn, the yellow of larch and birch and poplar relieving the comparatively sombre green of spruce and fir; the rich afterglow of the setting sun giving a crimson tinge to the snowy ridges of the Mealy Mountains; the fairy blue of the river ice in the twilight hour and the deeper blue, changing to indigo and then to black, of the forest lands. More and more, we felt that here was a goodly heritage indeed.[174] The lure of the Labrador was no longer a mere catchphrase but a deep reality. From the ridge of Sunday Hill, the weekend promenade ground, a glorious panorama could be seen in two directions, eastward away down Lake Melville for fifty miles to the islands, westward across Little Lake, and on through the rapid for another fifteen miles up Grand Lake, where the forty-mile lake took a turn around Cape Ca[r]bou,[175] so that its further reaches could not be seen. One of our favourite relaxations in the late autumn or early winter was to make a "brush-house" of spruce and fir boughs interlaced with upright poles, with a roof over the back portion and no front wall. Here we would go for the sunset and twilight hour, boil our kettle, and have a picnic tea beside our campfire, sitting on a thick carpet of brush.

The northern Christmas seasons retained their charm. As Santa Claus's little friends became more and more numerous, the preparations naturally became more extensive. On one occasion, a little hoax added to the gaiety around the tree. The proceedings were interrupted by a tale of woe and an appeal to the hearts of the adults present. The story was that of an unfortunate infant without parents or any funds available for food and clothing. Was there anyone present with a fatherly or motherly heart who, despite a well filled quiver, could find room for one more? There was a certain amount of whispered conversation. In a small community where everyone knows everyone else's affairs pretty intimately, there was natural speculation as to whence this infant had come. Also, the prospective foster parents might well want to know more of what they were undertaking. Within three minutes, however, a volunteer foster-father shuffled forward to receive a china cupid with an engaging squint and a yellow china curl and undeniably destitute of clothing.

The emergence of the hunters from the woods always livened things up considerably. These men always exhibited a great hunger for sweet things, a natural consequence of restrictions endured away in the woods. They also longed to laugh, and the budding North West River Dramatic Society, while it might not satisfy sophisticated audiences, did fill a really deep need for entertainment, to some extent, at least. Some took away books into the furring grounds, and a little lending library was much appreciated both by these nomads and also by the people of the village. During the years of the Great War, it was of course extremely trying to go without news for nearly eight months at a time.

After the New Year, there was another round of the suburbs, including a run across to Kenemich, and then it would be time to prepare for the two months or more of more distant travel. Occasionally, I would make a trip up Grand Lake, where two families lived at the head of the lake and two more a mile or two up Naskaupi River, but this was not a routine addition to the winter programme. A hundred-mile round trip without any good reason, perhaps, seemed hardly justifiable, but the people there knew that they could always come for help if really needed.

Now that I knew there to be so good an unqualified practitioner as Mr Hettasch at Nain, it seemed needless for me to go there unless specially summoned by him, so I proposed to make Davis Inlet my turning point on the northward leg and Cartwright on the southward leg, again unless specially called on south. Dr Grieve had resigned his position at Battle Harbour and had taken other work in St John's, so that I was the only qualified practitioner north of Belle Isle straits except for a short-term man at Okak who was to leave after one more year. Of course, it was an impossibility for one man to cover seven hundred miles of indented coast; the only thing to do was to concentrate on one district, making such excursions outside it as circumstances might dictate. At Cartwright, I should be sure to hear of any urgent cases within a fifty-mile radius.

The winter of 1915–16 was a grim one. True, the fur market had risen with a bound, but fur-bearing animals come in well-marked cycles, depending on the bait they feed on rather than on any human depredation. Voles form the staple diet of foxes and lynx, while many grouse and rabbits also fall a prey to them. This year was a bad one in the cycle, with the bait not recovered and the predatory animals only just on the upward grade again. In such a year, distressful scenes were sure to be met with, and I had a good reason for making a careful investigation into conditions, as in my capacity of justice of the peace it was one of my duties to issue relief to remoter cases of distress, out of reach of the official dole administrators. The prevailing system was cumbersome with many loopholes.

In one case of this year, an unsuccessful fishery had ended with an application for relief which had been disallowed. The wretched man, who had a wife and children to suffer for any shortcomings of his own, had gone to his winter home just before that period, when travel is impossible either by water or ice, with practically no means of subsistence except what he could get from nature. There were a few rabbits and an occasional grouse, but they were short of ammunition as well as food, and when the rabbit snares were empty, the family mostly went empty too. At the risk of their lives, some kinsfolk crossed the bay while the ice was still far from safe and reached them with supplies before they were quite starved. While there was defective administration, there was also unquestionably a defective personal equation too in many cases. Unless the problem were to be faced and energetically dealt with, there must be an endless succession of tuber-culosis, beri-beri, scurvy, rickets, and minor disorders as well as of stunted, defective children. The only form of administration that offered any hope of real success at this time [1915–16], as I have heard more than one governor of Newfoundland admit, was that supplied by the type of district commissioner so widely employed in other parts of the British Empire, men who despite bureaucratic red tape study intelligently their people and problems and with a mixture of common sense, humour, and thrift, make a little go a long way, whether of money or human initiative. Needless to say, neither the intelligent study nor the work could be done by travellers on steamers or residents for a few weeks each summer.

One day, I shot a traveller seal intended for my dogs, but at the very next house that I came to, a hungry family, although they did not fall upon it raw, did not lose much time in cooking part of it and making a satisfying meal for a change. We had taken our own supplies as usual, but it is simply impossible to sit at a table of a hungry host with a hungry wife and children looking hungrily on without sharing. However, once the surplus was gone, at least we could all go hungry together, without envy or compunction. If someone in authority had shared such experiences, possibly something might have been done, but correspondence was of little use any more than was "seeing red" and employing invective. This creation of a class of professional paupers, without turning out one really marketable product or one more employable man, was distinctly depressing.

Under the circumstances, I had to return to North West River to restock with food supplies before going on north. The bay was fast outside Rigolet this year, so that I had been able to go direct instead of making the detour via Back Bay. On my way south, I had been requested to make a call to see a patient a few miles outside Rigolet. Arriving at the house, I saw a very comfortable man, incidentally the one well-nourished-looking person in the house. It appeared that his legs had shot out from under him in a boat while fishing the previous October, and with February imminent he was still playing the invalid before a gullible and sympathetic group of relatives. It is extremely doubtful if he had ever suffered from anything more than a bruise, but he "thought he might have a touch of pleurisy." I assured him that he had nothing of the kind and prescribed outdoor exercise twice daily, without arousing the faintest enthusiasm.

As I returned from Cartwright to Rigolet, this man followed me in there to make one final, desperate effort to extract a dole allowance. All night he rolled and groaned in the "comers and goers kitchen" of the post, keeping the other occupants awake and scaring them not a little. Of course, he took care that a highly coloured report should reach me next morning. After a preliminary word to the agent, I sent for him. "Mr B[udgell],[176] you see a very sick man before you," I said, and the patient almost beamed. "I know of only one thing that can do him much good," I added, "and that is for him to cut a thousand turns of wood." J. sagged at the knees and his jaw dropped, but he cut the wood and earned some supplies as well as an honest appetite.

None the less, while there was a certain amount of co-operation as well as honest individual effort, the different agencies at work – politics, business, religion, and philanthropy – overlapped or clashed, and the more apt of the dole hunters played off one against the other with some skill. Co-ordination was badly needed, and only a suitable commissioner could achieve that. The relief diet, which consisted of white flour, tea, grease in the form of oleo or fat salt pork, sugar or molasses, and tea, was of course supposed to be subsidised by nature's bounties of game meat and fish, but all too often the dole candidates lacked either ammunition, nets, or initiative. Gunpowder and shot and twine to be paid for in produce would at least have taken away the excuse of not being able to get these auxiliaries to the semi-starvation dole diet, but there was no one to look into these matters and adjust them. It was so essentially a complex problem, to be studied and solved by combined medical, judicial, and legislative agencies. In every bay was unexploited timber. Small sawmills giving work to dole candidates under adequate supervision could have turned out marketable goods, improved the standards of workmanship, and greatly reduced (if not abolished) the drain on public funds. It is true that this year nature was not in a bountiful mood, but this only emphasized the need for well-organised work.

There were, too, some nests of chronic pauperism which from their very geographical position and the nature of their environment really held out no prospect of a good livelihood for inhabitants and which needed compulsory evacuation, or else an ultimatum that anyone who lived there would get no assistance from the government. There were also places admirably fitted for small-scale colonisation, granted adequate leadership, but it was useless to put people without initiative even into a Garden of Eden and tell them they had got to live by its resources. The experiments with Labrador fishing crews, drawn largely from people in distressful circumstances, had convinced me personally that the great majority of dole candidates were not beyond reclaim if only led instead of being left to drift. A further experiment, carried out later, served to emphasize this conviction. By getting a quantity of railroad ties cut around the head of Lake Melville, not only did we encourage dole candidates to produce something marketable but also gave enterprising but struggling men a chance to subsidize the income derived from fur-paths and fisheries.

A tragic illustration was afforded by this winter's tripping of the inevitable disappointments of such itinerant service by failing to arrive at any given place when most needed. As we passed old Lydia Tooktishina's shack northward bound, all was well. Within two days, she was almost shot to death. Once again, a loaded gun had been left about carelessly. Her little boy [grandson] started to play with it; off it went, and a charge of shot passed through the old lady's right thigh, miraculously leaving both the bone and the main artery intact. None the less, it was bad enough. With wonderful self-possession, old Lydia sat compressing the bleeding vessels with her fingers and trying to induce the demoralised child to cut strips off something or other for a bandage. The child was too bewildered, and her strength must soon have failed and her life probably ended but for the opportune arrival of a lone traveller on foot from far away south. Happily, this man could keep his head. The limb was soon firmly bandaged and the patient made as comfortable as possible. Then the rescuer set out on another forced march of fifteen miles to the nearest neighbours.

Thence, while one party came back to tend Lydia, a special courier made a rushed trip to Makkovik, hoping to overhaul me there, but I had already left. So the Reverend Mr Lenz, Moravian missionary at

Makkovik, set out in a wild storm over Kill-a-Man Neck and made all possible speed to Big Brook. He carried antiseptics and dressings, with the result that when I saw her on my return south the tough old soul was doing well, although there was still considerable discharge from the wound. However, a journey to hospital of over 150 miles at this stage was just as likely to do harm as good, so it was arranged that she should come only if fresh cause arose and should report at Indian Harbour the following summer. Long before then, she had resumed full activity.

A great feature of the spring at North West River is the hunting of the migratory birds as they fly north to secure a much-needed supply of fresh meat at a time when everything else fails. As already mentioned, the main breeding grounds in this latitude are in the eastern basin of Hamilton Inlet, amid waters enclosed by islands and also in ponds and marshes of the barren lands. While a few do breed around the head of the inlet, they are but a small minority, and most of the ducks and geese met with hereabouts are genuine birds of passage bound for more northern latitudes. Even those that stay have not paired when they arrive, and ducks' eggs are an unknown dish to the majority of the people of this district. Hunting is a real battle of wits in which the birds have a good chance. The hunters go out in camouflaged canoes, painted white to resemble bits of pan-ice, and the occupants wear white coats and hats and crouch behind white screens. The canoes are much lighter than ice, of course, and bob about in a most suspicious manner in anything but smooth water. Almost every group of birds has its sentinels, posted wide to prevent a surprise attack, and the gulls are allies most helpful to the ducks and most exasperating to the hunter.

To go off in the twilight of morning, to see the sun rise over the mountains; to hear the honk of geese or the sounds of various ducks and divers; to spy the quarry and experience the thrill of the stalk; to land and make a glorious driftwood fire and listen to the sizzle of a frying pan and the song of a kettle; to fill the aching void in surroundings which add a flavour to any meal; to renew the chase and land again and enjoy a mid-day siesta on the warm sand or sod under the May sun; to hunt again and then to camp and fight the day's battles over again after supper in the glow of the campfire; to sink to rest with the distant plaintive call of the unsleeping gulls for a lullaby – such a combination makes a delightful relaxation from the daily round ashore. And, homeward bound, to visit a spot where great cracks in the ice on the shoal gape wide enough not only to permit the downward passage of hook and sinker but also the return of the said hook with trout of from one to three pounds wriggling a protest against the involuntary exit from their natural element – this again adds both profit and interest to the expedition.

The spring fair, the first of a long series, was also a great occasion. People gathered in from the suburbs till the little capital of the district was crowded to capacity. The sale of work was subsidised by competitions of various kinds, and following an entertainment the proceedings wound up with a basket social. This is a method of raising funds that I have never met with elsewhere. The women and girls decorate baskets, or the best available substitutes, which often include model canoes, tents, log houses, etc., and into each basket goes supper enough for two persons. The baskets are supposed to be secrets as to ownership, but the Intelligence Department is busy, and the jealous husband or swain must pay for the privilege of supping with his better half or his Juliet by outbidding all competitors in open auction. It causes a good deal of fun and is only rarely carried to excess. On this occasion, Red Cross reaped a nice sum.[177]

Another great spring feature was the inspiration of a moment. Empire Day, May 24th, was imminent. How could it best be celebrated? Why not have a canoe regatta? So races were organised, men's singles and men's doubles and mixed doubles later on. At such a time, the river was rapid, and real watermanship was called for. If conditions were too bad in the channel, there might be better facilities in the bight around the river point. Everyone turned out to see and share in the fun, and if only the weather was kind the occasion was both picturesque and full of excitement. Later on, a recreation ground was made and soccer football matches added to the programme.

About the same time, the ice would begin to drive down the lake, and the bay seals would come up. Before the ice gets too rotten, parties go out darting [spearing] seals at their breathing holes, but by far the greater number are caught in nets. There are different varieties. The bigger ones, which weigh from two hundred or three hundred pounds each, are known as *harps* when mature and *bedlamers* (is this a corruption of *belle de mer*?) when in a more youthful stage of existence. The smaller variety of bay seal is the *jar*. In the eastern basin of the inlet is found the handsome *ranger* seal, which much resembles the fur seal of Asiatic waters. There are also *hood* seal and the great *square-flippers*, which yield the thickest hide for boot-bottoms, and one or two others. The sealing season is a time of great activity and much mess, which needs public spirit and co-operation to prevent it from becoming a real nuisance.

Unfortunately, this industry has a real surgical danger. Any scratch or cut becoming contaminated with seal oil is apt to behave in a most unpleasant manner. If only it will form an honest abscess which can be opened and evacuated, it is something to be thankful for. All too often, a swelling appears, often at a distance from the wound, and possibly a second. These subside with rest and hot fomentations and elevation of the arm in a sling. Then, just as the victim gets to work again, the whole process lights up a second time and perhaps a third. Amputation is by no means unknown as the only ultimate recourse. So far, I have only had to remove one finger, but that is one too many. The bacteriology of the infection is quite obscure. A deputation from the Rockefeller Institute of the United States came here one summer to do certain work, and I asked these experts kindly to undertake an investigation, which they willingly did, but they could find no organism which did not also appear in the lesions of the skin disease known as impetigo, of which there were several cases active at the time. It seems as if a virus rather than an organism must bring about this painful and crippling condition [known popularly as "seal finger"[178]].

This mention of seal infections recalls an amusing incident. Anyone living and practising in remote regions is apt to receive enquiries or requests from enthusiasts in research work who live in more developed communities. Some are perfectly reasonable as well as interesting, while others commend themselves less. I received one summer through a third party a package containing a preparation made from the noxious weed known as poison ivy, which produces intense discomfort as well as disfigurement on those susceptible to its effects. With it came a letter from an American professor who shall be nameless, asking if I would inoculate from fifteen to fifty of our Montagnais Indians with the preparation and observe results. There was no insurance policy for my life or my scalp attached to the letter. I replied that there is an old adage that "one good turn deserves another." We also had an interesting virus contained in seal-oil whose effects on Eskimos and mixed stock were known to us but not its effects on American professors. If he would inoculate from fifteen to fifty of the latter with seal-oil and tabulate results, I would then give a *quid pro quo*. I noted that he was in no hurry for his returns, while I found it hard to restrain my impatience. I also pointed out that they had Indians in the United States, while we had no American professors in Labrador. So far, I have never received my report from Professor H.,[179] and until I do, our Indians will not even be asked to submit themselves to inoculation with the virus of poison ivy.[180]

The spring, before the coming of the winged pests of Labrador, is a delightful season. Not only the migratory birds but also a few songbirds arrive, and nature dons a garment of freshest green. Boats are caulked, painted, and then launched, and there are rumours and speculations as to when the first steamer will come. Of course, the advent of radio years later was to dispel much of the uncertainty of our frontier life. It was on my way out to Indian Harbour in the spring of 1916 that I was called to see the worst case of beri-beri that I have ever seen recover. The only one that I recall seeing and fatally was the deadly "wet" beri-beri, which developed in that case involving dropsy of the lungs.[181]

Arthur Newell was in a truly shocking state. Both legs were completely paralysed. Both arms were so far gone that they could barely be raised two inches from the bed. Only the dark eyes, looking out from the emaciated face which topped this corpse-like body, seemed to be alive. In addition to all this, he had a tuberculous condition which necessitated an operation if and when he recovered enough to stand it. Seldom was there a more hopeless-looking case or a more gratifying transformation. Within six weeks, with only dietetic treatment and massage, he was so much improved that the operation could be done, and before the summer was ended he could walk from the hospital to the waterside. To send him home would have been to doom him, so as our accommodation was too limited for chronic cases at North West River, if any other solution of their problem could be found, once again I sought and received the co-operation of St Anthony, whither Arthur went for the winter. He returned home thence a new man, and for many years he has served the difficult sector of coast with winter dog-team mail service, which his unfortunate uncle, Steve Newell, so long supplied, but he has never been without brown flour, having learned his lesson in a hard school.

That same summer brought yet another case of tubercular wrist in the skipper of a fine banker-schooner from southern Newfoundland. He not unnaturally preferred to go south to St John's for the operation, where he would be within easy reach of home and friends, but despite an all-night vigil the steamer when southward bound made such a brief call, with so little warning, that he missed her, and rather than wait for another two weeks, he asked me to operate. So a fourth [patient's] hand was removed with part of the arm, after which the patient made a good recovery and before very long was again at the wheel of his beloved vessel. Sad as this was, the biggest tragedy of the summer for me was the death at Indian Harbour hospital of poor Jim Andersen, my first pilot over Kill-a-Man Neck in the winter of 1913–14. Poor Jim, one of the gentlest and kindest of men, though by no means lacking in hardihood and courage, was yet another victim of the white plague. He came with his upper arm and shoulder badly diseased as well as lung involvement, and his case was hopeless. He was conscious to the end, and the closing hours of his life it was my privilege as well as my sorrow to share. A measles epidemic was another feature of that summer, a visitation which laid low six of our seven maids and laundresses at one time when the hospital was crowded. However, the storm was weathered, and to offset this on the debit side of the ledger, the arrival of the first real live dentist to visit Indian Harbour and Hamilton Inlet marked an epoch. He, unfortunately, came in complete ignorance of what his facilities would be, and so his scope for utility was diminished, but he could at least make out a report for his successors, and what he had he made to go a long way.

In the early autumn, we received our first official visit from a governor of Newfoundland when His Excellency, Sir Walter Davidson,[182] came with Lady Davidson as far north as Indian Harbour. Unfortunately, they could not spare time to visit North West River. It was in this year too that I was asked to serve as military commissioner for a large district of Labrador. It was not a matter of conscription so much as selective recruiting of the best manhood available. I can honestly say that no single man in that district who, in my opinion, could and should go refused to do so, which is far more to their credit than mine. Nurses were now hard to get and doctors impossible. Once more, my wife had to agree to stage a comeback as winter nurse at North West River. There are vivid memories for me of that winter's travel.

George and I now travelled with a single komatik, sixteen feet in length. The first stage of the journey, as usual, was to Cartwright, where I received a call on to Sandy Hills. Old Sol Burdett of the golden heart and the fiery tongue was no more to be seen there. The case I had to see was just another of those where an X-ray would clear up a doubt and where for lack of such a verdict the patient must choose between prolonged inactivity and the possibility of aggravating a condition which rest might check. The former was not to be thought of unless the need could be convincingly shown in the case of a man to whom activity was a main factor in livelihood, and happily the latter did not happen.

Before we had finished supper, a teamster from further south arrived in hurried search of me. A case of haemorrhage after childbirth twenty miles to the southward demanded attention. Night was already coming on, and neither George nor I knew the way, but it was the work of a few minutes to get a fresh team from a neighbour of my host's, who also consented to go with me himself. It was a wild ride in the dark. It was blowing hard, and on a number of ponds that we had to cross, there was bare ice. Here it was impossible to keep our course, and we simply blew away to leeward, dogs and komatik and men, till we hit the lee shore, which we then had to follow round till we could pick up the path again. At one point, my leg was almost broken by being jammed between the komatik and a big root which stuck up through the snow. However, we arrived in time, and it was soon a case of "both doing well."

Within forty-eight hours, however, when northward bound again at North River, I had to fight perhaps the most desperate battle for a woman's life of my whole career hitherto, though two others have run it close. On my arrival there, a young expectant mother was in labour with her first child. The dreaded complication known as eclampsia was in process with violent convulsions, and it was also a case of obstructed labour that really needed a proper equipment of obstetrical instruments and at least one skilled assistant. Of two native women present, one was a nervous wreck and the other calm but completely inexperienced. There was just a possibility that there might be some equipment at the Hudson's Bay Company's post at Cartwright, where the wife of a recent manager had been a nurse who did much midwifery work, though it was very unlikely. Still, in such an emergency no faint hope must be ignored, as I was very doubtful if the woman's life could be saved without such an asset.

So I sat for three hours controlling the convulsions with chloroform while the husband did a desperate drive in search of the hoped-for equipment. When he came back without it, I had to tell him that his wife might be dead in half an hour. Nature's efforts had long since ceased, and a life depended on what a knife and two pairs of hands could do. Besides the native woman, I had the husband's brother in reserve to help deal with the inevitable haemorrhage after delivery, if delivery could be achieved. After a grim struggle, a dead child was delivered, and powerful drugs, combined with manipulation, checked the furious bleeding. And then the patient proceeded to make an uneventful recovery, and she is now the mother of an average-sized family.

After a return to North West River, I followed well-meant advice to my own discomfort. I had several times been assured that I erred in making the northward trip in January or February and that I incurred much needless punishment by doing so. March, it was urged, with its longer days and milder weather, was the right time for that trip. So this year I was trying the new plan. Just as I was ready to leave, who should turn up but Father Henry, just about all in with a bad attack of tonsillitis acquired while on his travels. Even apart from this delay, the result would have been the same. The frost had already broken between Makkovik and Hopedale on the way north, but it never struck us that it was anything more than a temporary break, and we held on and completed our journey to Davis Inlet.

The mild weather continued. The snow went as if it were late April; the ice panned up and the brooks became raging torrents. By the time that we reached Makkovik again, it began to be very doubtful if we should reach home before open water. For the next twenty-five miles, there was solid ice or land, but once we passed Seal Cove we got onto pan-ice. It was that or nothing. The shore was too irregular as well as precipitous at times to follow slavishly, added to which much of it now consisted of bare rock. Near the shore, the pans were smaller through being pounded against the rocks by the tide and the sea which hove in before persistent inshore winds. Further out, the pans were bigger, but any shift of wind might soon cut us off from the shore, an occurrence which had almost cost Dr Grenfell his life many years before.[183] With a big team of dogs, each with his own trace, in this scrambling work some traces were bound to hook up on ice at inconvenient moments. The komatik would come to a standstill on a pan incapable of supporting it, which meant a hurried jump onto a bigger pan or ...? To go in between the pans meant either drowning or severe injury, as the heavy masses rose and fell in the swell. It was nothing to what the Newfoundland seal hunters do in the great spring hunt in icebreakers as they leap from a moving vessel from pan to pan, though there was a certain handicap in being attached to a komatik and team instead of independent.

Frankly, two days of this was enough, though with experience it would soon become a matter of indifference. When we took to the land to cross the peninsula back to Hamilton Inlet, it was far more tedious, if less dangerous. Alternately, we helped our straining dogs to haul the komatik over bare mud or waded waist-deep in great ponds of melted snow with our team swimming beside us. When we came to brooks, there was no means of either fording or bridging them. They must be followed to their mouths, where there was either shoal water or a bridge of ballicatter ice. Then we must needs follow the other bank back to a point opposite where we left our line. It took us a week of dour struggling to make seventy miles of headway, but how many extra miles were covered in detours I have no idea. During all this week, we never saw the sun. Rain and fog added to the wretchedness of our progress and to the difficulties of pathfinding. Each night, we doffed our saturated shift of clothing and donned our dry shift. Truly, it was a relief when we were once more on the ice of Hamilton Inlet. From now on, the portages were few and comparatively short. There had not lacked Job's comforters,[184] who with perfect sincerity and a good deal of reason assured my wife that there was no hope of our return, and our arrival at North West River on April 18th was as much a surprise to the inhabitants as a relief to ourselves. Ever since then, I have taken whatever January and February could do rather than risk another early break-up in March.

13

Pestilence in the Wilderness:
The Challenge of Disaster

The end of the war came without our knowing of it until January 27th of the following year, when the first of our returning volunteers [Murdoch McLean and Robert Michelin] arrived home on snowshoes. It did seem a bit hard when these unrepresented citizens had given all that they had to give and (when a party of timber cruisers could be sent to Rigolet in December, if required) that our volunteers should be dumped ashore at Battle Harbour, over three hundred miles from home, and left to pay their own board till ice travel began and then their own transport back home. It took me five years to get them the just refund, but the colonel of the Newfoundland Regiment backed me up, and eventually it was paid. And then came a destruction far, far greater than that which was wrought by high explosives and chlorine gas.[185]

On October 25th, 1918, the little schooner *Rigolet* was seen scudding before a strong easterly wind and seabound for North West River with the last open-water mail for the season and a consignment of late cargo. She crossed the heaving bar, ran up the river channel, anchored in the stream, and warped into the Hudson's Bay Company's wharf. On jumping aboard, I immediately noticed that her crew looked extremely sorry for themselves. Our old friend Sam Pottle, sailing under new colours, looked as if he had lost his last friend, and Captain John Blake, Sr, seemed to lack the usual twinkle in his eye. There were also two men from Rigolet who had to make their way down Lake Melville in a small boat, as the schooner was to be hauled up for the winter at North West River. John Blake and Sam Pottle had to get on to Mud Lake and naturally wished to use the fair wind before it gave out. All they said was (and they knew no better) that there had been "a wonderful bad cold" on the mailboat and that they had caught it. They were feeling better now and would not hear of delaying their return home.

That was a Friday. On Sunday morning, I woke with a splitting headache and severe nausea as well as excruciating pain in back and legs. It was Tuesday morning before I felt any interest in such things as mail, and then it was very lukewarm. And now the nurse reported a number of people ill in the village and one that was causing her anxiety. This was Tom Blake, elder brother to Fred and John, the most beloved man in our community, who had wrestled with tuberculosis from young manhood, always active to the limit of his capacity but never robust. I got up and went to his bedside. All that day and far into the night, the nurse and I fought for his life, but in vain. He was dead before morning.

And then came a long, wild nightmare. There were about one hundred people in the growing village at that time, but fortunately all the long-distance trappers had long since departed for their furring grounds. There were seventy-five of us left, of whom sixty-seven went down with the Spanish Flu, as we now read it to be from newspapers brought on the *Rigolet*. Fortunately, the nurse, a very efficient Swedish-American, Miss Selma Carlson,[186] proved immune as did my wife, who was also a nurse. But for this fact, our mortality of two would have been greatly increased, I feel sure. Besides poor Tom Blake, who died of a rapid, cerebral type of the disease, we lost old widow [Mary] MacKenzie, whose son Billy had already died on Flanders fields. She was an extremely stout old lady who contracted pneumonia when apparently convalescing. It just illustrated the weakness of our available manpower to mention that when one leg of the rude wooden bedstead broke through a rotten plank in her floor, we lacked the strength to hoist it back again. My teamster, Jim Pottle, was down, also our new handyman, John Bird.

The main objectives, of course, were first and foremost to maintain the morale of the community under this staggering blow, and it speaks well for the material we had to work with that only a single case of panic can be recalled. With the last of their failing strength, the sickening ones did their bit, and with the first of their returning rigour the same willingness was manifested. The second thing was to maintain nutrition, and the third was to maintain ventilation combined with warmth. Nourishment was quite a problem. The two nurses went from house to house with hot soup, but the first thing in case after case that could be tolerated was a raw apple cautiously nibbled. We happened to have had two barrels of these come by *Rigolet*, and they met the

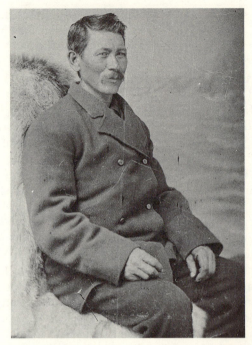

Thomas Blake (*Them Days* Archives)

need as nothing else did. Of course, the appropriate drug treatment
was carried out, though this could only be symptomatic. Following on
the early nausea and headache came, in most cases, an intense, irritable
bronchitis to which no drug but opiates gives any relief, and these
naturally had to be employed with great caution. Having to do a daily
visitation from house to house, as well as a fair share of outdoor work,
I soon found that fresh air was the best palliative. A racking spasm
on rising, even after a night in a well-ventilated room, would be
followed by almost a cough-free day if spent in the open.

Other factors intensified the grimness of the whole experience. For
upwards of a week, the sun was obscured by heavy clouds, and
repeated easterly and northeasterly winds raised great flood tides which
carried away much firewood from the riverbank and also swept away
no less than four boats, three of which were never seen again. (One
motorboat was subsequently recovered.) In the river channel were
three decked boats waiting to be hauled up for the winter. These were
Yale, Rigolet, and *Dolphin,* the latter a small schooner belonging to a
third fur-trading company [Charles S. Porter, New York] which had
appeared to liven up competition at North West River. One morning,

I saw that *Yale* was adrift. Jim was just beginning to get about again, and the two of us had to go off with six inches of snow on the deck, put out a kedge anchor on a long line, get up the main anchor and thirty fathoms of chain, and then reset the latter. We could just about row ashore after the ordeal. Had we driven out of the river, I doubt if we could have got back. The digging of the grave for our two funerals was a dour job in the rapidly freezing ground, and we could just make up enough coffin bearers for the transport of the two bodies. And as if the flu were not enough, we found that we had smallpox also to contend with, fortunately of a mild type, the modified or "new world" pox.[187] Most of the cases were ambulatory, and very few of the white and mixed stock showed a pit after it, but as soon as it got among the Eskimos they both pitted and died.

As soon as we could muster enough manpower from hospital personnel, trading posts, and the few short-distance trappers available, we were extremely concerned to make our little fleet safe for the winter as soon as a high tide came to our aid. We had no proper slip for hauling up vessels at North West River at this time. Round logs with block and tackle were all our facilities, and before the first high tide came, in swept a great field of "slob" ice, a creamy, cheesy mixture of snow and ice which forms after a snowfall when the water is really cold, and threatened either to cut us off from the vessels or perhaps to carry them away from their anchorages. However, the high tide came behind wind and slob, and the latter drove on up into the lake. As soon as there was clear water in the channel, every boat was manned and, with all sail set, driven ashore as high and dry as was possible. On that tide and the following one, the salvage work on the entire little fleet was completed.

While only two had succumbed, many had been near to death in the past three weeks. While we, with a doctor and two nurses, had escaped much better than might have been the case, what of our neighbours, from whom we had been cut off alike by our weakness and stormy waters that could not be passed through? As komatik travel opened up, we began to hear news. At Mud Lake, there had been but three deaths and those all in one house. John Michelin had lost his wife, and his son Donald had lost his young wife and their infant child, prematurely born through the sickness. With a number of others, it had been a fight to the last ditch, without the nursing care and hygienic routine that had relieved so many at North West River, and convalescence was greatly prolonged in some that did survive. The smaller hamlets, Traverspine, Goose Bay, and Kenemich, escaped infection because of their isolation, but Sebaskachu had a harrowing experience, and Hugh Campbell lost his wife at Mulligan River.

However, it was when news from further afield began to drift in that we realised, grim as our experience had seemed, how very lightly we had escaped as compared with others in Labrador. From Cartwright came the news that Father Henry had lost one-quarter of his entire congregation and that over seventy orphaned children were being housed by kinsfolk, many of them bereaved. From the Moravian Eskimo territory came figures which simply dwarfed these. At Okak, out of a population of 270, every man had been wiped out, and thirty-nine women and children had emerged alive. At Hebron, further north, with a population of 170, again every man had been wiped out. It sounded like the death knell of the Labrador Eskimos.

Yet one more drop in our cup of bitterness (and it was a big one) was the fact that it was one of those game-free years. The fur-bearing animals had just about exterminated all the "bait" – grouse and rabbits as well as their staple food of wild mice – and were themselves disappearing to fresh hunting grounds, leaving famine in their wake. So not only was there a scarcity of game meats but there was also a scarcity of fur, and only the "distance men," as they were called, who had got away before the plague struck, were able to hunt before Christmas in any case. So hunger was a potent ally of disease in that black year of 1918, which brought the Armistice but also the flu. Christmas! It seemed to many a mockery to celebrate. Gaiety would be but a mask. However, others felt that the children should not be robbed of their birthright, and when we gathered round the tree, a good many of the older ones possibly regained the faculty to laugh on that occasion. It was essentially a year in which to get on the move early once January arrived. There would be much to do.

As far down as Pearl River, which had escaped without loss of life, the worst was already known and seen. At Valley Bight, the usual contest in fiction was abandoned by mutual tacit consent; there were other things to talk about this year. It was there I found awaiting me a young itinerant school teacher, a mere girl. She had started her devoted service at Ticoralak the previous autumn, at the comfortable home of Jerry Flowers, and it was there that she met the flu. Her chief recollection of the nightmare was the kindly but lugubrious countenance of the lengthy and lean host peering in at the door of her room and mouthing the cheering question, "Is you worse, miss?" From there, incompletely recovered, she had gone to less comfortable quarters and grimly carried on till she could bear it no more. She had been brought to Valley Bight to head me off. I felt the rapid, weak pulse and applied a stethoscope to her chest. Hers was a clear enough case of an influenza heart as well as ragged nerves. Prescription, first and foremost: to get away from work. A trip to North West River, with rest and nursing, good food, and oblivion in sleep. In a few weeks, she was in fighting trim again, though she needed to be careful where she went and how she lived.

The next day brought me to a scene that I never shall forget. We drove up in the sunset hour to the one remaining shack at Pease Cove, now the home of Sam Wolfrey. As I entered in the half-light, I almost tripped over a pathetic bundle on the floor by the stove. It was a small girl about ten years old. She was the picture of misery. One side of the face was all puffed out, due to a great abscess of her jaw, this again being due to a carious tooth. For days together, the poor mite had had no appetite, which was perhaps as well, as there was nothing to eat but a morsel of dry bread. Sam himself, involved in a chronic fight with TB, had been unable to hunt that winter. The one "rising" of flour that they had was "borrowed" from neighbours who could ill afford the loan and who had little hope of repayment. Added to famine had been loss of sleep. For a week, the poor kid had known nothing better than fitful dozes, always with a background of semi-conscious pain. And even the relief of light was denied them at any time during the sixteen-hour nights, as they could afford no oil. Abject, utter dumb suffering. Demoralisation in the parents and stupefaction in the children.

The first thing to be done was to get all hands fed and the other children away to sleep with an unwonted sensation of repletion. There was only a room and a half, and the rickety dining table was the only one available for the little operation. Then, by the light of two flickering candles taken from our grub box, the patient was anaesthetised. It had to be chloroform. The safer but more explosive ether could not be risked. The abscess was evacuated, but that was incomplete work until the offending molar was also extracted. It was a simple enough little job for anyone with a hospital training, but few major operations could have been more of a conscious blessing to the little victim. She did not wake for twelve hours and then woke with some appetite.

We sped on down Back Bay next day, and night found us at Jim's home but without Jim's father to welcome us. He was another victim of the flu. The scattered units of this neighbourhood had all been hard hit, and out of consideration for Jim we spent a day here, sleeping at Woody Point. Next day we went ahead. Just south of Cape Porcupine was another tragic wreck of a home of which a real funeral pyre had ultimately been made. Herbert Earl was a quiet old recluse with a wife and two children. A timid man, he was no successful trapper or fisherman, though he rubbed along with occasional relief. He had a flair for fine mechanical work such as mending watches. The previous autumn, Herbert had gone into Cartwright for supplies, just after that fateful call of the last steamer, and had brought home the infection which forthwith laid low the entire family. Herbert and the daughter died and froze on their bunks. The widow and the little boy survived and existed, but no more, for a time. Running out of supplies and also dry wood, they had to tear up the floor for kindling for the stove. They scavenged on the landwash for mussels, starfish, jellyfish, anything that would make a little broth, and even ate their one husky puppy. Finally, they were rescued and the remains of the shack burned over the two corpses.[188]

Seven miles further on, we came to North River. It will be remembered that there was a single house on the north shore of this stream and three more on the south shore. From these four houses, eleven corpses had been gathered up and cast into a common grave since there was neither sufficient lumber for separate coffins nor manpower for separate graves. At the house on the north shore, poor old Aunt Liz [Elizabeth (Painter) Williams] had had a truly shocking ordeal. She had seen her husband [Jim Williams], two sons, and another woman [a daughter] die in succession, leaving her in absolute isolation. Unable to risk a fire because of the unburied bodies, she had lived for eleven days on raw flour and berries. It was well that the water barrel had been filled before the men all perished, as a great team of wolf-like huskies were bitterly resenting the neglect of their usual meals and were trying repeatedly to break their way into the unprotected house. After eleven days, she was rescued too, alive, sane, and amazingly resilient.

We left on the last stage of our journey to Cartwright, nine miles distant across Sandwich Bay, and about halfway across I ran into Father Henry, a changed man since I had last seen him a few months previously. If ever a young priest had been through deep waters, this one had, struck by a pestilence of which he and others who shared his problem knew little or nothing, the necessary mainstay of the village morale, himself struggling with the infection but simply refusing to succumb, comforting the bereaved and administering the last sacraments of the church to the dying, heading the gravedigging parties as they worked at the icy ground, and then conducting the solemn, beautiful, but too oft-repeated ceremonial. He left his own record, a humble, paper-covered printed journal called "A Winter in Labrador,"[189] published not for his own profit but for the good of the victims.

He had been northward bound but turned right back, opened up the parsonage, and entertained me for three unforgettable days which were to bear solid results. His parishioners were my patients, and unless his grim tragedy could be capitalised for the welfare of all, unless the community's greatest disaster could be made to produce its greatest blessing, then indeed the experience was a total loss. How could he preach a gospel of love? And of what good were my pills and potions and scalpels? Every cloud is silver-lined if a man has the vision to pierce the outer gloom, and every disaster is a challenge which can result in a full measure of compensation, if accepted. He was veritably a voice in the wilderness[190] and I a rusty wilderness practitioner, but we had some powerful friends, and we had a story to tell.

Then and there, we registered a vow that those seventy and more orphans were going to have a better home than those that they had lost; more than that, the whole rising generation of Labrador was to have improved educational facilities if it could be managed at all; and itinerant teachers were no longer to be submitted to such ordeals as that which I had recently witnessed, but they should meet their pupils under conditions far more advantageous to both. We even christened the new enterprise the Labrador Public Schools (not *school*, for the first was to be the first but not the last), and I recounted how the one and only Bill Shepperd, in trying to talk of denominations, had succeeded in calling them "abominations." Father Henry was in no mood to reject an orphaned Methodist because his parents had committed the crime of worshipping God in some other way than his own. He was even prepared to lay aside his parochial work, if he could get permission, and give the new enterprise a start by becoming warden of the first school. And these visions proved to be no empty dreams.

After three stimulating days, which included a house-to-house visitation of Cartwright, Father Henry made a fresh start and went once more to Paradise, which had lately been much more suggestive of Dante's inferno.[191] Here again, houses had been made into funeral pyres as the only possible way out. Families of children bereft of both parents had cowered in darkness, misery, terror, hunger, dread of ravening dogs, and in an atmosphere that can be better imagined than described. If one parent were spared, was it better to lack a mother's care or to depend on a half-crazed woman bereft of her man? Here had been no outstanding personality to command or direct. Much heroism and self-sacrifice, doubtless, but more confusion, greater inexperience of sickrooms and principles of general treatment. And so on round the bay that had suffered a 25 per cent loss of its population.

Next, northward to Eskimo land, now decimated. I was meeting with a fair amount of smallpox but always mild. The worst case I saw among the white and mixed stock was another young itinerant teacher, a man this time, in a tiny shack away at the eastern extremity of the north shore of Hamilton Inlet. He was just in the eruptive stage and really miserable: no bed but a sleeping sack, no invalid diet, no one with any idea of nursing. He had but one request to make to me. Had I a can of fruit to spare? Thank heaven I had. The next memorable occasion of that trip was my arrival at Makkovik, where I heard the tale as fully as it could then and there be told of the ravaging of the Eskimos by the flu. Forty per cent of the twelve hundred surviving Eskimos of Labrador were wiped out? Could they, diseased as the remainder were to a considerable extent, recuperate after such a blow and multiply again? The stories surpassed all that I had yet heard.

One little summer fishing community, away on some outside islands, was only awaiting the coming of the supply ship *Harmony*,[192] an old clipper reinforced with a steam engine, before retreating into winter quarters. *Harmony* came and brought the supplies and the flu. Unless she came, the Eskimos must starve; because she came, they must die a speedier death. Within a few hours of her leaving, such is the susceptibility of the aboriginal, the whole community was stricken except one little girl of seven years of age [Martha Menzel]. There was here too a horde of wolf-like dogs, and with no one to feed them they speedily reverted to wolf-like, predatory life, tearing up and devouring bodies, perhaps hastening death in some cases. The child, like old Aunt Liz at North River, was limited to a diet of raw flour and berries, but unlike the old woman she could not barricade herself against the dogs; she had no fuel left, and on cold November nights the only way to keep herself from freezing to death was by admitting these man-eating beasts to sleep on the floor of her shack and to nestle up again their shaggy bodies for warmth.

For some reason, they never touched her, perhaps because there was abundant scavenging outside, though the lust to kill might well have burst forth at any time. For three weeks, this ghastly existence went on. Then friends ashore, wondering at the failure of these fishers to appear in winter haunts, came on a tour of investigation. Horror-stricken, they beheld the ravening dogs and the mutilated corpses. That there could be anyone alive never entered their heads, and when the child appeared and ran towards them, they fled in terror. Once more solitude and suspense, day after day, night after night, week after week, for three long weeks more. Then the ice began to form strongly between the islands and the mainland. Those ashore realised the menace of a great pack of wolf-like huskies with an acquired taste for human flesh, and a strong party came out, well armed, to exterminate the dogs. Then at last they found the girl to be a living reality. She grew to womanhood and motherhood.

In just such another case of a summer fishing community, supplies and pestilence came together. By the time that *Harmony* had left and the supplies were shipped in a motorboat for transport to winter quarters, there was just one man in fit state to run the engine and one young woman to steer. The rest were already dead or dying. Human bodies and dogs were hastily added to the load and the engine was started. For a while, they made good headway. Then the engineer collapsed, the untended engine sputtered and ceased work and the little ship of death drifted on with its one human survivor and the dogs already nosing at the corpses. Had the wind been offshore, there would have been one more victim, but in course of time the boat drifted right ashore on another island. Here the woman was fortunate enough to find a little flat hauled up, in which she escaped from her ghastly companions. I travelled on to Hopedale. In many places were numerous bodies of dogs lying unburied. Many had been hauled away out on the ice and sunk through holes, and many more had been soused with inflammable oil and cremated, but still there were all too many. I have seen dogs suffering from tuberculosis, and I suppose that many of these animals may have caught the flu infection, though many undoubtedly resisted it.

Nain was now become the rallying point for the few survivors of Okak and Hebron. Mr Hettasch was there, and the troubles were over. Flu and smallpox had done their worst. I turned back therefore from Davis Inlet. Old Sam Broomfield had weathered the storm without loss and was as hospitable as ever, but Tom Evans was nearing the end of his allotted span.[193] As he said, "One eye is blind and t'other one no good." I was to make with him the last trip to Hopedale that he ever did make. It was a good run north, but we struck a hard storm with high wind and drift on the way back. I had to describe anything that I could see, and he had to guess what I was describing. In this way, we struck the south shore of Kaipokok Bay, about three-quarters of a mile from his house. When the old fellow died, Aunt Harriet survived him only a very few weeks. It was better so.

By this time, we were able to get occasional pilots across the Big Neck when conditions suited. It was a good cutoff if things went well. It started with a three-mile walk up a frozen brook, reminding one of Kill-a-Man Neck, then a diagonal crossing of Tuchialick Pond and a further ascent of a shoulder of hill. From here on a clear day, it was possible to see a prominent hill on the south side of Hamilton Inlet between Back Bay and the eastern basin outside Rigolet. Then across undulating barrens for twelve miles or so, with a sudden descent onto Big Brook, along the brook for a mile and then up a woodland portage path to the remains of Wilson's tilt. A little way on was the usual mug-up place. Then up the long slope of Half-Way Hill, from the crest of which in clear weather could be seen the north side of Rocky Cove Hills and an important little landmark, Clefty Hill, for which we must aim. To the right of Rocky Cove Hills could be seen a wide span of the inlet. Down through scattered woods to the Clefty Hill, then a swing to the westward through a series of woodskirts and ponds with a dive down onto Fox Cove Brook, on which the traveller might emerge to the bay or cross intervening barrens, according to the going. All very fine in good weather but a bad place in a storm, as many have found to their cost. Each time I have crossed, we have been fortunate enough to complete the trip between dawn and dark. Once we were hunted for most of the last twenty miles by the harbingers of a blizzard which broke on us in the last hour, and we got out all right.

Back in Hamilton Inlet, we still had Double Mer to clean up, and at last there was to be a little comedy to dilute endless tragedy. We had a fifty-mile run that day, and we were hungry, Jim and I. Always the same old story: no meat (no fur), dry bread and tea (if the tea), hence always the extra mouths to feed from our supplies. Not that we begrudged it. We were going back to plenty, at least, but for those we left behind it was a return to hunger after a very brief taste of paradise. It was a cheering thought, as we plodded along, that at old Tom Oliver's rested a box of travelling supplies awaiting our coming. After a hard day's travel, we reached the house famished. Old Tom lay on the floor, a bundle of griefs and groans, with a flourishing crop of smallpox disfiguring his kindly face. He apologised profusely because during the plague the dogs had broken into his store and raided my box. Heavens, surely they hadn't got the lot? No, it was only a piece of bacon. The rest was all safely bestowed in cans.

Out came the box, and meat, vegetables and fruit were soon thawing out. Then came supper. I knew that it would be torture to old Tom, half starved on bread and tea, to lie there and watch us eat, and yet our spread was hardly in accord with the normal diet issued to smallpox patients. Mind and matter proverbially interact and I thought it worth taking the risk, so Tom was invited to join the banquet. Up he popped like the proverbial jack-in-the-box, and he plied a knife and fork worthy of a hungry athlete. Tom has always maintained that that meal was the best medicine that he ever received from a doctor in his life. And so back to North West River.

Talk of possible boarding schools had already caught the imagination of our near neighbours. Since the first winter of village life at the young village, when our nurse had taught right through the winter, the best that the people had been able to get was two months of a teacher's services for their children. Their ambitions were awakened, and hopes were beginning to take shape. If boarders were taken, surely day scholars would get a chance too, and there would be a guarantee of all winter service. And now they were challenged to think of others first, of those seventy orphans of their fellow countrymen in Sandwich Bay. To their lasting credit, the little community at the head of Hamilton Inlet raised that spring at the fair nearly $700 as the nucleus of a

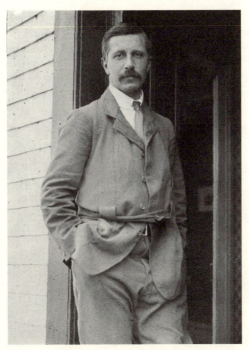

Dr Harry Paddon, c. 1920 (Paddon Family Papers)

combined orphanage and boarding school for the Sandwich Bay orphans. We now had quite a good piece of land cleared and were beginning to raise some of our own vegetables at North West River.

During my absence, the nurse had received an urgent summons from away up Grand Lake to a hamlet near the mouth of Naskaupi River because of a severe outbreak of dysentery in the children of three families. Unfortunately, a blizzard delayed her progress, in spite of heroic efforts on the part of herself and her guides to get ahead under great difficulties. She spent a most exacting period nursing the survivors, but in one house three of four children had succumbed before her arrival.[194]

During the following summer at Indian Harbour, arrangements were completed for Father Henry and myself to go on lecture tours, in England and Newfoundland for him and the United States and Canada for me, to try to raise a fund for the first of the Labrador Public Schools. My wife and I had been for four years continuously in Labrador, since substitutes were simply not to be obtained till the war was over. Now, at last, it proved possible to get not only a nurse but a doctor to keep things going at North West River during our furlough.

Yes, it was sad to be "one of those who did not go," but to have missed that period in Labrador, and especially the winter of 1918–19, would have wrecked the whole plan of campaign and any success associated with it, and more than ever did I feel that Colonel Driscoll had made the right decision so far as he was concerned. The vindication had yet to be completed. We had the experience behind us and the story at our fingers' ends, but what was to be the result? This winter of 1919–20 was just as critical in its way as the winter preceding had been on the Labrador coast.

14

Campaigning for Funds: The Founding of the First Labrador Public School and Beginning of Child Welfare Work

It is a far call from Labrador to New York, Boston, Ottawa, Montreal, and Toronto in more senses than one, and financial campaigning was quite a new experience. I was extremely fortunate in my instructions and in the opportunities afforded me. I visited famous institutions and met or listened to men of international repute in the medical world. Also, the campaign for funds gained me access to many interesting places and people. The salesmanship aspect of this work was repellent, but its social side led to much interest, wide acquaintance, and some friendships that have survived for a score of years. The cause at stake offset the commercial aspect to a great extent, and there proved to be a real psychological interest in the contacts with so many individuals and audiences.

Boys' and girls' schools and men's and women's colleges, men's and women's clubs, drawing rooms, and even pulpits – all these were included in the programme. But the most exacting of all were the brief interviews with businessmen in their office strongholds, many of them considerably fed up with philanthropic drives during the war and the beginning of its aftermath. Such interviews were almost a matter of form. Questions rained like shrapnel. "What is your budget? Whence does it come? What is the cost per head per month in your institution?" And many et ceteras. Subconsciously at first but later consciously, businessmen resolved themselves for me into fairly well classified groups with characteristic viewpoints. It was a matter of quick diagnosis in the first minute of contact and the recital of one of a small series of gramophone records kept on file to suit the individuals encountered.

One of the bright spots was a brief reunion with Frank [Babbott] of Indian Harbour memory, and another was a visit to the home of Dr Little, who had resigned his position at St Anthony and was building up a most successful practice in Boston. Sad to say, he was not long to survive. He died at the all too early age of forty-eight with a very successful future still before him and with a personality such as always leaves a big gap when removed. St Anthony was fortunate to get a successor in Dr Charles S. Curtis,[195] who while he would be the first to do homage to Dr Little, has maintained high standards of institutional service as well as executive ability at St Anthony.

I have many happy and grateful memories of this first visit to the United States and Canada, which has been repeated during four subsequent winter sessions. Thanks largely to the introductions given and the openings offered on either side of the Atlantic, Father Henry and I found ourselves in possession of sufficient funds to build and to operate for some years to come the first of the Labrador Public Schools. The building was erected during the summer of 1920 on the shores of Muddy Bay (not to be confused with Mud Lake), five miles from Cartwright. Father Henry gained permission to reside there in order to become the warden for a term of three years. There were an English nurse-matron and English teachers, and there were forty-four children in residence for the first school year, most of them being orphaned victims of the great Spanish Flu epidemic. Thus was a second foundation laid for permanent constructive work in the backward dependency. Needless to say, I could not rest content till a second of the Labrador Public Schools should be built, and that at North West River. This was to take seven long years to bring about.

A deputy had been found for me during my winter's absence in Dr Philip Place.[196] As he was also to be available for the summer, there was a golden opportunity to extend *Yale*'s itinerant service, and with a special reason. For the second time, I had the service of a dentist for my district, and this time he was far better equipped than the previous dental adventurer. Together we visited the head of the inlet, and at Kenemich the household of old Malcolm McLean afforded quite a dental clinic in itself. It was then the height of summer, and the welcome of a host of sand flies, together with myriads of mosquitoes, was more vociferous and impressive than that of the kindly old Scot and his partner. As might be expected, the welcome of the younger generation was tendered with some reserve. The man of the hour soon got to work, and ere long victims lay about in varying degrees of goriness and pallor. The exact proportion of blame to be borne by the dentist and the insects was hard to assess. For three torrid hours the carnage continued. When we left, the philanthropy of the visitation was clearly more apparent to the leaders than to their juniors.

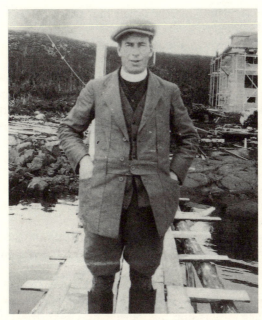

Rev. Henry Gordon at Muddy Bay during construction
of the residential school (Yale University Library)

Another memory of that summer is of entering Pack's Harbour, ten miles from Cartwright, on the outskirts of Sandwich Bay, mainly for a night's anchorage. It was already twilight, but we had hardly anchored when a boat bumped alongside and a harassed Labrador father asked me to go ashore and to have a look at one of his sons. By the light of a smoky lamp, I saw as convincing looking a diphtheritic membrane as I could wish not to see, covering soft palate and tonsils. There were also the rapid pulse, the enlarged and tender glands, and the generally toxic appearance associated with "dip." As soon as it was light, he was rushed across to Indian Harbour. Bacterial examination confirmed the bedside diagnosis, and antitoxin was given. The patient soon improved, and happily there was no further case reported at Pack's Harbour.

It was about this time too that we received a second official visit, this time from Sir C. Alexander Harris,[197] who had succeeded Sir Walter Davidson as governor of Newfoundland. As the charting of Lake Melville was still very defective, I was invited to pilot SS *Seal*[198] from Rigolet to North West River. Not having visited Cartwright yet but only having seen the granite shell, His Excellency reached Rigolet in somewhat pessimistic mood. "This is all very picturesque and interesting in a way, but what future can there be for this country and people?" Having been through a somewhat similar mental process a few years previously, I merely asked him to suspend judgement for twenty-four hours.

The following day, we left at dawn, but Lake Melville was not in a hospitable mood. The *Seal*, of only three hundred tons, developed a liveliness that surprised some of the passengers disagreeably. It was getting towards sundown ere we anchored off the river mouth, and it was altogether too rough to attempt an official landing that evening. However, one boat with three men in dripping oilskins came alongside with an urgent enquiry if there was a doctor aboard, as no one was aware of my presence on *Seal*. When we landed on the "Frenchman's side," I found one of the youngsters of Monsieur Thevenet of Revillon Frères down with a sharp attack of pneumonia. Fortunately, it was to be as brief as it was sharp, and I was able to leave him with an easy mind when the *Seal* was ready to leave.

The following day, after breakfast at the little hospital, Sir Alexander made a tour of inspection and attended a little ceremony where an address of welcome was read. He also saw a little expedition of trappers leave for their distant hunting grounds, the youngest member of the family being a lad of thirteen, proud to be accompanying his father and uncle on his first big journey up Grand River. He also met Gilbert Blake, a local guide who had already made a name in the literature of the country by taking a party up the Naskaupi River, across Lake Michikamau, and down the George River to Ungava Bay.[199] Then by invitation a few of the individual trappers met His Excellency, who talked with them as man to man about some of their problems. As we left the river mouth, I ventured to ask if he still held the pessimistic viewpoint which he had voiced at Rigolet. He replied, "I have received an entirely different impression."

That winter, we were to have a patient whose case brought into relief the dangers as well as the romance of a trapper's life. It was Judson Blake, the eldest son of our old friend Fred, who underwent this terrible experience. Emulated [stimulated] by the example of one-armed Willie Goudie, one of his brothers, Charlie planned a raid into new hunting grounds in the same remote regions. He secured two willing companions in his new venture in Judson Blake and Mark Best, Jr. Leaving while the summer was still hot, they paddled up Grand Lake and up Naskaupi River for ten miles, where they took the Red River portage. It is gruelling work portaging food and other equipment as well as the canoe over high hills from water to water. Charlie, of course, was an old hand. Judson was physically stronger and more experienced at this kind of work than Mark, and the latter fainted dead away under his canoe on the final journey. One of the others, returning to look for him, found him just coming round and offered

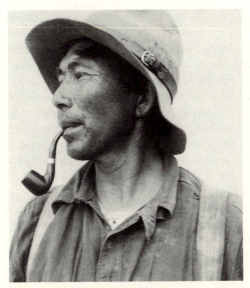

Gilbert Blake (Fred C. Sears)

to carry his canoe the rest of the way. Not a bit of it. Mark was going to get that canoe across alone or not at all, and he eventually completed the task.[200]

When they reached the end of their long journey, three hundred miles from home, they had to build tilts and plan out their respective paths. These men are strict Sabbatarians, and they planned to have weekend reunions at the most central tilt, which was Charlie's property. One Saturday, as Judson was going to keep the tryst, he was ploughing along on snowshoes after a recent storm when he trod on a "blown-up place," a great icy bubble where compressed air had separated the ice from the surface of the water while still thin. He went through into the river, and encumbered by his snowshoes he had considerable difficulty in getting out.

Having escaped from drowning, he was next in danger of freezing. It was the dead of winter, with short days and long nights, when the temperature was apt to be −30° F or more. He had to travel hard to keep the circulation going with an icy shell formed on his outer clothing. When he reached the tilt, hoping no doubt to find Charlie with a good fire in the stove and kettle hot, there was not a soul there. Both Charlie and Mark had been held up by the storm; and worse still, some Indians had used the tilt and characteristically burned up all the ready chopped firewood without troubling to replace it. So the exhausted trapper had first of all to go to work and provide fuel for himself. By the time he had a fire going, he was too weary to care to eat. He stripped off most of the wet clothing, which he hung to dry on wires stretched between the stovepipe and tilt walls, and stretched himself out near the stove to fall almost into the sleep of exhaustion. His awakening was a rude one. He was aroused by a choking sensation to find himself in a cloud of smoke with flames leaping around the blazing clothing, which had ignited as it dried. Instinctively, he plunged for the door and ripped it open. A gust of wind rushed into the little hut, spreading the flames everywhere. As he leaped to comparative safety, he was bombarded by the entire contents of his rifle magazine, as the weapon, which had been left loaded, had its cartridges exploded by the heat. Again he escaped unscathed. None the less his troubles were only beginning.

He now stood in the sub-arctic night, clad only in underclothing and moccasins with nine miles to go to the nearest tilt. His snowshoes, which were always hung out of doors, were still available; otherwise, his doom was sealed there and then, but his feet, so inadequately protected, were bound to suffer seriously from the snowshoe lashings. It was no time to dwell on difficulties and risks. It must be a race with death. At first, the bite of the frost on the exposed flesh was painful. Then followed that deadly numbness with an almost overpowering desire to lie down and end it all, but this was resisted, and about dawn he reached his own nearest tilt.

There was still much to be done before he could thaw out frozen extremities and seek relaxation. He must reckon on two days of isolation before relief might come, and fuel must be provided for that period. This meant the felling of trees and the chopping of the trunks into short billets and the splitting of these for the stove, also the transport of the wood into the tilt or alongside it. He was already so crippled that he had to crawl with his hands on the snowshoes instead of his feet, and his task took him pretty well the whole of the short winter day. Then at last, after a meal, he started to thaw out his feet in a mixture of snow and ice-cold water. It was torture almost worthy of the Inquisition as circulation started up again in such areas as were still visible, and part of that night he spent in delirium. Another miserable day followed, and when this ended without help coming, Judson resigned himself to death. Scribbling three farewell notes with a rifle bullet on some fragments of paper, he lay down for what he expected to be his last sleep.

Morning found him still alive, and at last a hail was heard. Charlie Goudie had arrived at where his tilt had been, interpreted the signs and hurried to the rescue; but so doubtful did he feel of finding Judson alive that he hesitated to approach without some reassuring answer to his shout. The meeting must have been dramatic. Judson began to apologise for burning the tilt, in which some fur had perished, and Charlie, laughing unsteadily, told him not to mention it. Charlie proceeded to attend to the injured trapper's needs, and when Mark arrived a council of war was held. The nearest settlement was Hopedale, about 120 miles away, but with no hospital, doctor, or nurse. North West River was about three hundred miles distant but with better facilities for treatment, and the vote was cast for North West River. So the crippled man was packed onto a hunter's sled, and the human team of two began to haul their load along a trackless path.

Days passed in weary succession. On upgrades, when the flow of blood was towards the head and away from the feet, there was comparative relief, but on downward slopes, suffering reached its peak, and nights offered little compensation for the ordeal of the days. The sufferer opened one abscess with his own razor, thereby gaining some ease. Then supplies began to run short, and Mark, the youngest and least strong physically, began to flag. Another council was held, and it was determined that Charlie should push on alone to the hamlet on Naskaupi River, where were two settlers' homes and also an Indian encampment at this season, while the other two stayed in camp. All supplies were meticulously rationed out, flour by the cupful and ammunition by the cartridge. Only of tea did they have any abundance. So Charlie passed out of sight and the other two began their anxious vigil.

Then from the void came one-armed Willie Goudie, into whose trapping territory they had now penetrated, and a new problem had to be settled. Mark was now rested, and it was decided to resume the journey, hoping to meet any relief party coming from Naskaupi River, so they started off anew and failed to connect, with the result that the pair completed the task. At Naskaupi River, dog-teams were waiting to rush the patient to North West River, and the three-hundred-mile nightmare came to an end. The whole ordeal lasted from the burning of Charlie's tilt on the night of January 27th to the arrival at North West River on the evening of February 11th, a period of fourteen days, and if anything about the whole tragedy could be described as fortunate, it is that the journey did not take a great deal longer, as it might well have done. When the patient reached hospital, I was far away on my main winter trip, and my wife was the only nurse at the cottage institution. She had to administer anaesthetics for one of the two minor operations and do them. On my return, the patient was convalescing well. There was an area of exposed bone on one heel, so large that I thought a grafting operation would be needed, but eventually nature did all the repairs, and the following autumn saw Judson back on his beloved fur-path.

One other adventure of this same trapper's which he shared with three others is worthy of record while it does not come within the sphere of medical practice. One spring, a party of four was homeward bound down Grand River. The frost had broken, and the woods were impassable, with several feet of half-melted snow. It was the river or nothing, and the areas of open water grew daily bigger and the rapids fiercer and whiter. The party travelled both with canoes and sleds. On the ice, the canoes were hauled on the sleds, while down the rapids the sleds reposed in the canoes. On one occasion, they halted at the head of a long, fierce rapid and deliberated. It was an ugly-looking enemy to face, but impatience won. Judson, as steersman, with John Michelin (a nephew of old John of Mud Lake) in the bow, Fred Goudie, a brother of Charlie and Willie, steered the other canoe with his nephew Harvey in the bow. Before the leading canoe started on its wild ride, Johnnie wrapped a waterproof cape round his waist and nether limbs. This little precaution against a bad wetting almost cost him his life.

All went well until the light craft reached an eddy by a great rock. Here were some ugly curlers. Into one, the canoe dived and emerged half filled. A second dive completely filled her, and but for the extra buoyancy afforded by the sled, they must have sunk. With gunwale awash and the crew sitting immersed almost to their shoulders, they whirled on down the rapid. They were near the edge of the downward stream with a fierce eddy tide boiling alongside. To get across the double current meant death. It was little that the pair could do towards helping themselves. With their paddles whirled from their grasp in the moment of foundering, they spread their arms like swimmers, treading water to preserve their balance as far as possible. It can have been but for a few moments, though it no doubt seemed far longer, when they were swept round into the eddy tide and began to pound against the edge of the ice near the shore. With a shout to Johnnie to jump, Judson lunged for the ice, gained a good hold and hurled himself out of the water. Seeing the canoe threatened with destruction, he salvaged that before turning to look for his companion, of whom there was nothing to be seen.

A moment later, however, he spied a hand reaching from under the ice and grasping a little prominence on its edge. With a leap, he seized the hand, then the wrist on which he hauled till Johnnie's head emerged. It was no time for standing on ceremony. Nature had endowed Johnnie with an abundant thatch of hair which afforded excellent holding qualities. Taking a generous handful while keeping firm hold on the wrist with the other hand, Judson gave a mighty heave, and Johnnie lay gasping on the ice, protesting against being scalped rather than drowned with a gurgling, sputtering shriek. The other canoe was also swamped, but her crew got ashore with less difficulty. Camp was pitched, a great fire kindled, and the drenched and chilled men dried out while the kettle boiled. Ere the journey was resumed, Fred, who was the veteran of the party, looked back and shook his fist at the baulked foe. "If I live to come up the river again," he vowed, "I'll show that old rapid I can run him without upsetting."

Misfortune seems to run in some families. I have already told of the mishap which crippled Judson's father, Fred Blake, when far away on his fur-path, and Judson's two narrow escapes have now been chronicled. But that by no means exhausts either the trappers' adventures or the medical and surgical history of this family. Another brother, Graham, was brought out of the country suffering with ulcer of the stomach, which might easily have left him with health impaired for life and dependent on a dietary which could not possibly be maintained in the woods. However, by this time we had started poultry keeping, and there is one treatment for gastric ulcer with which we have had some very successful results, known as the Lenhartz treatment,[201] in which the diet consists mainly of eggs and chilled milk. The eggs we could manage, seven dozen at least being required within a period of a fortnight, but we had no cow yet. At Mud Lake, however, between seventeen and eighteen miles away, a brother-in-law of the patient, Robert Best, who was a son of old Mark, did keep a cow, and two brothers of Graham's took it in turns to make the thirty-five-mile round trip on snowshoes and hauled back blocks of frozen milk to the hospital. By these means, a complete cure was achieved. Graham stayed out of the woods for a term of winters and then went back trapping again.

Yet another brother, John, who was the baby of this large family, was due to go off to his fur-path when he came to me complaining of a "sore side," not very bad. Examination revealed undoubted appendicitis, the appendix being removed a day or two later. Yet another brother developed an appendix abscess at Indian Harbour after I had left on a furlough, and Dr Place operated. Poor Fred developed cancer of the intestine, and so weary and apprehensive was he of operating rooms, after all that he had been through, that he endured what must have been agony for a long period and only came to hospital when he was almost moribund. We hastily explored in the hope of relieving if not saving, but the condition was hopeless and the end came very soon. His wife had died a few years before, also in Indian Harbour hospital, of broncho-pneumonia.

One of the most terrible tragedies of our North West River community life has been the burning of the home of one of Fred's married daughters, which included the loss of the mother and five children.[202]

The husband and father was away as well as the eldest son. The wife and mother slept on the upper floor with the girls, who ranged in age from infancy to about fifteen. The mother awoke in the night and smelled smoke. Her cries aroused the second son, who was asleep on the ground floor. He found the fire already beyond his control and dashed for help to his uncle's house a few score yards away. The mother, hampered by the younger children and probably failing to realise in time the rapid spread of the flames, was trapped in the upper room. When the rescue party arrived, the house could not be entered. Dry as tinder, it simply disintegrated in flame in a few minutes. It was a terrible homecoming for the father and eldest son. Even as I write, the brother who was the victim of the appendix abscess nineteen years ago is again in hospital with a serious though not hopeless surgical condition. An association over a quarter of a century with a family history of tragedy and triumph such as this naturally forges a link which nothing can break.

That spring, *Yale* presented us with a difficult salvage problem. Lacking a proper haul-up slip, all that we could do in the autumn was to haul her up onto "ways," great beams laid on the shoal by the riverbank with block and tackle and all the manpower available. This was liable to strain the boat and was very arduous work. The previous autumn, at old Malcolm McLean's suggestion, we had moored her in a quiet creek where the ice just melted out in spring and no running ice could harm her, even in Kenemich basin. At the time, when the bay ice was giving out fast and Sandy Point run presented a wide tidal channel, we received a message to the effect that *Yale*'s engine room and cabin were half full of water, that the ice around her would soon cease to support her, and that she would then sink in four fathoms of water, which would necessitate a wrecking tug at great cost to salvage her. There was no time to be lost.

With Fred Blake, George Pottle, and Gilbert Blake, I crossed the run and went to view the situation. It would need a canal eighty yards in length and cut out through ice still from two to three feet thick to get *Yale* out of the deep water. This canal must be fourteen feet wide, and all the ice in it must be dispersed under the surrounding ice. To achieve this, three parallel cuts, each of the full eighty yards in length, must be made with lumbermen's gang-saws from the old abandoned mill. Crosscuts must be made every two feet, and the resulting blocks of ice, each seven feet long by two wide and from two to three feet thick, must be spiked and shot away under the surrounding sheet-ice. Moreover, to achieve the best results of all this labour, it must be completed before the next spring [maximum] tide at the full moon. It was a heavy task, but it had to be done.

We secured one extra recruit, Duncan McLean. The days were now nineteen hours long, and we worked about seventeen hours a day. We were ready, and only just ready, for the spring tide, but there was still a hitch. Unfortunately, the change from deep to shoal water was not gradual but consisted of a very steep mud bank. Most of the weight being aft in *Yale*'s engine room, we could not get the heaviest part of her ashore at all, and she overhung the bank. All that we could do for the present was to put an anchor out on a very long line stretched across the shoal to hold her where she was till open water.

We re-crossed the run to North West River. As soon as the bay was open, we heard that *Yale* had slipped back off the bank into deep water, that only at low water was the tip of her bowsprit exposed and that Malcolm feared that no local facilities would float her. All we could get for the next salvage operation was the old schooner *Rigolet* of about thirty tons and with only a hand windlass. However, plenty of men were available. What we really had to float was three tons of cement ballast and two tons of iron keel and two empty tanks for water; besides, two empty oil tanks would be helping us with their buoyancy. It should surely be possible to dive to her keel astern and pass a line between rudder and sternpost, after which our old dodge of hauling down oil drums should exercise powerful leverage as the tide rose. Crossing the bay, we passed old Malcolm's house at about two o'clock in the afternoon, and within eight hours we triumphantly anchored *Yale* off that same house.

Rumour, as ever, had exaggerated. It was at high water that only the tip of the bowsprit could be seen. At low water, the foredeck was clear of water. False coamings were rapidly built around the hatchway leading to engine room and cabin, and bailing began, as the pump was choked and it was at present impossible to clear it. To our surprise, we could hardly gain at all on the water. We had concluded that the ice had formed sufficiently thickly in the creek to press on the shaft and dislodge the packing from the stuffing-box. A moderate leakage we were expecting but no such in-rush as would necessitate bailing. Then, in a moment of inspiration, we sought and found a porthole [open] under water. Once that was closed, we soon had her afloat and the following morning regained North West River, where she was put into condition for her new season's work.

Our arrival at Indian Harbour that early summer was memorable. It was a late year for navigation, and it was July 1st before we arrived about six o'clock in the evening. We were devoutly hoping for two or three quiet days to get the hospital ready, especially as the ice was far too heavy for schooners to get through. But just one hour after our arrival, the first steamer blew her siren. All that we did that evening was to get ourselves ashore and our own quarters prepared for the night. Soon after dawn next day, the steamer was back with a serious case. An unfortunate man had been caught in the anchor chain and had incurred a compound fracture of both bones of one leg. Shutters had to be ripped off, fires lit, bedding prepared, instruments sterilised, all in a hurry. The skin was cleaned, the patient anaesthetised, and the limb set, but there was a very grave risk of infection following such an injury. Happily, this complication was averted, and the patient made an uninterrupted recovery.

15

Fire and Friends, Sidelights on the Physical Problems of Trappers, Founding of the Second Labrador Public School

The pendulum was swinging more and more. The decline of the cod fishery in the aftermath of the war grew more pronounced. The war-stricken countries, and especially those to which most of the Newfoundland fish usually went, had lost their purchasing power. The cost of the salt and the remuneration for fish were out of all proportion to the cost of living. Smaller and smaller grew the host of invading fisher-folk and ever fewer our Newfoundland patients. It is true that the Labrador quota had increased but not to such an extent as to maintain the former [medical] activity.

Our school at Muddy Bay was now sending an annual contingent of cases. These were largely cases of enlarged tonsils and adenoid growths which interfered with health and development not a little. But it was no ordeal of terror for the youngsters. In fact, no one was quite of the élite in the school who had not made the pilgrimage. The anaesthetic was made an attraction rather than a horror by prize competition. The anaesthetist counted by the watch as he administered the drug, and the little patient counted after him. The boy or girl who reached the highest figure before becoming inarticulate received a quarter of a dollar.

The winter of 1923–24 was another furlough season and was memorable for two reasons. First, it was during this winter [sic] that the final settlement of the boundary lines between Canadian and Newfoundland territory in Labrador was made by a committee of the British privy council.[203] Technically, it was a model of fairness and thoroughness in British justice. Practically, it seemed as if Newfoundland

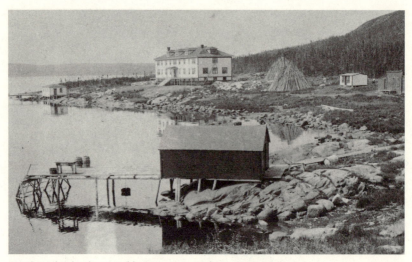

Residential School at Muddy Bay, 1924 (Yale University Library)

was rather unlucky. In the old days, when the Dominion of Canada was formed, long after Newfoundland had become a colony, a very loosely worded agreement was made in which Newfoundland retained the coast for her cod fishermen and Canada took the rest of the great peninsula, the value of which was not in the least realised at that time. When whispers got abroad of immense water powers, great forests, and vast deposits of ore, competition tightened up. Newfoundland contended that the coast must follow indentations, while Canada replied that the coast was the cod-fishing zone along the granite shell of Labrador. Finally, after many years of bickering, both governments agreed to submit the case to arbitration. The definition of *coast* was the crucial point.

In the summer of 1923, the Canadian government tender *Acadia* had charted Lake Melville in a manner far superior to anything done before, and tidal survey parties had demonstrated the evidence of river water as far east as a point twenty-five miles outside Rigolet.[204] Harking back to scriptural literature, it was decided that *coast* included all the terrain drained by rivers flowing out to the sea from the height of land, and Newfoundland, which had now assumed dominion status, gained a dependency three times the size of the mother colony. I was in Canada doing publicity work when the verdict was announced.

The other event, while of no interest to any wide public, affected me far more deeply. I had crossed the boundary to the United States, still campaigning for funds, and had been invited to address the Medical Club of Rhode Island on the occasion of their annual banquet.

There were about 150 present, including the staff of the hospitals as well as practitioners of the little state. Just before I rose to speak, a telegram was handed to me which read, "North West River hospital burned to the ground. One patient perished." It was a hard blow. Poor Will Montague! He had been paralysed, and life held for him little activity or happiness perhaps, but it was a shocking end.

And the work?

There was a moment's temptation to capitalise on the occasion to the full in the address that had to be given. Almost as quickly, there came the conclusion that there was one above all others who had the right to hear the first news of this tragedy, and that was the lady who had financed the founding as a memorial to her mother. Of course, insurance would cover some of the loss but only a certain fraction. For the moment, the only thing to do was to put the matter on one side and carry on, so rightly or wrongly the audience heard no word of the tragedy that night.

Once again, a black cloud was to have a silver lining. The sweetness of disaster lies in the friendship it evokes, and friends were to prove more potent than fire. It was bad enough. A life lost, all our treasured possessions gone up in smoke as well as much equipment and a considerable sum of cash, but ... The lady donor [Mrs J.S. Lockwood] at once expressed a desire to make everything good that insurance did not cover and also urged that something finer and more resistant to fire should rise from the ruins. It was a great chance to correct realised errors in the construction of the old building. The two main floors were lined with fireproof material throughout, which has since spelt salvation on more than one occasion. The old lofty rooms were replaced by lower ones. The contents of the walls included two layers of wind-proof Cabot quilting, reaching from roof peak to foundation sills, and cold passage space was reduced to a minimum.[205]

"Your hospital burned down, doctor? Why, then, we must all get together and build it up again," declared a veteran *habitué* of the Labrador coast in summer, a keen yachtsman and sportsman. And since the reconstruction was bespoke, he contributed an electric plant for lighting the new little institution. Many other friends followed suit, according to their capacity to help, and we returned to Labrador with good reason for gratitude and encouragement. That summer at Indian Harbour witnessed the arrival of the United States round-the-world fliers with the unusual addition to the normal summer population of a squadron of warships and fourteen hundred naval men besides journalists and photographers. But for us, even that interesting spectacle could not bring quite the thrill that we received from the completion and occupation of the new cottage hospital at North West River. To

commemorate the event, we launched a new campaign against our arch
enemy TB by forming a definite Association Against Consumption, in
which local members pledged their cooperation by doing everything
possible in their own homes towards preventing its onset or spread.

The trapping industry, with its many perils, continued to supply
occasional patients. The family clans being few, there was sure to be
a number of namesakes. I have mentioned three John Blakes, and it
was a second Willie Goudie who underwent a hard experience on the
occasion of his first independent trapping venture. His mother had
migrated to Canada with her husband some time after their marriage,
and Willie and his brother Walter had spent just those years out of
the country when they should have been acquiring woodcraft. After
the husband's death, the family returned to Labrador. The widow did
all she could towards the family budget with work such as laundry,
and the daughter entered domestic service, while the boys lived largely
by their axes, cutting endless firewood for anyone who would take it.
Apart from these assets, they lived mainly on nature's bounties. It was
a dour struggle and a life that suffered so greatly for lack of interest
as compared with the romantic trapper's life, which was the lot of
most of their acquaintances. So it was a great event when Willie was
offered a chance to go on another man's fur-path, the owner to take
one-third of the proceeds.

The preparation was a time of great anticipation. Would it be a good
year for fur? It was fine marten land, and prices were good. The
possibilities of improving the family circumstances seemed so bright.
But ready cash was scarce and credit limited for so inexperienced a
trapper, and Willie had to consider what he could possibly do without
rather than what he would like to have. One detail omitted was a
watertight matchbox.

An experienced trapper accompanied Willie up the river to where
his path began and then went on to his own, but it was agreed that
the man who furred the nearest path should keep an eye on the raw
hand to some extent. And so Willie was left on his own. It was still
early in the season, and the snow was wet after a new fall. As he
hauled his loaded sled through the snow-laden woods or forged ahead
through falling snow, moisture penetrated to his precious matches, and
Willie was left in the heart of the wilderness alone and without the
means to make a fire. He could not boil the kettle or bake his stove
cakes or cook a bit of meat; and worst of all, while he could keep the
circulation going when on the move, he had to sleep at times.

The lad tried every resource that he could think of to produce a light.
He made a lot of fine shavings, extracted the powder from several
cartridges and fired a bullet into the powder, hoping to explode it, but

without success. And so despite all that he could do, frostbite attacked his feet, and his strength would not long hold out on a diet of raw flour. These misfortunes delayed his return to the river, and his neighbour grew uneasy and went to seek him. He found him toiling painfully along on snowshoes but still sticking to business, for he had not neglected to tend a single trap on his race for life, and he was actually removing a dead marten from one of these traps when found. It was a sad setback at the outset of the new career, but his plucky struggle gained him sympathy and respect. I had to trim up or remove sundry small portions of his anatomy, but he was still able-bodied and able to walk without a limp, and perseverance has not been without its fruits.

Willie's experience was put into the shade by the ordeal through which his brother Walter was to pass a number of years later. Walter, in a bad year for game, became the victim of a severe attack of beri-beri, which penned him, a helpless cripple, in his tilt for many weeks. It was the self-sacrificing devotion of a brother trapper that saved his life. His transport to hospital was delayed by the fact that his fur-path was away near the head of Grand Lake, and Grand Lake is very late in freezing, owing to the great depth of its water and its long, wind-swept shape. It was not till Christmas Eve that a poor wreck of a man, moaning with pain and helpless as a newborn babe, was carried into the ward. It took months to restore to him even the power to walk, and his hunting days were probably ended.

The trapper's diet is a real problem. Tea, flour, and sugar are the basic manufactured constituents, together with lard, which is preferred to butter because it will not freeze. Rice is also used by many and some baking powder. Fish and game figure very largely, and when these are scarce, particularly the game meats, there is real privation. Sometimes a fat black bear is killed in the autumn or the hunter gets a chance at a caribou. The meat of porcupines is highly esteemed, and the flesh of beaver and lynx is also excellent. Only in absolute emergency will fox be eaten. Even the husky dog disdains fox, but when grouse and rabbits fail, the protein elements of a balanced diet are defective. During a series of bad years for meat, after the biggest horde of foxes ever known had devastated the country, I had no less than four cases of young men, normally hardy, courageous, and self-reliant, who were simply enervated wrecks from lack of their normal supplies of fresh meat. There was no sign of beri-beri or any other disease about them, but they had lost self-control. They could not go into the country, as of old, unaccompanied, and the humiliation was well nigh intolerable. Since the game returned, there has been considerable improvement in their condition, though once self-confidence is lost it may be a long and painful process to re-establish it.

Apart from disease and major disorders such as those described, minor disorders of digestion are fairly common, and these of course may at any time become aggravated. Also, as is well known, physical conditions react on the psychic, and on the long forced marches, especially when groups of individuals are racing home, the tilts are overcrowded, there are too many kettles to be boiled at one time, and everything combines to put overtaxed human nature on edge. They frankly admit the occasional breakdown of the personal equation. Yet let any one of their number be the victim of misfortune, and there is no limit to the self-sacrifice and service of his fellow-trappers. It is a real freemasonry.

The komatik travel still offered comedy, tragedy, and some degree of adventure. George had volunteered [for the army], but a slight deformity had caused his rejection. He had remarried and settled down with the Hudson's Bay Company, and his cousin Jim Pottle was my teamster for a period of seven winters of travel. On our return journey from Davis Inlet, we had an experience on the Pottle's Bay barrens that might easily have ended disastrously.[206]

Lydia Tooktishina had remarried, her second husband being Simon Shuglo. We came to their house about noon on a stormy day following a big snowfall. The wind had been rising in a deliberate, businesslike fashion all the morning. It was going to be bad on the barrens, but unless we crossed that afternoon it might mean two or three days of inactivity at Big Brook. Also, Simon himself was anxious to cross that day on his way to Rigolet after supplies. So after the mid-day meal, we started. Simon had a good leader, used to this route, and left to himself the intelligent beast would doubtless have found his way. It was only about ten miles to where old Steve Newell's house used to stand on the shores of Muskrat Pond, but the previous autumn Steve had moved his house to a less exposed and better wooded spot on the margin of a bigger pond, Tilt Brook Pond, about a mile and a half further on. We coasted along till we reached the mouth of the brook where the crossing began. After topping the first rise, it was almost like plunging into breakers. Alongshore there had been little drift, as the wind was a bit off the sea, but on the barren lands it was a smoke of drift. We hit a small pond at the bottom of the slope all right, but a moment later I knew that we were off the track. We were tearing a way through low, scrubby bushes which had no right to be there if we were on the right route.

After a brief halt, this first error was corrected, and we ascended the next rise and ran down onto a big pond. To pick up the way again on the far side of this was perhaps the crucial point of the whole crossing. When we reached the far shore, there was a short ascent, without much

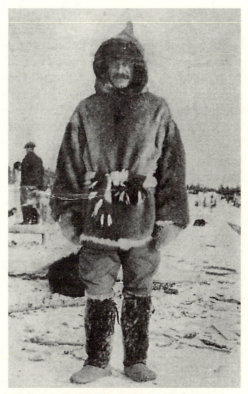

Dr Harry Paddon on the winter trail
(*Them Days* Archives)

to tell a stranger whether he was right or wrong, but on reaching the summit of the rise we were soon in trouble. It was a maze of rocks and scrub timber in which our dogs' traces continually hooked up. Soon there was a sharp crack and one trace parted; almost simultaneously, two more went and three dogs were loose. We could not see some of our leading dogs for drift; Simon had completely vanished, and the three loose animals were excited and difficult to recapture. By the time that we had hitched up the truants again, Jim and I found ourselves alone with our team in a raging storm, not knowing if we were on the right route or where lay the best way out to Pottle's Bay. Moreover, the short winter afternoon was fast slipping away.

It was no use sitting still, at any rate, so we started up the team, hoping that our leader's sixth sense would enable him to keep on Simon's track. Simon no doubt had been too fully occupied in steering his own komatik amid the many obstacles to notice just when we failed to keep close up to his rear. Suddenly, to our surprise and relief, we found Simon coming up astern. He had missed us and halted his team. We had passed him without any of the men being aware of it, but his dogs must have sensed our presence and bolted on our track. It was something to be in company again. Simon forged ahead and led the way down a wild descent. His komatik upset, and it was fortunate that we found and retrieved his axe and gun as we followed in his wake. He arrived at the bottom of the bank considerably shaken and bruised and also bewildered. When we came up, he admitted that he was lost and wanted to dig into a snow hole and camp. This did not at all appeal to Jim and myself. When I asked when last he had known where he was, he explained that he had forced his leader off the track on coming off the big pond, hoping to get more shelter by travelling on the lee side of a hill than on the windward side. The dog, like many others who are overruled, was now inclined to intimate, "It is up to you, gentlemen." So long as a pilot has any idea of what he wants to do, I have always tried to give him fair play. Too much trouble has occurred through interfering with the pilots. But when he is at his wits' end, something must be done.

Some things were clear enough. Our general course was south: we had sheered away to the southeast. To regain our line as quickly as possible, we must go about west, which was right into the teeth of the wind, with some pretty heavy punishment in store for the dogs and ourselves. The danger lay in our crossing the line of march without seeing any sign of the track. Disregarding a further plea by Simon to dig in, we started to punch to windward. It was almost impossible to get the dogs to face it, but we did get ahead gradually. That was the second and the last time in all these years that I have personally seen husky dogs want to quit work.

Presently, we came out on a pond. Both Jim and I hailed it with relief as Muskrat Pond, and I was practically certain that a prominence in the shoreline was the point on which Steve's house used to stand. Simon, however, declared that it was too big for Muskrat Pond and again urged digging in before nightfall. I remembered only three ponds in the neighbourhood – Muskrat Pond, Tilt Brook Pond and a big pond away to the eastward, which we were now leaving steadily behind us – and Jim pointed to a spruce stump which bore signs of an axe as additional evidence that this was a spot where someone had cut wood. Simon still doubted, but Jim and I started out to find the narrow neck of land which separated Muskrat and Tilt Brook Pond. In a few minutes, we saw another sheet of ice and our last doubts vanished. We had a bitter stem of a mile, which finally froze all our faces, and just as the twilight was fading, we saw the light in old Steve's new abode.

We had hardly unharnessed our dogs when Father Henry and his teamster emerged from the drift, coming before the wind from a house a few miles away. It was a two-roomed cabin, with two families already living there, and with five new arrivals there were no lack of inhabitants; but Labrador homes are very elastic, which is as well as the whole eighteen people were confined there by the raging storm for three days. It was well indeed that we had refused to give in to Simon. Short of food for ourselves and without feed for the dogs, and with all the discomfort already described in connection with a somewhat similar adventure in Back Bay on the part of others who did dig in, it is more than doubtful if we should have survived. As it was, I had a deposit of food supplies at Steve's, and he had dog-feed, so apart from the overcrowding we might have been worse off.

Pushing on to Cartwright, I went round Sandwich Bay before visiting Muddy Bay in order to give Father Henry time to get back. There were again over forty children in residence. A scout troop had been started, and I witnessed a game of soccer football on the ice. They were certainly a jolly, healthy looking group, and I felt my conviction strengthened that herein lay the solution of some at least of Labrador's problems. I set them a prize essay competition on "What I would like to be and why," and the imagination and ambition displayed in regard to careers quite outside trapping and fishing was refreshing. It was a great satisfaction to patch up a breadwinner's body, but with the parents of the next generation it might be hoped that one was investing at compound interest. Fifteen years later, one at least of those children [Millicent Blake] is a graduate nurse and a silver medallist into the bargain; another [Stella Williams] served for three years as housemother at our second Labrador Public School at North West River; a third is also soon to graduate as a nurse; a fourth [Florence Michelin] has been a nurse's aide and showed considerable ability. Others have done well in domestic service; others again have become wives and mothers in homes that are far superior to those in which they grew up. Truly, child welfare work brings returns.

Another line of service giving great satisfaction to the victims as well as to the doctor was restoring of sight to failing eyes by the simple means of spectacles. Without being an eye specialist or skilled ophthalmic surgeon, it was possible [for me] to help many middle-aged women who were straining their failing sight to do the family mending and to whom reading tended to become a forbidden luxury. There were also many who from childhood had had errors of refraction of the simpler varieties; and these could be afforded the comfort so long denied of full and perfect vision. There were some cases, of course, that needed the specialist's experience and treatment. A few years later,

I was to have the interest and pleasure of taking an eye specialist [Dr Frank Phinney] for a cruise along hundreds of miles of the indented coast, but that will be told later.

The more outdoor life lived by many women as well as by children of tender years, or even months, was having its effect, as were reforms in diet and clothing, but now at last was to spring into being the second child welfare institution as Yale School at North West River. During the summer of 1925, I received a telegram from a volunteer colleague of five summer seasons at Indian Harbour, guaranteeing $500 a year for five years towards a boarding school at North West River. This document, preserved in our archives, may be said to have really inaugurated the new venture. I already had nearly $2,000 salted away for the same purpose. Then, with little delay, came the welcome deluge.

A lengthy Yale senior student, six foot, six inches in stature, possessed a fine baritone voice, and having a genius for photography as well as being born Varick Frissell,[207] had been seized with an urge to be one of the first two white men to reach the Unknown Falls, which are on a tributary of Grand River and so near to Grand Falls that the spray of the two falls can be seen from a single hill, standing between them. (Another young American who had spent a winter in Labrador had visited them on snowshoes in company with two trappers. The little party had almost starved on the way out, striking a very bad time and region for game.) Having planned the expedition with a fellow student, Frissell had written to ask me to secure local guides, which of course I was glad to do without the slightest idea of what was to follow. Frissell stayed at North West River on the way in and again after completing his ambitious trip successfully. He and his companion had renamed the falls, which happened to be Y-shaped, after their university.

A few months later, I was staggered to receive an offer from the Yale Board of Charities through Frissell to provide a partial endowment for our projected boarding school at North West River with the sole proviso that the school should be named after the university. Needless to say, this generous offer was thankfully accepted, and in September of 1926 Yale School was formally opened. And so the third foundation was laid, and the fourth was added the same year. It consisted of the addition of a barn and cow to our ever-growing garden and poultry house; the establishment of a definite enterprise in agriculture and livestock farming was to assume a community aspect. With cottage hospital service, two child welfare institutions, and a farm, we were ready to launch out into the stage of construction already heralded in a modest way at Muddy Bay School.

PART THREE

Construction

16

The Passing of Yale *from the Service*

The satisfaction over the birth of Yale School was somewhat clouded by the loss of Father Henry [from] Muddy Bay School. This had occurred in 1925. After a decade of notable service, this fine padre and warden had felt it necessary to resign on the ground of health. His going left a gap hard indeed to fill. But he left fine foundations for others to build on and a memory which is still fresh to many. While he had naturally formulated the general plan of campaign in regard to educational policies, although giving me free scope in the department of health at Muddy Bay, Yale School was to be the real starting point for working out a comprehensive policy of my own.

In the first place, while fully realising that every system has its merits and that no honest effort fails to produce results, I very much prefer the small group, the model home to the big institution, for child evolution and supervision. It is obviously far more likely to be an inspiration to the young homemaker of the future, besides allowing for far more individual observation and development. Secondly, I had been much impressed by reading the work of another pioneer in frontier education. This was *A Winter Circuit of Our Arctic Coast*, by the late Archdeacon Stuck of the United States Episcopal Mission to Alaska. This gentleman had rakingly criticised the institutions of his own organisation of that time for being hidebound and impractical. He quoted the case of a young man who had frittered away his boyhood at a mission school over book work which in no way fitted him for effective citizenship in Alaska. He could not grind his own axe, make his own sled, net his own twine, or do any of the hundred

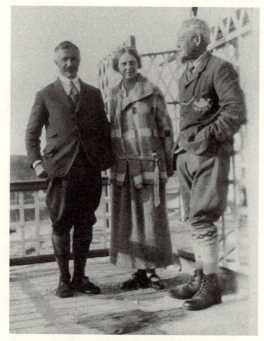

Harry and Mina Paddon with Dr Wilfred Grenfell
at the Indian Harbour hospital, c. 1925 (Paddon
Family Papers)

and one things that go to keep a frontiersman independent and successful.[208] I registered a vow that this reproach should never be made
against Yale School if I could help it. Father Henry and I had discussed
these matters together freely, and the policy of Muddy Bay School had
been directed towards the same ends. But Muddy Bay was not the
cottage type of institution for which I craved, much as I loved it and
admired its work.

The competitive element lends such a stimulus to life, especially a
young life. I desired at least two cottage model homes, each with its
garden and poultry yard, with a continuous competition in production.
The housemothers, young women of the country with some outside
training, were to be allowed a dietary at once liberal and restricted.
No canned, imported food was to be used at all if it could possibly
be avoided, except tomatoes. Native fish and game meats, native
berries, home-grown vegetables, and eggs with milk from the home
farm were to be the mainstays, together with such imported staples as
dried beans and peas, flour (mostly brown), sugar, butter, cocoa, and
salt pork. Some dried fruit was admissible, and home canning was to

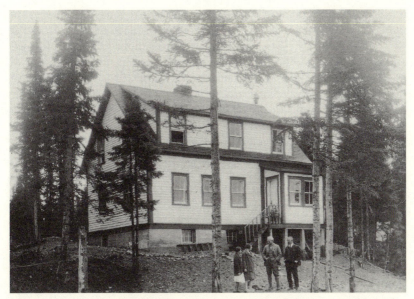

Dr Wilfred Grenfell and Dr Paddon with teachers at Wood Cottage, North West River, 1929 (Yale University Library)

be stressed. For animal fat, when otherwise scarce, there was always unlimited crude cod oil besides the milk content. On such a diet, there would certainly be no malnutrition at the school, and the more it could be standardised or copied as nearly as possible in the homes, so much the better for the younger generation of the community as a whole. It had been a mistake, as was afterwards realised, to segregate the Muddy Bay children five miles from the nearest settlement. There had been strong reasons, but they were outweighed by others. In the village, day scholars could attend, which doubled the classroom utility of the school, and also the school could act as a popular example and stimulus. And within a year, another outright gift supplied a second boarders' cottage with the desired element of competition.

Monthly records of all children's weights were kept, and every child received a routine physical examination on admission to the school, with an annual checkup. The housemother was not to be thanked for any economy at the expense of a child's welfare, but records were kept of the cost per head per month for food, heat, light, and service. The older children, of course, did much of the work, and individual interest in poultry and agriculture was encouraged. Until the boy scout movement became firmly established at North West River under a capable scoutmaster, I used to conduct first aid classes at the school, and the nurse held home nursing classes. Some youngsters aspired to help in the barn as it grew in size and the cow gave place to a herd; and it was not to be many years before Yale School supplied us with a farmer, and we also got another lad placed in a similar capacity further south.

There is no doubt that this child welfare work brought us nearer to the people as a whole than any other branch of our activities. Their delight in exhibitions of the children's work at the end of term and in the really excellent entertainments given by school members was marked. As far as their means allowed, parents were invited to help in the maintenance of their children at school, and where cash failed, contributions in firewood, berries, fish, and meat, etc., were made in many cases, and the people bore the cost of school equipment and the heating of the schoolhouse. Many of the children came from poor homes, though this was true of a smaller proportion at North West River than at Muddy Bay. I always felt that even in cases of apparent mental defection, unless gross, a chance should be given for two years under favourable conditions and experienced workers before a child should be condemned as hopeless, and many transformations have been truly startling.

For a youngster who had been underfed, under-ventilated, and under-disciplined and had suffered from lack of clothing and insufficient sleep, the school life offered a completely new existence. There were often physical defects to be dealt with – throats, eyes, teeth, or some little deformity. We saw one slender maiden almost double her weight within three years after removal of infected tonsils and obstructive adenoids. We could not get a dentist quite as often as we should have liked, but there was at least a great improvement in dental hygiene. And if bodies doubled in weight or thereabouts with physical treatment, something analogous went on in the mind. "The first thing I must teach these children is to laugh," had been the remark of the first head teacher of Muddy Bay School, and youngsters, especially from isolated homes, who had never possessed a toy or played a game were not apt to be hilarious. Prematurely aged by becoming the drudges of the less worthwhile parents, they were little old men and women in manner while still of tender years. Manual training for the boys encouraged any natural talent in that direction too.

It was the rather sudden scope for expansion offered by the second cottage that resulted in the wildest cruise of old *Yale*'s career with us, and the story may be told as her farewell to this record, for the work was getting beyond her capacity, and it was not to be very long before her successor was to appear.[209] To cope with the extra children expected, we had had to send out a supplementary order for supplies of various kinds which could not arrive in Rigolet till late in October [1927]. We had resigned ourselves to the task of a series of freighting trips between Rigolet and North West River in the late autumn when we heard that a steamer was actually coming to North West River in early November, bringing a survey party to cruise the forest lands around the head of the inlet on behalf of a powerful paper company [Bowater-Lloyd]. We could hardly credit our good fortune. It was the old *Meigle*, a Newfoundland government steamer, that was coming, and her capacity was such that there would be no lack of space for freight besides the company's. She was sure to call at Rigolet, and it never struck us as conceivable that the freight would not be accepted.

It so happened that the Hudson's Bay Company were making a change at Rigolet by substituting a powerboat for the old schooner that had long done duty for that post. *Rigolet* was long since scrapped, but *Thistle*²¹⁰ had succeeded her and was now condemned to be broken up before the new *Fort Rigolet*²¹¹ came the following summer. As the company also hoped to get freight to North West River on the *Meigle*, we loaded our whole consignment ourselves onto the *Thistle* within the space of two hours and a quarter. With the *Meigle* winches and other facilities, it could be taken off the *Thistle* in one and a half hours at most. Having done everything that we could do, we went back to North West River, leaving a message for the captain of the *Meigle* that we would keep our scow and *Yale* in the water to help in the unloading of the steamer at North West River. On November 10th, *Meigle* arrived off North West River without a single package of our freight aboard, although she had been at Rigolet long enough to ship it four times over. Comment is best omitted.

We were now in a most awkward predicament. We had the choice of shutting down part of our school, although the children were already assembled, or getting that freight up somehow. It was far too late for a series of trips with *Yale*, if indeed we could do one, but there was just a chance of success if we could tow the old *Thistle* up Lake Melville with all the supplies aboard. A free wind would almost certainly mean a blizzard of snow at this season, but if we could only get a calm spell lasting twenty-four hours or so, it could be done. Another difficulty was for crews for two boats. For *Yale*, the engineer and myself and one other hand would do, but the *Thistle* would need four, making seven in all, and there were not seven men left in the little village who were used to cruising in a decked boat at all.

It happened that a generous friend had supplied our first radio outfit for North West River station, and we had secured the services of an employee of the Marconi wireless service in Labrador. John Watts²¹² was a versatile being who had not only worked at wireless but had skippered fish crews and acted as clerk in a store and as bosun on a schooner. He was a most valuable recruit as a sailor but knew nothing about the inlet. He came as skipper for the *Thistle*. I had with me a young Englishman, a graduate of Cambridge University who has since gone far in the Sudan civil service, and we filled up with three other local men. This did not give us the two experienced crews we needed for such a job as this, especially as *Thistle* was not seaworthy. Her hull was good as yet, but spars and canvas were rotten, or at any rate not to be trusted in an autumn gale; and worst of all, her windlass was defective, as we were to learn very much to our cost.

Still, "never venture, never win," so we set out on November 11th, fully realising that our return by water was problematic in the extreme. The wind was strong and so far ahead that we had to pinch her as close as possible, and it was the engine that kept her going when the sails flapped. It was frosty, and the foredeck was soon a sheet of ice; icicles hung from the booms, and ice had frequently to be beaten off the staysail. After we crossed the two big bights, Sebaskachu and Mulligan Bight, and got under the long, straight shore of the lowlands and highlands, things improved considerably, and we made much better progress.

We reached Rigolet that evening and spent much of the night in preparation for catching the morning tide. On November 12th, when the tide began to run up about nine in the morning, we set out on our final venture. The weather was overcast and it was stark calm. All day there were no more than faint puffs of wind from an easterly direction with flurries of snow. All the indications seemed to be for in-winds with probable snow. It took us all the rest of the day to tow our ponderous consort about twenty-five miles to St John harbour. As it threatened to be a dark night, we anchored there, hoping to get out about midnight with a free wind and get well up the bay next day, if not all the way. If once we could get *Thistle* to any safe haven anywhere near North West River, we could even get the freight home by dog-team, if we could not still make a series of short trips in *Yale*.

Our anchorage was almost landlocked. Less than a cable's length [two hundred yards] ahead was a low wooded point. The shore on our port side was so handy as just to allow swinging room if a shift of wind should tail off *Yale* in that direction. The other shore was so near as to prevent any choppy water forming that could worry us at our anchor. Only to the east was there any open road to the wider waters outside. *Thistle*'s anchor had held her when riding, bows under, to a northeasterly gale at Rigolet. If ever a boat seemed safely moored, it was *Thistle* that night. *Yale* lay alongside, tied to *Thistle* with an engine ready to go at a moment's notice.

We did not set an anchor watch under these circumstances, but Watts was up several times during the night and found not the slightest cause for uneasiness. We were as much surprised, therefore, as disquieted when a grinding and bumping aroused us in the darkest hour before dawn. When we got on deck, it was to find both boats driving out of harbour in the one direction that they could drive out, before a strong northwesterly wind which already came in heavy squalls. It turned out later that in some obscure way, the stock [crossbar] of *Thistle*'s anchor had broken, so that it readily turned over and dislodged the flukes. Otherwise, this could never have happened.

We were in a bad plight now, for just when speed was of vital import, the old worn-out windlass kept jamming, and it took us an altogether excessive time to get our anchor up. Until that was up, we could only drive helplessly. But for the windlass, we could easily have made into another cove, which under present circumstances offered even better shelter than the anchorage from which we had driven, and *Thistle*'s spare anchor, with a line ashore in addition, would soon have rendered her safe from any further drifting. We were but a score of yards from safety at one time, but after that we rapidly drove out into the bay.

Once we got the anchor stowed, we had to get *Yale* clear of *Thistle* and keep clear, but with a towline between. As we got further out into the open, the wind was more westerly and right down Lake Melville. Three miles from St John Island is another island anchorage in Pelter's Cove, but it was away to the northeast, across wind and sea, and we knew there was no chance of towing *Thistle* there. Safety must be sought on the south side and towing downwind. About two miles distant was Trout Cove, which bore a good local reputation for an anchorage, though I had never been there, but we drove past the entrance to the cove before it was light enough to see our way in.

There remained one chance and only one, so far as I knew, of finding any safe anchorage above the mouth of Back Bay, and Back Bay was an uncharted problem which might bring disaster to anyone venturing to meddle with it. On my winter travels, I had several times visited a lone Eskimo shack on the point of a snug-looking cove at a spot called Peter Lewis' Brook.[213] If we could get in there, all might be well. As we rounded the point referred to, a grinning array of rocks greeted our eyes, with broken water playing over shoals still submerged. We had now shot our bolt as regards finding safe anchorage for both boats. Wind and sea were rising, and by keeping on we should run into the unknown dangers of Back Bay. The only thing now was to moor *Thistle* in such shelter as the outer part of the points afforded, take off her crew, and run for shelter on *Yale* into Rigolet Narrows run. A new stock had been improvised for *Thistle*'s main anchor, and by manœuvring with *Yale* we got the schooner's two anchors fairly well spread. It was already too rough to row between the two vessels against the wind, but we let down on a line and hauled the quartet to safety, and I think they were not sorry to get off *Thistle*. Then, under reefed mainsail and the engine's power, we simply romped across the lower end of Lake Melville to the entrance of the run and entered Caravalla Cove.

It blew a fairly stiff gale all day, and we lay comfortably enough in an anchorage that we had often used. The run was so narrow and the area of the cove so limited that it seemed impossible that we should meet with anything to hurt us there. About four in the afternoon, a snow squall came roaring down the highlands, and then came the hurricane. From hills from seven hundred to eight hundred feet in height, white squalls leaped at us in endless succession, so that when the snow ceased, the shower of spindrift could hardly be distinguished from it. With wind and tide contributing their quota, the most amazing sea hove in through the narrow entrance from the raging bay. The strain on our chain and warp [line ashore] became so great that we feared for our holding gear and started up the engine.

At first, we steamed at half speed on our anchors, but that was not enough. Even at full speed we could not gain a yard, and hour after hour we kept punching away to ease the strain. The clouds dispersed, a brilliant moon shone, and hard frost added to the discomfort of the anxious watch on deck. At last, between three and four in the morning, the warp of our kedge-anchor parted, and we swung and sheered on the main anchor and chain alone. We could not risk losing that, so with six men at the anchor chain and windlass and one at the wheel, we got the anchor up and went out into the run. Unless we could find a secure anchorage within the Narrows run, our chance was a slender one. Only a mile below Caravalla Cove was another and smaller cove which made an excellent harbour in any ordinary weather, but could we punch into it against the wind?

We had to give the upper point a good berth, as it runs off shoal for some distance, when we turned in. Happily, the configuration of the high land here was in our favour. The wind off the hills swept diagonally across the cove, leaving almost a dead space in the upper part. We ran on into the very edge of the shoals before we dropped anchor. The relief from the tension of the last twelve hours was great, but there was still the *Thistle* to be thought of, and we had very little hope of finding her where we left her. For the moment, however, it was sufficient to get a hot drink and forget our troubles in sleep. November 13th had indeed proved an unlucky 13th. When the 14th dawned, the hurricane had subsided, but it still blew a hard gale. From a hilltop with glasses, we could make out the *Thistle*. She lay about three-quarters of a mile from the point off which we had anchored her, a gleaming mass of ice, rigging and all, and obviously hard ashore. At least she still held together, which held out a hope of salvaging her freight.

The 14th continued stormy without any improvement, and the 15th was similar. Our chances of returning by water steadily dwindled. That day, we received a visit from old Peter Mesher, our Eskimo [mixed breed] woodcutter at Mud Lake in 1912, who assured us that there was a fine anchorage under Long Point, at the head of Back Bay, within two or three miles of the wreck. He added that Mark Mucko, the resident at Peter Lewis' Brook, could pilot us in there. As it would be a great advantage to be on the same side of the bay as *Thistle* and a few hours saved might make the difference between success and failure, we reached [sailed with the wind abeam] across the bay on the morning of the 16th. Though it still blew far too hard to attempt any salvage work, Mark came aboard when we rounded up under the point and confirmed Peter's report, so we squared away before the wind and ran down for Long Point. As we approached the point, I could see one small island outside it and another above that and a little outside it, so that we were running into a cup-shaped cove into which wind and sea were driving. The only possible harbour must clearly be on the far side of the point, and we were heading right for the little channel between point and islands. Still, our pilot stood impassive.

"We need two fathoms of water at least, Mark. *Yale* draws eight feet," I reminded him.

"All right."

Meanwhile, the water grew more and more muddy looking.

"Where do we anchor, Mark?" I enquired rather anxiously as we came abreast of the upper island. The tickle looked horribly narrow and the water suspiciously shoal.

"Anywhere here," was the laconic reply. We were almost in a death trap and things happened fast.

"Let go!" I yelled to Jack Watts, who stood by the anchor, at the same time putting the wheel hard over. Crazy as it sounded, fortunately Jack reacted immediately and obeyed. Had we run on another half minute, it might have been too late.

Round came *Yale*, and the anchor brought her up with a jerk. It risked the anchor, but it was the only way to save the boat. As the chain came tight, the heel of her keel struck bottom, but the jerk of the chain pulled her clear as she rose to the next wave. With several hands at the chain and the engine backing their efforts, she was hauled ahead till the anchor came off the bottom. Then the engine had to fight it out with wind and sea, and the engine just won – and only just. It really looked like a deliberate attempt to wreck a second boat, though I am sure it was nothing of the kind, just sheer stupidity. We got rid of Mark as soon as we could and ran back again to our anchorage in the Narrows. The weather was at last moderating, and we expected a change on the morrow.

The wind came round to the eastward in the night, and long before dawn we left the Narrows and made for *Thistle*. We collected all the Eskimos that we could to help in the salvage work. We anchored *Yale* as close to *Thistle* as we dared, and a party boarded her. Her sternpost was almost ripped out of her, and the hold had some feet of water in it which rose and fell with the tide. It was bitter work, working waist-deep in the water. On *Yale* another party stowed freight as it came aboard, and the boats did the ferrying between the vessels.

On *Yale* we barred up the door between engine room and cabin, dismantled the bunks, took down the table, and made a hold out of the cabin. There were over forty barrels of fresh vegetables for the winter consumption of hospital and school. (Later on, we were to be independent of imported vegetables.) The barrels were too bulky to stow well, so we emptied out the vegetables loose onto the cabin floor, where they made a level layer over two feet in height. Onto them went crates of onions, sacks of dried peas and beans, and many other supplies till the cabin was filled to the hatch. Then, any spare space in the engine room was used up, and finally the deck was loaded as much as could be risked. We instructed the Eskimos to make a shelter out of the sails of the wrecked vessel, as well as some steel drums of gasolene, and put into it any dry goods or hardware that would suffer from exposure. We explained to them their salvage rights and promised them fair play if they played fair on their side. With snow beginning to fall and a rising easterly wind, we set out in the early afternoon of November 17th to try to reach North West River.

Thicker fell the snow and harder came the wind. We could not trust the compass, as there was so much metal on deck, and had to steer by wind and sea. We picked up Pelter's Island all right, and so bad was the outlook for running on that I was in two minds whether to go in and anchor, but there was a lot of ice in the cove, and I feared that we might get frozen in there. So we held on and, clearing Pelter's Island, turned northwest to pick up the north shore of the bay. We made our landfall, and about that time it cleared up for a while. The sun appeared before it set, and long after dark we were abreast of the eastern point of Mulligan Bight, about thirty miles from home. It was no night for running the shoals and entering the narrow river channel. Dense masses of cloud overhung the land ahead, and the snow was evidently not finished with, so we ran a few miles into the bight and anchored under the eastern shore.

The morning of the 18th dawned, and a worse day could hardly be imagined for the task that lay ahead of us. It blew a hard gale from the east, with a blizzard of snow blotting out all but the immediate foreground. We had to sail on several different courses, with miles of islands and shoals running out from the north shore and the big shoals out in the middle of the bay. If we missed this fair wind and had to punch a headwind, the boat would speedily become an unmanageable iceberg, together with more and more ice forming off the land and around the river mouths. It seemed insane to put out and madness to remain, so we went. The next four hours would settle the fate of *Yale* and possibly of ourselves.

Our first task was to pick up Mulligan Head, on the west side of the bight, distant about four miles from our anchorage. This was successfully done, but it was far less difficult and was done in far smoother water than what was to follow. From here, we had to make a ten-mile run across the mouth of a wide bight to pick up a little island on the outside of four or five miles of shoals. If we got inside it, that was the last of us. If we got too far outside it, we were more than likely to miss the channel leading to the point of North West River bight and to be pounded to pieces on the big shoals in the middle of the bay.

Our objective was Edward Islands. I reckoned that *Yale* was making about eight knots, running almost dead before the wind and sea on her engine and reefed mainsail. We had therefore an hour of comparative security. Then it must be a case of "eyes skinned." As the hour ended, we were on the lookout not only for any sign of land but also for signs of shoaling water, as evidenced by the steepness of the swell and colour of the water. With seventy minutes gone, we changed our course so as to run out further offshore. At the same time, two men were told to hoist the jigger, or rearmost sail, to steady the boat as she rolled most wildly on the new course. Several items of the deck load started to shift and threatened to go overboard, but this was quite a secondary consideration, as another three minutes might see us ashore if we were too far in the bight. Just as the sail was sheeted home, I caught sight of a dim silhouette of a small island on our quarter. We had scored a bullseye on Edward Islands, running blind on a ten-mile course, steering by wind and sea and guesswork. If we had held our course for another two minutes, we should have perished. Had we turned two minutes earlier, we should probably have failed to see Edward Islands.

Our next task was, if anything, even more difficult, for to reach John Bull Island, between seven and eight miles on, we could not go on a single course, as very foul water intervened. It had therefore to be a two-legged course, and once again there was the double risk of running either too far out or too far in, and the channel was less than two miles wide at John Bull Island. First we had a hard thrash to clear the long shoals that ran for half a mile to the southward of Edward Islands. Then we eased her considerably, while keeping wind and waves on our port quarter; then at last we ran in for the land again, wondering what we should see first. If we saw the wrong thing, it might well be the last thing that we should see. At last, snow-laden woods appeared right over our stem. It was John Bull Island, and we had scored a second bullseye when our lives depended on straight shooting.

This is written in no spirit of brag. The odds were tremendous against us, and we could only do our best. I would not expect to hit on Edward Islands so accurately under such sailing conditions three times in fifty, and I should think three times in a hundred would be a fair estimate for finding John Bull Island successfully on such a day. Call it luck or call it Providence. It just was not our day for getting drowned.

We still had one problem to solve: to get into the river without any [leading] marks. We skirted along a little group of four islands and turned into North West River bight, four miles from home. The bar at the river mouth was one line of breakers in such a sea, the channel indistinguishable from the shoals. Without being able to see the position of familiar buildings and flagstaffs, still less the hills beyond the channel, we charged the line of breakers and got through. In a few minutes, we were being greeted by friends who had had no idea of seeing us that day, if indeed at all before ice travel began. After a meal, unloading was rushed, and on the following tide *Yale* was hauled up for the winter.

We had saved our winter's fresh vegetables and many other valuable supplies and in the end lost only a very little of our whole cargo, so the last voyage of the *Thistle* had not been altogether in vain. After another season's uneventful service, *Yale* was sold. A year later, she changed hands again, and after a few seasons with her new owner she drowned him, the only man ever lost from her in twenty-eight years. She is now engaged in summer salmon activities. It would be hard to find a finer little seaboat or one that has had a more knockabout career.

17

Further Developments in Child Welfare Work, More Wayside Comedy and Tragedy, Another Staggering Blow

The child welfare work naturally had its anxious side as well as much interest and satisfaction. One winter, a scarlet fever epidemic reached Muddy Bay School, and it was only the efficiency of the nurse that limited the outbreak to nine cases in a group of between forty and fifty. At North West River, in the second year of Yale School, we had another influenza epidemic which, though not so severe as the Spanish Flu, was far from being a joke. Three youngsters were seriously ill, and many anxious days and nights were spent before anxiety gave way to relief. Nothing succeeds like success, and whatever the vindication for mishap, evil repute spreads rapidly and public confidence is shaken. So far, in nineteen years of public school history in Sandwich Bay, at Muddy Bay and Cartwright, one child has died of tuberculosis, which has been the only case of fatal sickness, and in eleven years of Yale School's career we have a clean slate. Another terrible blow was in store for us, as will appear later in this chapter.[214]

As soon as communication by ice travel opened up that winter, I heard rumours of serious trouble in another direction. Of all tragic cases in a country like Labrador, no type is more so perhaps than mental cases. At home, they are a nightmare and a menace, and it is simply impracticable to bring them into a tiny cottage hospital to mix with other types of cases and to add to the already heavy responsibilities of a single nurse, especially when the doctor is so much on the move. If the trouble develops in late autumn after the close of navigation, with the whole winter to be faced before there is any chance of removal to the mental hospital in St John's, the problem is difficult in the extreme.

Poor Jim, one of the kindliest and cheeriest of men normally and a real trier at his trapping and salmon fishing, lived in a solitary cabin with his wife and several small children about twenty-five miles from Rigolet. The nearest neighbours were five miles away. Jim's brother had ended his life under restraint some years previously. Jim began to act queerly early in the autumn, but the family was so solitary that little was known about it, except at his home. The first real alarm was caused by his suddenly threatening with a gun two chance visitors who lived fifteen miles above him in Double Mer. They fled for their lives, and the affair was reported at Rigolet. It was the men on either side of him, whose trapping ground adjoined his, towards whom he was especially hostile, and one in particular, whom Jim called "the long-legged devil," was marked out by him for injury or destruction. His wife, terrified of what might happen, hid all his heavy rifle ammunition, but as the family depended on powder and shot for much of their food, he had to be left a shotgun. His nearest neighbours on either side of him left their homes for fear of him, and a council of war was held at Rigolet.

A strong armed party went to Jim's house but came away without achieving anything but to leave Jim convinced that the world was his enemy. He repeatedly expressed his regret at his lack of ammunition for his .303 calibre rifle and his determination to "shoot it out with the long-legged devil" at the first opportunity. One day, Jim's brother-in-law decided to visit his sister and approached the house on snow-shoes. Unfortunately for himself, he was long and spare, and Jim saw, as he believed, his arch-enemy advancing to battle. Seizing his loaded shotgun, he gave chase. John did the best long-distance run of his life and made good his escape, and now it was up to me as doctor and justice [of the peace] to deal with the situation.

I reached Valley Bight, where Bill Shepperd was no more to be seen. Bill, of all people, had overloaded a small boat with salt and had drowned himself and two others in a sudden squall close to his summer salmon place. Bill's son Peter reigned in his stead at Valley Bight, but there were two other relatives, nephews, to share the paternal estate, and unfortunately the whole place underwent a speedy transformation for the worse. The old days of prosperity simply perished with the founder of the home. From Valley Bight, a three-mile portage led across the intervening peninsula to Double Mer, which must be crossed diagonally for about twelve miles to reach Jim's house. Frankly, I did not in the least believe there was any danger to myself if Jim once saw who I was. He would look to me as justice to give him what was due to him from his enemies, and we had always been good friends. Of all things, any display of force was to be avoided.

With a single companion, I drove across the portage and most of Double Mer, and a quarter of a mile from Jim's house I left the driver and komatik behind and walked towards the house, taking care to keep well out from the shore so as not to appear suddenly and provoke a hasty shot, perhaps. The anti-climax was rather absurd. The house proved to be empty! Evidently, Jim had run out of supplies and had left for Rigolet with the whole family. There had been no sign of him as we crossed the bay, which meant that he had a long start and would reach Rigolet before we could come up with him. There would certainly be plenty of men to handle him there, and after recent events there seemed no doubt that he would be put under restraint. For the moment, there was nothing to do but to return to Valley Bight, where my own team was enjoying a rest. But what to do next?

I had planned to go right for Cartwright by the Back Bay route without calling at Rigolet, and there seemed to be a good deal of reason for still carrying out that plan. Whatever was to happen would have happened, surely. There was ample manpower there, and a similar case had previously been put under restraint without any medical intervention whatever. I should only be south a few days and should call at Cartwright, in any case, on my way north. I finally decided on this course, and the following morning we left Valley Bight to make a long diagonal crossing of the bay to Pease Cove, between twenty and twenty-five miles away. It was a bitter day, the coldest of the winter, and whereas it was calm when we left, a hard westerly wind breezed up, and recent light snow was whirled into a blinding cloud of drift. We had one canine member of our team, of a kind already referred to, born foolish and growing more foolish each day that he lived. Many young dogs are apt to run out wide in youth, hooking up their traces on any projecting hummock of ice or any stump or rock if it be on the land.

On this particular morning, we ran into a bad patch of rough ice, broken up by some early winter gale and then packed in and frozen together while largely standing on edge. In such cases when a dog hooks his trace, he is jerked off his feet by the pull of the rest on the komatik, hauled backward by his trace as it slides round the obstruction, and brought up with a bang against the hummock. Either his neck or the trace has got to go, unless teamster and doctor can bring the komatik to a standstill, and so far as my experience has gone it has never been the neck yet. A few such experiences usually knock some common sense into the offender, but this animal was incapable of learning by experience. He was in particularly good (or bad) form this morning and took full advantage of the opportunities afforded him by the rough ice, loudly calling on heaven and earth to witness his wrongs at each fresh bump that he received.

Then, on one occasion, instead of the single trace parting, the "bridle" (a strong, long loop of thick sealskin onto which all the hinder loops of the traces are threaded) parted with a loud crack, and away went all of our team except the canine idiot who had caused the trouble. We were in a nice pickle now. To shout was as vain as to pursue. The dogs were not in love with their job that morning. The drift and the rough ice and the frequent stops annoyed them, and no herd of Gadarene swine[215] was ever more diabolically possessed than those nine fleeing huskies. Jim [Pottle] and I, with the canine malefactor who with fatuous tail-wagging vented his satisfaction over the salvage of his worthless neck, were left in a raging storm with a heavily loaded komatik, five or six miles from anywhere.

Something had to be done, and the most important thing, of course, was to recover our team if it could be done. Otherwise, the whole trip was wrecked as well as a lot of valuable livestock gone. There was one other consideration of importance. With wind and drift like this, if we once abandoned the komatik it might not be so easy to find it again, and when the storm finally subsided a mound of snow might be all there was to indicate the whereabouts of komatik and load, and amid rough ice there would be many mounds of snow. We knew there was a small island not very far from us, and if we could find it and haul the komatik close to it and under its lee, all would be well. So with the unpopular dog gambolling playfully about us in ecstasy at seeing the fruits of his labours taking such an entertaining form, we hitched ourselves to the bridle and started hauling. We soon had had enough of that. It was a heavy load for two men, and if it was cold when going along at five or six miles an hour, it was much colder going at between one and two. Despite our hard work, the wind seemed to blow right through us as we almost stood still, so we decided to abandon the komatik, even at the risk of not finding it again.

Next came the problem of the dogs. There were three things that we could think of. Needless to say, the dogs had thought of one or two more. The first hope was that they might have run on together to the house at Pease Cove, where we were bound. The second was that on reaching the south shore, they might find the house at Peter Lewis' Brook, a few miles above Pease Cove, and run there. The third prospect was of their separating, wandering about and getting in traps. The first thing for us to do was to seek them at Pease Cove, so we set out to walk there.

We had not left the komatik two minutes when a big team of ten dogs came right on top of us out of the drift. It was a Rigolet team with two men in search of me. ["Mad"] Jim was talking slaughter at Rigolet, and no one cared to take the responsibility of putting him under restraint. We simply had to do something about our team before I could go to Rigolet, so Jim [Pottle] and one of the newcomers went back to our komatik, intending to make two small teams out of their ten and our one and get our komatik and load to safety. The other man and I walked towards Long Point, near the scene of the wreck of *Thistle*. Off the point, we came on three of the truant dogs playing around seal holes. We caught the rascals, took them onto the narrow tickle between a little island and the point, and hitched them to a stump where Jim and other teamsters were sure to see them. Then we held on, and when the other overhauled us we all went on together to Pease Cove, where nothing had been seen of our remaining runaways. After a meal, I directed Jim to spend the afternoon with our four dogs and two that Sam Wolfrey could lend him in looking for the missing six. I then left for Rigolet, where Jim was to report on the morrow whatever he found or did not find.

It was after dark when we made Rigolet, and poor old ["Mad"] Jim was asleep. The agent, Mr Cobb,[216] was in no way scared of him, but he had not cared to take the responsibility of treating him as a mental case. On the whole, it did seem best perhaps to treat it as a judicial case for the present, enough at least to spare Jim any idea that he was regarded as insane. So next morning, I put him under arrest for breach of the peace, without any fuss, and engaged a candidate for the dole as special constable or warder, using the customs house as quarters for the pair. Jim was considerably restrained by a modified straightjacket. I told him that if on my return from Cartwright I heard a good report of him, I would allow him greater liberty.

Most fortunately, Jim [Pottle] turned up with the full team next morning. The weather had moderated after I left, and within half an hour of leaving Sam Wolfrey's house Jim came on the whole six missing dogs having a glorious and prolonged siesta under the lee of Long Point. We must have passed quite close to them in the morning without being able to see them. So we were able to resume our trip, leaving our patient under the supervision of the agent at Rigolet. Mr Cobb undertook to win his confidence and befriend him in every way possible, and he achieved a great degree of success. On my return from Sandwich Bay, I found that he had quieted down a great deal and showed signs of uneasiness only when teams drove into Rigolet.

Passing on to Ticoralak, [we found] there was another familiar face missing, that of Jerry Flowers. Jerry, like old Steve Newell, was afraid of little except an operating room, and he endured the torments of a gastric ulcer till the mischief had not only become incurable but at his age the associated haemorrhage became uncontrollable. When he was finally rushed to hospital at Indian Harbour, two of us operated on

an almost moribund man, and he succumbed shortly after. At Rocky
Cove, gruff old Arthur Rich was no more to be seen, and further north
old Willie Wolfrey had vanished from the homestead at Bob's Brook.
Could the younger generation live up to the traditions of the best of
their elders?

I have already referred to the fate of Johnnie Lloyd, one of my first
two surgical cases away back in 1912, and the story may be told here.
Johnnie had grown to be a fine young man, the mainstay of his foster-
father, Austen Flowers, brother and next-door neighbour to Jerry, and
he was also on the eve of marriage when the tragedy happened. One
day early in the winter, Johnnie left Ticoralak with Austen's smart little
team of able huskies to visit friends at Rocky Cove. There was a strong
northerly wind with threatening snow, and his foster-parents were
rather apprehensive about his leaving, but youth must be served.[217]
Why, for the first six miles it was all along shore and also for the last
five. There was only a six-mile crossing across the mouth of Fox Brook
bight, less than an hour out of sight of land. So off he went. It was
the old story of steering by the wind and the wind shifting without
the teamster being aware of it.

Off the Rocky Cove hills, the wind was tripping off from the
northeast, so that the further he went across the bight the more Johnnie
sheered away to the southeast. He must have wondered at the long
delay in sighting Jewel Head, and the first land he saw was not that
bluff cliff at all but a low-lying island four miles out at sea. Out here,
the wind was still more easterly, and a nasty sea was making and
bending and cracking the ice, which was still far from thick. Had there
been any shelter on Cato Island, Johnnie might have been tempted to
stay, but on the other hand, if the storm continued long the island
might be cut off from the mainland for many days. Realising his peril,
he turned in for where he knew Rocky Cove must lie, and he no doubt
urged his dogs to put out all they had to give.

He reached a tiny islet, Gull Island, just one mile from the houses,
but the ice broke up too fast, and it is possible that he got in the water
before he landed. However, he got ashore only to find himself in a
death trap. He was on a narrow ledge of ice stuck to the island rocks,
but the shore consisted of an unscalable cliff, and there was no ice on
which to get round the point of the cliffs to the shore nearest the
mainland, from which a safe bridge of ice still communicated with the
land. So within a few yards of safety, he was to perish. He opened his
grub-box and made a cold, cheerless meal so as to fight to the end. It
was a matter of time how long life could hold out against the pitiless
wind, snow, and frost. Fuel there was none, nor any shelter. Even had
he escaped immersion in the salt water, the wet snow of early winter

would seep through dickey and overalls till he was wet to the skin. His one chance, if chance it was, lay in the snow stopping, in which case he might have tried to drive a dog to where it might be seen from the shore. No miracle occurred to save Johnnie Lloyd, and there was nothing to indicate how long the ordeal of a lingering death had lasted. At some time in that bitter stormy night, or early the following day at the latest, the end came, and another good man was lost for lack of the simplest of precautions.

As we traversed his route that same winter, we had it far colder and every bit as rough as poor Johnnie had it, but we steered by compass from the point outside Ticoralak and made the land well inside Jewel Head, as we planned to do, without the least difficulty or danger. How many victims will be offered up on the altar of tradition and stubborn pride before the lesson is fully learned?

When the storm ended and Johnnie did not reappear at Ticoralak, Austen borrowed dogs and hurried to Rocky Cove, only to learn that nothing had been seen of his adopted son. Search parties combed the shore all around the deep bight in vain, of course. No doubt they thought of his having gone away out from the land, but the hidden shore of little Gull Island never entered into their thoughts in their search. With the shift of wind, it became more frosty, and a calm night caused young ice to form again on the open water. One morning, people at Rocky Cove saw dogs running to and fro on the ice just off Gull Island but never going far away. Then they knew. They found the boy, fallen forward over an ice-covered rock to which the body was so fast frozen that they had to chop it away. It seemed as though he had tried to keep moving to the end and collapsed from numbness and exhaustion. Once again, starving huskies had refused to violate their young master's body.

Back at North West River, spring was coming on. With the advance of our farming venture, this had become the most interesting season of the year in many ways. The possibilities were almost unlimited. Early came radishes, and hardy rhubarb came sprouting up through the snow. No finer iceberg and cabbage lettuce ever grew anywhere, surely, than in this sub-arctic Garden of Eden. Soon, a greenhouse was to speed up our early growth, and many thousands of young cabbage plants were brought along for transplanting by the end of May. Later, many would be taken from the ground weighing from ten to fourteen pounds. Turnips of several varieties, weighing up to a maximum of fifteen pounds, beets and carrots, spinach and chard, chives and kale, cauliflower, squash, tomatoes, cucumbers, and melons under glass. Peas of the best, vegetable marrows, strawberries. Also a wealth of flowers. Messrs Sutton & Sons[218] of Reading, England, sponsored this venture in

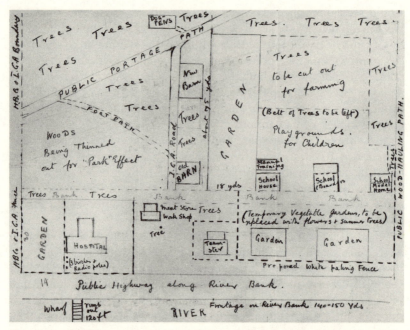

Plan of Grenfell Mission property at North West River, 1928 (Richard Paddon Papers)

generous fashion by annual donations of first-rate seeds. A garden competition caused judges considerable worry to decide on the respective
merits of a number of excellent displays. Moreover, the inspiration
radiated widely. Orders for greenhouse plants came from Rigolet and
Cartwright, and seeds went out from North West River as far north as
Davis Inlet and south to Sandwich Bay.

A single hen-yard has produced over five hundred eggs a month on
more than one occasion, and it was found that with all the overhead
expense of imported concentrates and a certain proportion of good
hay, the cost of fresh milk was lower than that of imported preserved
milk. With garden, barn, poultry yard, nets for trout and salmon, and
home-canning activities, it was possible to make living both good and
economic in sub-arctic Labrador, that "Godforsaken wilderness" of
one-time pessimists. I remember fatherly advice from businessmen in
Canada, feeling it was their duty to try to get a visionary fool to see
the error of his ways and to prove to him that the only hope for the
people of Labrador lay in their forcible deportation from the impossible wilderness where they or their forebears had been misguided
enough to settle.

As we learnt to know our neighbours better, we heard from them
many things about which at first they were reticient. The place of the

supernatural or mysterious in any community is not without its scientific interest. Traverspine supplied one story [the Traverspine gorilla] too well-founded to doubt ... Another story, also well substantiated and confirmed by different individuals at different places and times, is the following. At Bluff Head [at the mouth of Groswater Bay] one spring, the widow of John Oliver, whose tragic case was related early in this work, was off from home on a visit to neighbours a few miles away. She was expected home at any time, and one evening in the sunset hour a big team was seen coming over the marsh which was visible over a low skirt of scattered woods that surrounded the house. Clearly, their mother was coming, and the two sons and daughter made ready to welcome her. The elder son walked down the path through the skirt of woods while his brother waited by the woodpile near the house and the daughter came to the door. They heard the teamster shouting to his dogs, and their own dogs heard the commotion and uttered their usual greeting of long howls to a visiting team. And then, just as the elder son, seeing that his mother was not on the komatik, went on to bid the stranger welcome, teamster and team and komatik vanished. The home dogs continued much excited and very uneasy for a long time.

This team has been "seen" by several people, including two Hudson's Bay [Company] clerks who knew nothing about the story but who met a big team a few miles above Rigolet which passed by without any greeting, only to learn from repeated enquiries that no team had come up the Narrows run or called at any of the houses near Rigolet that day. This team was also seen at Ticoralak and followed by a puppy from a house there. The driver obligingly stopped his team and with a crack of his whip drove the truant pup homeward.[219]

Nor do the long-distance trappers lack their ghostly visitants, especially Indians. Two men, father and son, who have never had any troubles elsewhere, found an iron pot, old and abandoned but still quite serviceable, at a very old Indian camping place, which they adopted and took to a new tilt lately built by the younger man. They used the pot to cook a meal and lay down to rest. The younger man felt as if someone was trying to stifle him, and the elder man too was conscious of a sinister presence. Indigestion? Anyhow, they got out, but later on they tried again with the same results, and a barely used tilt has been abandoned and even part of the hunting ground, and no one will use it or camp near it. Later, they heard the story of that pot from some Indians. Many years earlier, a party of hungry Indians was struggling towards North West River trading post. A married woman gave out and was left in camp with one or more children. As soon as possible, the husband came back with food and found his squaw alone, insane and with abundant evidence of cannibalism. In terror he shot her, and

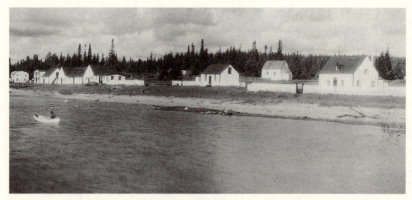

Hudson's Bay Company post at North West River, 1929 (Yale University Library)

the remains were buried nearby. The Indians would never use the pot which had been used in this ghastly tragedy, but the trappers had ignorantly taken and used it.[220] That is the only aggressive ghost I have heard of in Labrador. There are several others on record, but all of them are harmless, friendly visitants. One old Indian who objects, it seems, to a tilt being built too close to his last resting place disturbs the rest of sleepy trappers by chopping wood all night or part of the night. This is more by way of a joke or petulance than with harmful intent.

The end of komatik travel was again imminent when a big team drove into North West River, and to my great surprise I found the teamster was Charles Bird, our carpenter, engineer, and general factotum at Muddy Bay. He was the bearer of bad news. Muddy Bay School was burned to its foundation. Happily, there were no lives lost, young or old. Forty-four children had all been got out. Thank heaven, it was not in the night. It was a sickening loss of property, time, and service. It was to cramp our educational and health work in that bay and district for several years to come. In the reconstruction, when it came, at least one great fault was to be corrected by the shifting of the school to the shores of Cartwright harbour, to a magnificent location by a brook which offered various possibilities in hydraulic developments later on. It is only the addition of such innovations as sheetrock, rockwool, and asbestos shingles as auxiliaries to sub-arctic construction, especially where groups of irresponsible children are concerned, that have finally removed the perpetual nightmare of fire risks. Apart from a forest fire (and we have had sundry alarms of this kind at North West River), security is now possible if the price can be paid.

18

The Coming of Maraval:
Extended Medical Cruising

In the autumn of 1928, after more than sixteen years on the Labrador coast, I had the first breakdown in health, which took me out for a premature furlough. Once again, misfortune only brought into relief the worth of friends. I was taken ill on a late October cruise to Rigolet to connect with the last mail steamer and return to winter quarters. My wife and boys,[221] fortunately as it turned out, were off the coast for that winter, in any case. The condition was painful rather than serious but was aggravated by intense neuralgia which turned out to be due to an abscess at the root of a tooth. This would hardly have been detected without X-rays, so that the other condition was rather a blessing than otherwise, as it took me within reach of X-rays and a dentist to extract the guilty tooth. It was very stormy as we lay at anchor at Rigolet, awaiting the *Kyle*, and the old customs officer there insisted on having me brought ashore and installed in his own quarters. It was, of course, very upsetting to have to quit work without warning. Happily, the Australian nurse whom I had left in charge at North West River [Kate Austen][222] was an uncommonly resourceful, self-reliant woman, though she was to have a gruelling experience before I returned [see below, p. 232].

On the *Kyle*, the kindness and attention received were remarkable, and every effort was made to hasten her progress to St Anthony, as far as was compatible with the fulfilment of necessary duties. At Gready, the captain of a whaler to whom we had been able to be of some service at Indian Harbour came aboard and offered to steam right for St Anthony then and there in order to get me there more

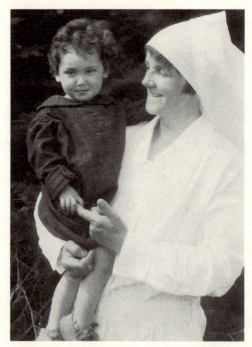

Kate Austen holding Ethel Sheppard (Fred C. Sears)

quickly. Encouraged by his kindness, I asked an even greater favour, although hating to do so. All my clothes and other personal belongings, except a few things I had taken for this brief, rough-and-tumble cruise, were at North West River, without any other hope whatsoever of recovering them for use that winter. It was a lot to ask for the whaler to go to fetch my trunks, but Captain Smith never hesitated, and I can only record with relief that he got a fine whale for his trouble. At St Anthony, Dr Curtis was also on furlough, but he had in Dr Mount[223] a deputy who was a real surgical artist, whose work was a delight to witness, and once I was convalescent, I was able to see some splendid operative achievements.

It was this winter outside that led up to *Yale*'s much-needed successor and the reorganisation of the whole itinerant medical service in summer. I received one day an invitation to go and inspect a family motor yacht, moored for the winter in a harbour in Rhode Island in the United States. The owner was thinking of giving her outright for service on the Labrador coast if she was acceptable. *Maraval* proved to be a seventy-five or eighty-foot powerboat with a gasolene engine and no sail at all. She had a fine strong hull and was naturally more elaborately fitted up than was necessary for the work in prospect.

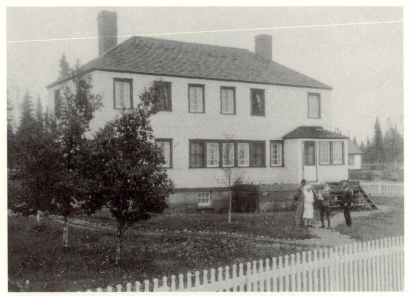

Dr Harry Mount, Kate Austen, Dr Wilfred Grenfell and Dr Harry Paddon at North West River hospital, c. 1930 (Yale University Library)

To rely on power only in so remote a region as Labrador is to take a risk. It is always well to have two strings to your bow in such cruising, and I did not like the prospect of being without sail. While *Maraval* possessed the merit of shallow draught, that very virtue was a demerit when it came to adding sail. She drew but four and a quarter feet and would be very top-heavy with canvas. It was certainly a boat that needed a certificated engineer in Labrador, while she was a beauty for coastal cruising along the United States littoral and had been safely to Bermuda and back. It was hard to refuse so generous an offer, and after consultation with those who had the right to decide, she was accepted.

When invited to take her north with a volunteer crew, I declined. I was learning a good deal about the Labrador coast by practical experience, but I had never studied navigation, and the Bay of Fundy, with its sixty-foot tides and fierce currents, added to the fogs likely to be encountered, which together put highly skilled mariners endless miles off their reckoning (to say nothing of gales which could only be dodged by knowledge of harbours and inside runs), seemed to me to call for experience and knowledge far wider than I possessed. An expert amateur was eventually secured to lead a volunteer crew with a certificated engineer, but as *Maraval*'s sailing had to be delayed, I went ahead after a visit to England. The next thing I heard of *Maraval*

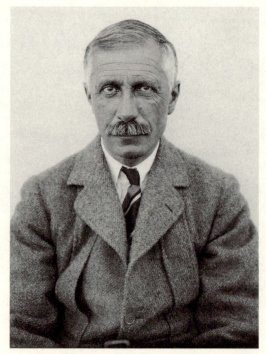

Dr Harry Paddon, 1929 (Paddon Family Papers)

was that she was a complete wreck, largely destroyed by an explosion of her day tank. Had it been the main tank (and it was a miracle that that escaped), boat and all on board would have been blown to dust. It was the heroism of the engineer, at the cost to himself of a broken arm and severe burns, that prevented the explosion of the main tank.

Yet again was disaster to bring sunshine. While I was, of course, most genuinely sorry to hear of the disaster and what those aboard had suffered in injury and shock, and expected that that was the end of a new opportunity, I was soon most happily disillusioned. The reaction of the donor was not by any means "Well, I'm awfully sorry, but that is the end of *Maraval*," but rather, "There must be a *Maraval II*, and she must be all the *Maraval* was not for that work," and I was actually invited to send in my views on her construction. After sixteen years of *Yale*, naturally I had some ideas salted away.

First, I desired a powerboat with auxiliary sail rather than a sailboat with auxiliary power. Where the season was short and the calls sometimes urgent, it was important to be sure of good headway, independent of favouring winds. Secondly, shallow draught: *Yale* drew eight feet and *Maraval* only about four. The first was too deep and the second not deep enough for a boat that was to carry sail. Six feet was to my mind the ideal draught. Thirdly, the mixing of passengers, patients, and crew in one small saloon cabin needs no comment. Fourthly, a little wheelhouse for the severe late autumn cruising especially would be an advantage while not essential. Fifthly and far more important than fourthly, crude oil instead of gasolene for safety and economy was my choice, with a good heavy-duty engine for wear and work rather than for speed. Eight knots would be a very good average, which could often be increased with sails. And so the masterpiece which is *Maraval* II was evolved from these rough notes by a master designer of boats.

With good steerage accommodation for doctor and assistant and two nice deck cabins for staff or other passengers, a fine dispensary where two bunks can be fitted up for patients and good fo'c's'le quarters for the crew as well as a useful bit of carrying space – and all these fitted into a seventy-five-foot hull – *Maraval* II, with her slightly old model 60-HP diesel engine, preferred to a more modern model for its output in work, had emerged as almost the ideal medical cruiser for the Labrador coast. Her stocky masts and moderate spread of canvas can add from two to three knots to her normal eight, given a good free sailing breeze. There were some early difficulties, the wrong bearing crippling her service for a while, but she had covered as much as five thousand miles in a three-month season of medical patrol work, and she has certainly proved herself as a seaboat. From Belle Isle straits to Hebron, five hundred miles to the north, she is known and looked for by Newfoundland fisherman, both planters and schoonermen, by Eskimos and Indians and the "liveyeres" [settlers] or by the white and mixed stock of Labrador in every bay along the stretch of coast. A few examples may be given of her service.[224]

It was the first season that I had her, and we had cruised as far as Belle Isle straits, taking some volunteer workers on their way back from summer service at North West River. We were northward bound, and my wife, returned to the coast, was on board as well as another nurse who was coming to work at North West River for the coming winter. We were intending to spend the night in Cartwright harbour, but before turning into Sandwich Bay I decided to call at Gready, where there was a wireless station, just in case there should be a message for me. And it was well that we did call, for there was a message and a very urgent one, sent in duplicate to *Maraval* and the *Meigle*, telling of a shooting accident away north in the Makkovik sector. The two patients had been taken to the Moravian Mission for first aid and then brought south as far as Holton, sixteen miles north of Indian Harbour,

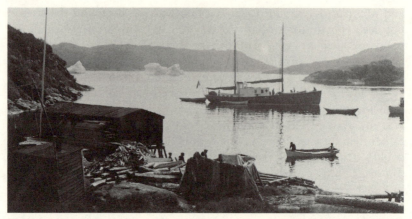

Hospital vessel *Maraval* in Labrador harbour (Faculty of Medicine Founders' Archive, Memorial University)

where there was another wireless station. Indian Harbour was already closed down for the season. It was an SOS to whichever vessel could reach the victims first. *Meigle* was at Battle Harbour, over a hundred miles south, and it promised to be a dirty night, blowing, and raining with plenty of wind. Holton is not an easy place to make at the best of times, and to try it in the night, unless exceptionally fine, was madness. So we went to Pack's Harbour, where we lay till three in the morning. By eight we were at Indian Harbour, where we dropped my wife and sufficient help to open up the necessary amount of accommodation at the hospital and generally to prepare for our return. The nurse accompanied me, and two hours later we reached Holton.

John Snow and his nephew had gone out shooting on a Saturday to try for a good Sunday dinner other than fish. A gun had been left loaded with the muzzle pointing straight down the boat from stem to stern. Hasty handling of the barrel resulted in the hooking of the trigger and an immediate explosion. John Snow, who had seized the weapon by the muzzle, had part of his hand simply blown away; and the charge passed on between his thighs and entered the chest, abdomen, and arms of his nephew, who crouched some feet behind his uncle. But for the latter's hand, the nephew would have certainly been killed on the spot, with heart and lungs and intestines simply riddled. Miraculously, not a single pellet had penetrated beyond skin and fat. I extracted between forty and fifty from the surface of his anatomy, and iodine and alcohol and dressings did the rest for him.

John Snow was in a far worse plight. To check haemorrhage had been the main objective of the first-aid treatment of Makkovik, naturally enough. The circulation cannot, of course, be stopped for more than a limited time without serious consequences. It was necessary to prevent his bleeding to death, but it was also necessary to tie up bleeding vessels and relax tourniquet or tight bandages and restore circulation as speedily as possible. There had been no one to do this, and when I removed the bandages I beheld an arm gangrenous nearly to the elbow. A high amputation was essential.

I had found a wireless awaiting me at Holton from Captain [Albert] Burgess of the *Meigle*, saying he was coming north direct from Battle Harbour and asking where to come. I had replied, "Indian Harbour." We reached Indian Harbour ourselves between five and half-past. The patient, who was far more jubilant about saving of his nephew's life than bitter about the loss of his own limb, was really heroic throughout. *Meigle* arrived about eleven that night, most fortunately with a doctor on board. At seven next morning, after a good night, the patients were shipped, both in excellent condition, and late that night *Meigle* landed them at Battle Harbour hospital. She then resumed her normal mail service, and on her return south the patients were both able to proceed on her to Newfoundland. John Snow, who was a merchant's agent rather than a fisherman, was back at the cod fishery the following summer, though he has now joined up with the chilled salmon activities. Needless to say, there was great satisfaction in such service to doctor as well as to patient.

Time after time, we would be headed off as the boat became better known. On one occasion, we entered Hopedale harbour and had hardly anchored when a boat came off with Reverend W.W. Perrett,[225] veteran Moravian missionary. Had we been spoken [hailed] by a motorboat as we came in? No, we had not. It seemed that the boat had brought in a case of a badly infected hand belonging to the skipper of a schooner fishing ten miles away. The hand was terribly swollen, and the case was beyond the capacity of a first-aid man to cope with. Within twenty minutes, we were heading out of harbour again, and barely an hour and a half [after] we heard the news, the skipper was transferred from his schooner to *Maraval*, which could act as a little floating hospital in such a case. He was with us for ten days, and while part of one finger had unfortunately to be sacrificed, it might have been a great deal worse. The grateful patient, apologetic that he could make no returns at the time, sent a voluntary donation towards the *Maraval*'s maintenance the following summer.

Many schoonermen used to beg us to follow the fishing fleet far north, where they were so terribly out of touch with hospital facilities, and it was largely on that account that we extended our patrol to Hebron. And never until we made this extended cruise had I realised the full grandeur of the Labrador coast. No one knows it who has not cruised in the vicinity of Cape Mugford. For several seasons, my skipper of the deck was Will Simms, once engineer of *Yale*. When he eventually aspired to owning his own schooner and doing coastal business, Captain Kenneth Barbour, one of the famous family of Newfoundland mariners, came in his place. Captain Barbour had the advantage of long experience of the coast north of Hopedale, which was just where Will and I became weak. (Besides the captain and medical officer, *Maraval* carries a certificated engineer, assistant engineer, and cook-sailor. The assistant engineer is a lad who is just graduating from Yale School, who has it in him to become an efficient diesel engineer.) Sometimes the ship's company included a dentist, which is of course a great addition to our efficiency, and one of the outstanding memories is of the time that *Maraval* carried an eye specialist, who also specialised in ear, nose, and throat surgery, for a period of three weeks.

It was Dr Frank D. Phinney,[226] of whose death we have but lately heard, who came and did this fine piece of service. Sacrificing the proceeds of a good practice in Cincinnati, Ohio, for three months of each year, he would come north for a long term of years, summer by summer, and work in northern Newfoundland at St Anthony. He had always wished to visit the Labradormen in their own homes and managed to arrange this trip with me. In twenty days, over the coast between Cartwright and Nain, he saw no less than 220 scattered eye cases, not 5 per cent of whom would have been able to see him unless he came to them. One morning at North West River, we sandwiched in seventeen cases of tonsils and adenoids. I had already done fourteen others that spring, but as I watched his speedy, dexterous, bloodless work, I had good cause to realise the difference of his technique and mine.

Sandwich Bay and Hamilton Inlet, both at [the] North West River and Indian Harbour ends, as well as a specially arranged clinic at Rigolet, reaped in succession the benefit of his coming, and we had gone as far as Hopedale when Dr Phinney felt that he must really turn south again, having a steamer to catch on a certain date. We had reached no further south than Indian Harbour when *Kyle* overhauled us, bringing a pitiful appeal from the Reverend P. Hettasch of the Moravian Mission at Nain on behalf of three Eskimos, all of whom were threatened with total blindness such as had darkened and embittered old Steve Newell's closing days, unless they were promptly and thoroughly treated. Dr Phinney gulped a bit when he read it, but there was no hesitation. "I cannot refuse an appeal like that," he said quietly, and *Maraval*'s head was turned north again for a rush trip to Nain and back of over 450 miles.

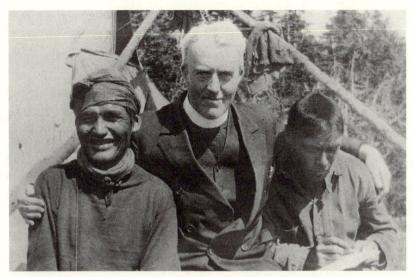

John Sebastien, Fr Edward O'Brien, and Joe Rich, Davis Inlet, 1930 (*Them Days* Archives)

At Nain was a little cottage hospital building erected by the Hudson's Bay Company and staffed with an English nurse. The use of this was gladly offered. On Sunday morning, three useless, sightless, menacing relics of eyes were removed, and three remaining eyes were safeguarded from the danger of sympathetic infection. (As I write, I have another such case awaiting operation in my little ward here.) Three other small surgical cases were also done, and as the nurse and Mr Hettasch (who is known as "Dr Hettasch" to all the neighbourhood) were quite competent to see to the after-treatment, we made fifty miles south to Davis Inlet that afternoon and evening.

Davis Inlet, where a number of Naskapi Indians spent the summer and whither *Maraval* had several times carried their priest [Father O'Brien] on his annual pastoral visit, seems to me about the worst place, if there be a worst, on the whole Labrador coast for winged pests in the fly season in the summer months. You eat, drink, think, dream, and talk mosquitoes and black flies. They are said to be even worse on the barren tundras of reindeer moss on the uplands, where they form a faint haze over the moss and have often been mistaken for the smoke of a steamer nearer the coast, but Davis Inlet is bad enough for me, and if there is worse may I never go there.

So far, all had gone well, but now came a series of baffling fogs, which just seemed bent on making Dr Phinney lose [miss] his boat after all that he had risked. A few miles outside Davis Inlet, we were hung up for twenty-four hours; at Indian Harbour, there was another prolonged delay which could not be helped. At Gready, fog again, and when we reached Battle Harbour, a bare sixty miles from St Anthony, where the steamer had to be caught, the thickest fog of all lay over the Strait of Belle Isle. It was also blowing hard, and the straits tides are strong. Our compasses were good, however, and we felt that it was up to us to get Dr Phinney to St Anthony if it could be done, though we did not wish to lose the boat, of course. Also, we were rather crowded. Finally, Will said if I would take her to Cape Bauld he would do the rest, and as it was the French Shore that I most dreaded and that was his native heath, we put out. At least there would be no steamers on the move. Neptune certainly reaped a harvest that day. I was especially anxious to pick up the western point of Belle Isle to give us our bearings for a straight run from there to Cape Bauld, but we never saw Belle Isle, though we felt its influence on the swell to some extent. This, at any rate, gave us a rough idea of how wind and tide were affecting our course by the chart, and we scored a bullseye on Cape Bauld, after which Will triumphantly took her into St Anthony, to the astonishment of those who witnessed her arrival.

Another great satisfaction lay in being able to clear up difficult diagnoses, in some cases at least, by taking them for X-ray investigation to St Mary's River, where these facilities were now available at a new little hospital which had sprung into being there in St Lewis Sound to replace the old Grenfell Mission hospital in Battle Harbour. This owed its existence, as did the little school associated with it, to the energy of Dr Herman Moret,[227] a Swiss by birth though trained at McGill University in Canada, who spent a decade of years on the coast in succession to Dr Grieve. A series of such cases travelled on *Maraval* to St Mary's River from various points on the coast, and Dr Forsyth,[228] who followed Dr Moret and whose brother installed the plant, was always glad to co-operate.

One youngster at Rigolet complained to me only of pain in one knee when kicking a football. That was all that worried him, though his gait was clearly affected. I was southward bound and took him along and was shown a beautiful negative of a detached head of the bigger bone of the leg, which overrode the shaft by a small fraction of an inch. A few months in plaster of Paris cured him without robbing him of all exercise. Then there were operative cases, frankly beyond me with my limited experience and practice and also small staff and other facilities, which I could now carry to another hospital and share in all the interest of the case, giving the anaesthetic or assisting at the operation.

The wife of an old employee of ours [Annie Bird, wife of John Bird] who lived at Cartwright had long manifested symptoms strongly suggesting ulcer of the stomach, just where it joins the intestine. She had grown thin from restricted diet and suffered not a little. The pair had lost their adopted son with a lightning attack of meningitis the previous year, and dread of cancer at last reconciled both husband and wife to surgical procedure. They came aboard together, and the husband willingly offered to pay his own expenses if he might accompany us to St Mary's River to know the worst, only it happened to be the best. For X-rays revealed some suspicious-looking shadows, and exploration revealed gallstones, which were successfully removed by Dr Clark, FRCS (Edinburgh),[229] who was deputising for Dr Forsyth for a time. When I saw the couple a few months later, the wife was a new woman with a fuller figure and a face that was no longer drawn with pain and anxiety. A little later, Dr Clark was able to accompany me on a short trip to Cartwright, where we had another deeply interesting surgical clinic, and the last patient's sister-in-law was successfully operated on for a similar gallbladder condition as well as chronically inflamed appendix.

Another little item of *Maraval*'s medical history is furnished by a northern Labradorman who had a very narrow escape from being shot to death through the heart by a rifle bullet. Happily, it was only a .22 calibre rifle, and the bullet struck some intervening obstacle, a book or something, in a breast pocket. It then glanced off and penetrated the skin and superficial muscles, hit a rib without fracturing it, and glanced on round the chest until it brought up against the margin of the scapula bone. It could readily be felt with the finger. I sat the patient with his face towards the back of the chair, over which he leaned, and injected the surrounding area with novocaine, and while he chatted nonchalantly to a friend the bullet was removed and with it the "rheumatic in the shoulder" which it was causing by pressure on a nerve.[230]

It was not only men that could be salvaged by *Maraval*. She had two floatings of stranded vessels to her credit. One was the schooner *Pauline C. Winters*,[231] a fine banker-schooner; the other was no less a prize than the icebreaker *Kyle*, which was herself rendering assistance to a distressed *Maraval* at the time. To take the case of the *Pauline C. Winters* first, on a grey October morning *Maraval* left Rigolet, bound for Cartwright. All through the summer, we are accustomed to see the glass go up for an easterly wind, even if there is a fog and some rain. It is usually in the autumn that the glass reverses its summer habit, and when the glass goes down with an easterly wind rising, look out! This was the case on the morning mentioned, and to Will Simms and myself came the thought, "Keep the north shore aboard [alongside]," for the north shore had a series of comparatively good anchorages as compared with the south shore, and on a sixty-five-mile direct run from Rigolet to Pack's Harbour, much may happen.

As we went outside into the wider part of the eastern basin, the swell increased as well as the wind, but although we reached Indian Harbour without much trouble, it was well indeed that we had not tried anything more ambitious. The real storm struck between three and four that afternoon and lasted forty-eight long-drawn hours, during which we might have gone adrift at almost any moment. In the outer part of the harbour, though hidden almost entirely and continuously from us by the whirling spindrift, four fishing schooners lay at anchor, the big *Pauline C. Winters* and three smaller ones. We heard afterwards that their crews had had all their belongings packed, ready to abandon ship at any moment, although they had all the holding gear in use that they could put out and were but a few score yards from the land. In one gust, the hospital chimney went down like an ear of ripe corn. Sheering [deviating from course] as she rode, *Maraval* would career to the squalls as they struck her, as if carrying a press of canvas. In all my seasons at Indian Harbour, I have seen no worse gale (if one as bad), though there was a worse one later in the same autumn which I am not sorry that we missed.

The morning after, while there was still a big tumbling sea and unsettled looking clouds, the *Pauline C. Winters* was getting under way. She was badly placed for this, as the other schooners were outside her. If she went off on the most favourable tack for clearing the land, she was likely to hit a smaller vessel, but if she went on the other tack there was a greater risk of running ashore. However, the captain thought that he had a better chance with the rocks than the vessel and got under way on the starboard tack. The wind failed just as she was coming about, and aground she went, though it was not so much a case of being on the rocks as jammed against them, as there was deep water right to a low cliff.

We were taking it a little easy after the long watches and with the weather still unsettled. There was plenty of time to go to Cartwright that day if it was fit to go, so instead of being under way about dawn I was still in my bunk when Will looked in about seven o'clock and said, "There's a banker ashore in Watering Cove and the captain wants help." In a few moments, we were off, and a mile's run took us as close ahead of the schooner as we dared go. She was in a bad fix. Jammed against the cliff, as described, her rudder was smashed, her sternpost broken, and she was already leaking aft. An hour or two more and she would be a total wreck, if not sooner.

Dories brought a stout two-line alongside, and it was made fast to us astern. Then we took the strain. She came away from the rocks all right, but we had to tow her out just about dead to windward for half a mile, and if there had been but a little more wind and sea we should hardly have done it. Then we had to turn broadside to the wind and

sea for something less than half a mile and next run in before the wind
for a final swing, almost at right angles, into the inner harbour. The
last was the ticklish turn. The banker was quite out of control, having
no rudder, and when we turned she ran straight on until the line
checked her and swung her onto a new course. If it had not been for
a fine high tide caused by the strong northeasterly winds, coupled with
a full moon, I think the *Pauline C. Winters* would undoubtedly have
gone ashore again at the final turn, but we got her in, and a wireless
was sent for a powerful tug to take her south to dry dock.

The affair with the *Kyle* was a two-sided one. Owing to the shaft
and bearing trouble referred to above, *Maraval* was lying disabled at
Rigolet for some days one autumn early in her career. Her engine could
work in dead smooth water, but with any rise and fall, the shaft
hammered on the after bearing in a manner that threatened wreckage
to the whole engine. I was feeling thoroughly fed up. We had been
there some days. We were right off the track of everything except *Kyle*
on her periodic mail trips. She was due within a few days, but we were
out of reach of news, and a few days was a long time. There was a
noise overhead, and an airplane circled over *Maraval*, spiralled down,
and landed gracefully on the water close by. In another minute or two,
Commander Donald Macmillan climbed aboard. A few minutes later,
we were flying to Indian Harbour. I knew that Sir Wilfred Grenfell
was cruising somewhere north in *Strathcona* and left a message to
inform him of our plight. I also learned that *Kyle* was due that very
night in Rigolet. In another thirty-five minutes, we were back at
Rigolet. In return for Commander Macmillan's help, though it was
hardly a *quid pro quo*, we were able to assist his little schooner
Bowdoin into the somewhat awkward anchorage at Rigolet with our
seldom-used searchlight when she also arrived long after dark. Then
Kyle came and Captain [John] Clark kindly agreed to tow us out to
Indian Harbour and put us in *Strathcona*'s way.

Close behind *Kyle* came a great fog bank. Next morning at dawn,
a light breeze from the southwest was driving the fog out of the run,
and point after point came in sight. Captain Clark ordered a tow-line
to be passed to us and we got away. Hardly had we gone a mile when
round chopped the wind to the east again, and in came the fog as
,thick as ever. Captain Clark was now in an awkward situation. He
was in narrow waters and a rapid tide-way. If he turned east too soon,
he might hit Man-of-War Rock, the badly charted bane of the mariner
in these waters. If he delayed too long, he would hit the north shore,
and this is just what he did, poor man.

He was further handicapped by the fact that if he went astern too
fast, he might sink or damage *Maraval*, though it was so thick that day
that I think he was ashore before he saw land. Anyhow, there was

suddenly a loud performance on *Kyle*'s siren, and grinning rocks showed on either side of *Maraval*. The steamer had headed right into a small cove and was in about as awkward a place for getting out again as could be found. Of course, she would not be hurt, as no sea could make, but unless she could get off by her own power plus *Maraval*, there would be a big loss of time and money. It was the mouse's turn to help the lion.[232] It was fortunate that we could still call on our engine in calm water. The tow-line was passed over our stern, and with engines full astern on *Kyle* and full ahead on *Maraval* – nothing happened. There was one other expedient to try. Gathering in the line over our stern, we hauled aft till we could venture no further. Then, with engine ahead, we went forward with a rush, and the sixty-ton *Maraval*, with her 60-HP engine, just managed to dislodge the struggling thousand-ton *Kyle* from her rocky and muddy bed. *Kyle* then anchored, and we went aboard. It seemed hardly the right thing to claim a quarter of a million dollars for salvage under the circumstances.

Such were some of the aspects of this interesting patrol work, though of course but a small selection is possible from many summers' work. In winding up this subject, I will refer to one feature of the autumn programme which always held a great charm and interest for me. This was the collecting and transport of youngsters for the schools at Cartwright and North West River from far-flung homes, whence they could many of them never come except for such help. There was no difficulty about collecting the old scholars returning to school, so far as the children were concerned, at least. In many cases, the new candidates were more than willing, having heard of the good times in store from older brothers and sisters. Occasionally, there was parental obstruction, but there, under the Children's Act, a justice had a strong lever. On one occasion, having determined to recover a bright young Eskimo whose foster-father was, I understood, opposed to his return-ing, I arrived at the encampment where a group of Eskimos were cod fishing, and finding the man in question away I kidnapped the wrong boy, who was more or less the double of the right one. However, when the irate parent protested and I challenged him to show that he could maintain the lad at home without government relief, he curled up [expressed shame]. So as Adam had been spirited away and could not be found, Allan had his berth.

Maraval went from house to house and hamlet to hamlet in the district around Rigolet during most of an autumn day. I remember going to a very distressful homestead on the south shore and collecting a boy and a girl whose mother was dead and their father completely inadequate. He just wandered from one place to another, working for his keep and parking the unfortunate kiddies with a young married couple who had quite enough of their own. The little girl was glad enough to come. She owned only a single garment, a rather porous cotton dress, but she pattered along cheerfully over the rocks, barefoot, to where our dory waited. Once on board, we had to do our best for her, as it was already well into September and apt to be cool. We draped a red blanket more or less artistically, with the help of safety pins, around her gaunt little body, and the heels of a pair of my stockings flopped droopily over the hinder ends of a pair of rubber-soled shoes not much more than two sizes too big. When we finally reached North West River, she had to wait on board until reserves of clothing ashore were tapped for a more seemly landing than she could otherwise have made. And how these youngsters could eat, in harbour or during smooth going! Our cook was a family man with a very fatherly heart, and he just loved to try out their capacity and tabulate results. To some, the experience of a full meal of nourishing food was a novelty.

The end of the season's cruising has ever been a sad occasion for me. The good fellowship on board; the endless variety of the sea, which to me is never monotonous; the contacts with patients, including the human as well as the professional interest; the changing scenes ashore; the adventures, at times, and occasional salvage work; the icebergs and northern lights and other beauties of nature – all these factors combine to make the summer patrol a delightful experience.[233]

19

Recent Developments
and Impending Changes

It has already been mentioned that during the winter of furlough which resulted in the coming of *Maraval* to the Labrador service, the nurse who was left in charge [Kate Austen] was to have a gruelling experience. Of this I saw the aftermath to some extent on my return from England. She saved one young man's life by successful manipulation of a bad rupture [hernia] which had undergone the deadly complication known as "strangulation."[234] She had also to perform a real obstetric operation at a case of childbirth which did not proceed to a normal ending. Both of these were very unusual experiences and very fine achievements of work quite outside a nurse's province, as a general rule. But I think the case of all others that will remain ever a vivid memory to that nurse is the case of Jane Williams.

When we started Yale School at North West River, it was a great satisfaction to be able to draw on graduates of Muddy Bay, not only for domestic servants but even for a house-mother for one of our boarders' cottages. Jane Williams, one of the first group of orphaned children to be admitted to Muddy Bay, was engaged as cook and house-mother's general assistant. And Jane developed a spinal condition that caused a severe degree of paralysis as well as much suffering, requiring constant attention over a period of months. When I returned, there was some sign of returning power in the wasted muscles and slowly regenerating nerves. Jane could at least be out in the sunshine all day and take a keen, co-operative interest in increasing the movements of fingers and toes and hands and feet and later the distance covered with the help of crutches or sticks.

Everything was progressive, hopeful, happy, when Jane went down with a severe broncho-pneumonia. It was a hard struggle, but once again she seemed to be convalescent when there came a relapse. The girl's courage and co-operation in everything asked of her were remarkable, but though fought to the finish, it was a losing battle this time. There came a night when the downward progress was marked to us who watched, and in the morning it was necessary to tell her the truth. I have witnessed a number of deathbed scenes but never a more quietly impressive one. Like a tired child relaxing after an overactive day, she thankfully abandoned the unequal struggle. It was just as if she settled down to sleep, and within a very few minutes breathing ceased. During the following winter, the same nurse had to handle an outbreak of infantile dysentery in the little hamlet of Traverspine, which now boasted three homes. There were two large families alongside one another. Anything more pathetic than utterly miserable, uncomprehending infants in the throes of persistent, painful diarrhoea and severe vomiting is hard to find; and the strain on a nurse, day and night involved in the tending of a group of such patients, must be well nigh unendurable.

A summer or two later, when there had been a hitch over the arrival of a new nurse for the cottage hospital, my wife had to handle a similar but bigger outbreak for seventeen days and nights single-handed. In each outbreak, the loss of life was restricted to a single child. For parents and nurses, it was hard to face the loss, but the salvage work achieved was a real triumph. Another vivid memory for my wife is that of an outbreak of influenza amongst about 130 Montagnais Indians, again at a time when there was no other nurse. Naturally, the demoralisation was frightful. To persuade people accustomed to live in tents, in an atmosphere that could almost be cut with a knife, that their lives might depend on fresh air and sunshine needed at once diplomacy and determination. A soup kitchen was established of which the Indians certainly tried to prolong the existence long after the need was ended. Judson Blake set off in an open motorboat and went day and night for Indian Harbour, and as soon as the news reached there, a relief expedition left within an hour and again went day and night back up the inlet. The worst was over when we arrived, though there was still plenty for the relief nurse to do. Not a single Indian perished in the main attack, though one nomad who returned after the rest were convalescent picked up the infection and unfortunately succumbed. The Indians presented my wife with one of the embroidered caps, similar to those worn by their own squaws, as a reminder of their gratitude.

I have told the story, so far it can be told, of the most desperate battle that I ever fought for a woman's life in childbirth at a lonely hamlet on the long winter trail when on my dog-team patrol. In that case, without proper instruments, if the worst had happened, there was at least every excuse. On the whole, the birth chamber is fairly free from serious complications in Labrador, and apart from the one case mentioned I went twenty years without a case that demanded instrumental interference. Then, within a period of twelve months, I had three cases, two of which provided experiences little less tense than that memorable night at North River. In both these cases, there was no hope of saving both mother and child, but the record of maternal survival remained unbroken after two very anxious periods.

The fight against tuberculosis was achieving very encouraging results. In the early years, it had been a constant dread of "Who next?" One family clan after another had lost its victims of the white plague. Tom Blake, while he had succumbed to Spanish Flu, had fought TB for most of his fifty-eight years. His son Douglas had gone under after a battle lasting five years. Willie Goudie and his son Matthew; two of Allan Goudie's daughters while still very young women; one daughter of Charlie Goudie's while still a girl in her teens; Josephine Hope, the one case to develop and succumb at Muddy Bay School; three young members of the Baikie clan; Peter Michelin, Jr, of Sebaskachu; Charlie Groves' first wife, who was another Montague; two daughters of old Malcolm McLean – here were fifteen killed by TB, and others had shown signs of activity at times. On the other hand, two young men, both of whom had been severely ill, had been trapping for a number of years without a sign of recurrence. As education in hygiene, co-operation on the part of the people, and the supply of fresh vegetables and milk all continued on the upward grade, there was an undoubted decline both in mortality and incidence. When in 1935 Jimmie Michelin ended his long conflict with tuberculosis, it could be truthfully said that there was not a known active case of TB within fifty miles of North West River.

Then in 1936 came a severe epidemic of whooping cough. I was in England at the time, where there was also an unusually severe outbreak of the same disease, and when I heard that it had reached Labrador I groaned, for I knew that the aftermath would be a reappearance of tuberculosis, and so it was. Most fortunately, it was limited to one clan in North West River district, though its ravages in that clan were terrible. A young wife and mother, already handicapped by heart trouble, was quickly overcome. Her husband spent half a year in hospital, and while he was in the little male ward his two-year-old child was also admitted and succumbed. One child lodged with relatives escaped, and the husband and father was driving dogs as vigorously as ever last winter. A sister of his also spent some months in hospital, where she too made a good recovery from the attack.

One discovery I can at least claim to have made independently out here, though it was discovered elsewhere about the same time. I had been reading in a number of the *Review of Tuberculosis*[235] of the direct bactericidal action of cod-oil on the tubercle bacillus. The long resistance maintained against consumption with no other ally but cod-oil, even by some of our poorest, had often impressed me. This was the first time that I saw scientific evidence of the significance of such events. The thought came to me that if cod-oil, when taken internally, could affect consumption of the lungs, why should not a more direct attack by using cod-oil as a dressing for tubercular sores be effective? Selecting a case with consumptive sores on both sides of the body, I used on one side dressing of crude local cod-oil, rendered out from the liver by fishermen's wives at Indian Harbour, and ordinary aseptic dressings on the other. The side treated with cod-oil showed far better progress than the other side, so that too was dressed with cod-oil, and rapid improvement occurred. This was in 1933.

A second experiment on another case gave similar results, and I reported these two cases to a Dr Goodwin,[236] who worked for a while on the Labrador coast in 1934. He also tried it out with results similar to mine, and he was so much impressed that he wanted me to publish the series of cases. I regarded the series as too small to be convincing. It was in 1935 or 1936 that I heard from him again, and he mentioned that a patented ointment, Gadoment, was now on the market in the United States, being a preparation of cod-oil for external use for tubercular lesions.[237] Since then, I have read in the *British Medical Journal* of the use of cod-oil for tubercular lesions as far back as 1843, also that it is now used as a general antiseptic for other infections than tubercular and that crude cod-oil is infinitely to be preferred to refined products.[238] So that while I make no claim, so far as I know, crude cod-oil was in use for external tubercular lesions at Indian Harbour, Labrador, before it was so used anywhere else.

Another great boon and convenience in the treatment of the ever-present fisherman's boils and one of the most valued items, therefore, in *Maraval*'s medical equipment is the comparatively recent product Elastoplast, which is manufactured by T.J. Smith and Nephew of Hull, England. This preparation combined antiseptic dressings and safely anchored bandage, all in one thin layer. It was again in the *British Medical Journal* that I read of its use in the British navy, where it greatly reduced the time lost off duty in case of boils. It is also invaluable for contagious skin troubles such as impetigo, since an occlusive covering can be placed on a sore which effectively prevents spread by contact, either on the patient treated or from him to others, so that school attendance need not be interrupted. It also has many other possibilities described in their place, but I just mention two in which it has been of great value in my own experience.[239]

Another recent development locally has been inoculation against diphtheria, long practised elsewhere, of course. Naturally, we have had antitoxin in case of the disease appearing, but we used to be so much shut off and usually heard well ahead of the approach of epidemics that there was not the same reason for it as outside, and also it naturally takes time to prepare the ground for such innovations in popular opinion. When I was in England in 1936, I received an introduction to Dr Stanley White of Messrs Parke, Davis and Company's staff,[240] with whom I discussed the problem of immunisation in Labrador. He introduced me to Dr Bousfield,[241] whose public clinics in East London I attended on several occasions. Through the good offices of Dr White, the directors of the firm have generously donated a liberal allowance of alum-precipitated toxoid for immunisation work on the Labrador coast, both in 1936 and 1937.

It is remarkable that in so unsophisticated a community as ours out here in the whole of North West River district, with about five hundred inhabitants, I should have met with only one single refusal on the part of parents to allow any child to be inoculated. Otherwise, every child of from one to fifteen years has received the treatment, as well as a number of adult volunteers. And through *Maraval*, the same facilities have been offered around Rigolet, Cartwright, Makkovik, Hopedale, and Nain. One torrid evening on last summer's cruise [1937], we inoculated forty-four youngsters, mostly Eskimos. A small succulent bribe to those who took the needle without any fuss soon popularised the treatment with the younger generation, and there were not a few applicants for a second injection on the same terms. Thus, little by little, progress was made in various departments of public health work.

During a number of years, our local agricultural enterprise received quite a stimulus from a series of visits from a real live agricultural professor from the state college of agriculture for Massachusetts, in the United States.[242] To receive personal visits from such an authority, who showed a strong and sympathetic interest in individual struggles with soil and parasites, lent undoubted encouragement to many who needed it. Another agency that has helped to balance the budget of not a few rather struggling homes has been the auxiliary Industrial Department. Out at Indian Harbour, sealskin mittens and boots and baskets and mats of native grass are the chief output, while further inland deerskin products predominate. Most of the deerskin is smoked, but the unsmoked white skin with the hair off make the daintiest of fur-trimmed mittens and moccasins. Some products are also made from imported textiles and wool. The market is largely local, although some produce is exported. For a number of years, this too was one of my wife's varied activities, but with expansion and departmentalisation it has passed naturally into other hands.

One disease in Labrador that has caused me not a little thought is appendicitis, such a household word elsewhere. Despite the smallness of our population, its rarity as compared to that of Newfoundland, up till very recently at least, has often attracted my attention. I do not know just how far appendicitis is a disease of civilisation or how free or comparatively free rice-eaters and vegetarians may be as compared to flesh-eaters or how far manufactured foods may have been suspected or shown to have any influence on its frequency. I have yet to see my first case in a Labrador Indian, nor have I heard of one; so far as I am concerned, I have seen but one case in an Eskimo, a woman, nor have I heard of another in a Labrador Eskimo. In twenty-four years, I came across or heard of but nine cases in the white or mixed stock of Labrador. Two of these cases were in Fred Blake's family in North West River district. Two were in the family of Charles Bird, our director of outside work at Muddy Bay and then at Cartwright, and both of these cases occurred, I believe, while the girls were being educated in Newfoundland. Two others were in one family in Hopedale district, and the other three were widely scattered. I have not the records of Dr Grieve or Dr Moret or of Dr Hutton, the Moravian veteran of seventeen years' service in Labrador, but considering my extensive travel and familiarity with the people of the coast, this figure is remarkably low.

In all these years, there has been the impression that appendicitis is quite normally common in Newfoundland, and I have certainly seen far more cases among the Newfoundlanders that I have met on the coast in summer than amongst all the Labradormen of my acquaintance. Then, in the spring and summer of 1937, I operated on or saw operated on as many cases as I had recorded in the previous twenty-four years, and I could not help paying some attention to the fact that it was after two almost game-free years, when the biggest horde of foxes on record had decimated grouse and rabbits, that this marked increase of appendicitis occurred. I have already referred to the effects of this sudden revolution in dietetics on other physical conditions and diseases.

Meanwhile, changes were occurring in Newfoundland that were bound to affect the dependency. This island dominion sank into such financial chaos that government by commission came into effect. Distress conditions in Newfoundland were appalling, and Labrador was, it appeared, Newfoundland's greatest asset. A pit-prop industry started up in Alexis Bay, a few miles north of Battle Harbour, by arrangement between the Commission of Government and a Welsh firm.[243] A powerful Canadian mineral corporation [the Iron Ore Company of Canada] received concession over twenty thousand square miles of Labrador territory for survey work, to be followed by something more than survey if anything worthwhile were found, and then in 1936 began the survey of the forest lands around the head of Lake Melville and the lower reaches of Grand River for one of the greatest of British newsprint firms [Bowater-Lloyd].

These activities brought North West River on the map as never before. Steamers came there, also members of the commission who were impressed alike with the agriculture and the forests as well as with the people. Rumour, of course, was rife, but at least there was for the moment a new sphere of employment for trappers in the summer months. A number of these were employed as guides and canoeists away on the height of land; others acted as compassmen for timber cruisers, and the owner of a motorboat stood a chance of a lucrative season. Four airplanes, two for each of the companies, had their cruising base at North West River during the summer of 1937. The winter population of the village now approached three hundred, with a school roll of over ninety. A new church, 80 per cent financed by the people themselves, who also gave much volunteer labour, had replaced the humble edifice of 1915. Considerable co-operation had been shown by the villagers in preserving the natural beauties of the place by replacing cut-out spruce and fir with transplanted birches and poplar.

The germ of administration also appeared in Labrador. A Newfoundland government ranger force was inaugurated, intended to be a replica more or less of the Royal Canadian Mounted Police, once the celebrated North West Mounted Police. The rangers, who were officially attached to the Department of Natural Resources, were not only to act as game wardens but also as poor relief administrators, customs officials and police constables. An experienced veteran of the Canadian force [Sergeant-Major Fred A. Anderton] came to Newfoundland to train recruits. As a justice, I was to have considerable association with the ranger force.

Besides the cottage hospital at St Mary's River, another such institution has lately sprung into being at Cartwright, the chief centre of the chilled salmon industry. While the cod fishery is once more in a very depressed condition after a gleam of hope last summer, the salmon markets are booming, and there is greatly increased competition, which may considerably affect both the relief bill and nutritional disease in Rigolet district and some other poverty-stricken areas. The new little institution at Cartwright is of special importance in proportion to the decline of Indian Harbour fishing and medical activities. Twice in one summer, *Maraval* breezed into Indian Harbour in the nick of time to pick up an acute case there and run it over to Cartwright, fifty miles distant, for immediate operation, and that same season, on another arrival at Indian Harbour, we found a case of acute retention of urine which would have proved fatal within thirty or forty hours.

It is hard to reconcile conflicting interests sometimes. Last summer, an old fisherman friend there came to me in great distress. His wife had had an apoplectic stroke and lay helpless in the crude summer fishing shack, needing attentions which they could ill render. Their fishing activities were almost hopelessly handicapped at a time when every hour, fish, and cent counted for so much. It was Sunday, and we were weekending in Indian Harbour with a dentist on board.[244] It was a perfect day for crossing the wide mouth of the inlet, and I told him to have his wife all ready at one o'clock, when we would run round to the cove where his stage was, ship the patient, and go right on. Just as we were ready to run for Cartwright, three motorboat loads of dental patients boarded us. "It's our only day, doctor." For four hours Dr Timmons worked away, but by the time that we could get under way, there was no hope of reaching Cartwright before nightfall. The approach to Cartwright is not of the easiest in the dark, the last seven miles being through a mass of shoals and low islands in narrow waters. I was particularly anxious to get the patient into hospital without delay, however, though it was a very dark night. We had rather a spicy hour, but we got through all right, and the dental patients were happy too.

What with surveys, new administrative forces, added medical facilities, the decline of one fish market, and the boom of another, the recent past and the present are times of transition and suspense. What will be the outcome of it all? The more thoughtful of our neighbours have mixed feelings. They know that they stand on the edge of a precipice, perhaps, or at best at a parting of the ways. And will it be for the better or for the worse? They hate to see old times, old customs, the old mode of life vanishing, while they realise clearly that furring has long since reached its saturation point as a main means of subsistence and that two bad furring years in succession would mean hard times for many. We who have known this little northern community so long also deplore the inevitable changes that time must work, while realising that they are inevitable and to some, at least, economically beneficial.

Conclusion

The hour has struck.

It was rather like watching the judge put on the black cap as we tuned in on St John's, Newfoundland, and heard the commissioner for Natural Resources announce concessions in forest lands of this region to Messrs Bowater, Lloyd & Co. and the impending erection of a lumbermen's town somewhere in this vicinity. Since then, there have been further negotiations between firm and government and a moratorium in regard to the Labrador while other big deals are being put through in Newfoundland by the same firm. It is only a matter of time. If this firm does not operate here, another will. The coming of Big Business will presumably mean another source of medical and educational service.

The questions to be settled are, first, where will such a town be located and, secondly, whom will the firm employ? And thirdly, what facilities will be extended, not only to employees but to other inhabitants in the neighbourhood? Notoriously, the cheapest and best woodsmen in the world come from Eastern Canada. At the same time, naturally, the firm will be urged to employ as much labour from Newfoundland and Labrador as may be compatible with their own interests. There will certainly be a considerable proportion whom they will not employ for various reasons, but it looks as if the end of the pioneer service may be imminent.

It is not for any man to estimate his own work, and in so far as I comment on it at all, it is to make it clear that if I hope there may be a credit side I am fully conscious that any credit must be shared with others, and also that I am well aware that there is a debit side. At least one may surely reflect with some satisfaction on the progress made, I sincerely believe, against tuberculosis. Twenty-five years ago, the lack of knowledge of hygiene alone was enough to maintain almost an epidemic stage of TB. The deficient ventilation, the common water dipper passed from hand to hand and mouth to mouth, as well as other eating and drinking utensils recklessly shared by diseased and healthy alike – all these, added in many cases to poverty and defective diet and clothing, were enabling tuberculosis to reap a ghastly toll. Around centres of work in Labrador, tuberculosis has unquestionably been reduced from almost an epidemic to a sporadic stage. In any community, alas, occasional cases are to be found. And this has been achieved in spite of the advantage to the enemy afforded by consanguinity, the intermarriage with cousins inevitable in a small community still further divided into well marked sub-communities. The strongholds of tuberculosis are now in outlying hamlets and lone homesteads where whole families are still decimated and almost exterminated by blind, deaf, non-cooperative victims alike of tradition and disease. Another real advance has been made against such nutritional diseases as scurvy, beri-beri, and rickets. Many of the people have an intelligent grasp of their causes and the way to prevent them, while around centres of work, with the exception of a few indifferent folk, shiftless individuals or families, these diseases have been practically put off the map.

The unbroken record of maternal survival in childbirth has very greatly helped to popularise better pre-natal care for the expectant mother as well as better treatment at confinements, and the welfare of the new-born infant has received a strong stimulus. The institutional work in the sphere of child welfare, which has naturally been shared by children of neighbouring residents, has also had a very marked effect on the diet, clothing, and general discipline of the younger generation as well as on the correction of physical defect. Further, educational activities directed towards self-dependence classes in first aid and home nursing have also had their value in effect. All these have subsidised the routine of wards and dispensary.

Finally, the auxiliary services – the school, the Industrial Department, and the farm – have all, to my mind, been practical forms of preventive medicine. The school, of course, has had another value. Unquestionably, numbers of the younger generation are better equipped for getting better jobs than mere rough labour because of their training in these little institutions. And even the production of a handful of nurses, teachers, and house-mothers for boarders, as well as a number of good domestic servants and promising homemakers, is something to rejoice over. In regard to these items on the credit side of the ledger, it is the

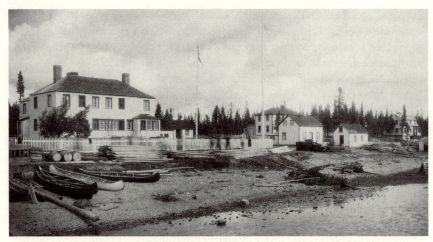

The new hospital at North West River, *left*, school at centre in the background, and Wood Cottage to the right (Fred C. Sears)

doctor's wife, nurses, teachers, and industrial workers, as well as a number of generous supporters, to whom most of the credit is due.

When it comes to things left undone or that might have been done better, there is admittedly room for regret. In the first place, obviously no one who wanted to make a successful career for himself by keeping abreast of the march of scientific progress outside would come to Labrador for more than a short period. Any surgeon knows that to do good surgery with speed, dexterity, and confidence and boldness, combined with soundness, constant practice is essential, an essential which is impossible for the pioneer in the back-of-beyond. And if this is true of surgery, what about the almost bewildering advances in many branches of medicine? For the frontier practitioner, without consultants and with medical literature arriving in accumulations after an eight-month winter, just at the time when he is most busily occupied during the short open-water season and with many strings to his bow, it is no easy problem to keep up to date. At the same time, it is always possible to do more, perhaps, than is done under such circumstances. When he emerges after more than three years of dog-team and small boat practice, as well as of the cottage hospital work in a centre with a population of barely five hundred, it is to find practitioners and students outside talking almost in a strange tongue. Some rest is essential and some renewal of ties of kinship, and then there is ever the problem of funds, which means more work.

It is given to few to do many things well. To a man like Albert Schweitzer, who can vindicate a doctorate in divinity, philosophy, medicine, and music, I can but pay my homage. Having tried myself to combine the roles of small institutional physician and surgeon, family doctor and friend, parish priest, amateur navigator and pilot, justice of the peace, promoter of education and agriculture, and finally, financial campaigner, I can only frankly admit that the task has been beyond me. None the less, there has been a good deal of interest, humour, and adventure in trying. I hope and believe that a portion, at least, of this northern community is better equipped for the great changes that are coming to their country and themselves than was the case twenty-five years ago.

And where I have tried to give credit to fellow workers, I must not omit the very real co-operation, friendship, and financial support supplied by the people themselves, which has been a considerable asset to the work. Nor do I forget the self-denial and devotion of junior members of staff, including many volunteers and also our auxiliary staff. I remember the spectacle of a diminutive Labrador cook, with one arm in a sling for a painful condition, carrying on with her catering for nearly sixty people in the old hustling days at Indian Harbour; and I also recall the one survivor of seven maids during the measles epidemic referred to above, trying to do as much as possible of the work of six others besides her own. I remember too an occasion when funds were particularly scarce and the prospect of being able to carry on as usual was a gloomy one, and I was handed a "round robin" offering of a month's service without salaries or wages from members of staff and domestic staff. Such memories have a very real fragrance.

Great changes are imminent, undoubtedly. Forests will contribute their quota, and the face of nature will be mutilated alike by woodsmen and miners. Great herds of domesticated reindeer will probably browse on the moss tundras and cause widespread repercussions in the world's meat markets. Developments in the fisheries may prove only to have begun. Sportsmen will fly to our rivers, and commercial planes will abound. Navigation will increase. The native races may be exterminated or put on reserves, and a new population may destroy the identity of the community that we have known. But at least one phenomenon of this sub-arctic belt will remain unspoiled, intangible, inaccessible, unchanged though ever varying, and that is the aurora.[245]

Notes

ABBREVIATIONS

ADSF *Among the Deep Sea Fishers*
BA Bachelor of Arts
BS Bachelor of Surgery
ChB Bachelor of Surgery
CM Master of Surgery
FRCS Fellow of the Royal College of Surgeons
HBC Hudson's Bay Company
HLP Henry (Harry) Locke Paddon
IGA International Grenfell Association
JPL Jessie (Paddon) Lloyd
LRCP Licentiate of the Royal College of Physicians
MB Bachelor of Medicine
MD Doctor of Medicine
MS Master of Surgery
MGP Mina (Gilchrist) Paddon
MRCS Member of the Royal College of Surgeons
RAMC Royal Army Medical Corps
RN Royal Navy
RNMDSF Royal National Mission to Deep Sea Fishermen
Toilers *Toilers of the Deep*
WAP William Anthony (Tony) Paddon
WTG Wilfred Thomason Grenfell

INTRODUCTION

1 WAP to WTG, 22 January [1940], Wilfred T. Grenfell Papers.

2 For historical details of the Paddon family, I am indebted to Raymond Lloyd, "Jessie Marian Paddon, 1877–1958" (1986).

3 Foster, *Alumni Oxonienses*, vol. 3, 1055.

4 Meacham, *Lord Bishop: The Life of Samuel Wilberforce*, 111.

5 Meacham, 113.

6 Foster, 1055.

7 Groves, *Historical Records of the 7th or Royal Regiment of Fusiliers*, 397.

8 When the Reverend Henry Paddon refused to settle anything upon his son, the bride's father, James Van Sommer, refused to settle an equal amount upon his daughter. However, Van Sommer paid the interest on the sum not settled upon his daughter and her children for life until, at his own death, they succeeded to their mother's share of the property (Paddon and Van Sommer Family Papers: transcription of letter by Elisabeth Van Sommer, February 1904).

9 Birth certificate of Henry Locke Paddon, 22 August 1881, Paddon and Van Sommer Family Papers.

10 Jessie M. Paddon [Lloyd], [Narrative of her early life, 1883–1902], 2. Milk fever: an infectious condition of the mother which if not treated immediately could be fatal. See Smith, *The Handbook for Midwives*, 151.

11 Groves, 397.

12 See Randolph Vigne, "The Van Sommers – A Huguenot Tradition," *Proceedings of the Huguenot Society of London* 24 (1986): 285–95.

13 Paddon [Lloyd], 13.

14 Ibid., 56.

15 Milward, *A New Short History of Wimbledon*, 18.

16 Paddon [Lloyd], 19.

17 HLP to Dr Frank Babbott, 10 October 1925, Richard Paddon Papers.

18 Messiter, ed., *Repton School Register, 1557–1910*, 379.

19 Thomas, ed., *Repton, 1557–1957*, 75.

20 *Reptonian* 25 (July 1900): 103.

21 *Reptonian* 24 (August 1899): 113; *Reptonian* 25 (July 1900):101.

22 High Court of Justice, Principal Registry, Family Division: Will of James Van Sommer, dated 12 December 1900, probated 25 April 1901.

23 See University College Oxford Admissions Register, 1863–1940, and Tutorial Lists, 1896–1914.

24 HLP to Elisabeth Van Sommer, 21 June 1925, Richard Paddon Papers.

25 H.L. Paddon, "Forty Days with Fleeters and Single-Boaters," 236–7.

26 Gordon, *What Cheer O?*, 90–1.

27 H.L. Paddon, "A Trip to the Great Northern Fleet," 167; "North Sea Wanderings in August and September," 256.

28 *St. Thomas' Hospital Gazette*, 18 (June 1908): 99; 18 (July 1908): 125, 126; 19 (October 1909): 149.

29 Ibid., 20 (November 1910): 193.

30 H.L. Paddon, "Adrift in a Fish-Carrier," 303.

31 *Annual Report of Dudley Guest Hospital*, 16. In the United Kingdom, before a medical student is registered, he must not only complete an approved course of study but work as a house officer for a year in a recognized hospital, six months in surgery and six months in medicine.

32 *St. Thomas' Hospital Gazette* 21 (February 1911): 71; Records of the Guest Hospital, Dudley: Minutes of the Weekly Board, 10 February 1911.

33 Records of the Guest Hospital, Dudley: Minutes of the Weekly Board, 1 February 1912.

34 Kirby to Colonial Secretary, 29 May 1912, Colonial Secretary's Correspondence.

35 Attorney General to Colonial Secretary, 5 August 1912, Colonial Secretary's Correspondence.

36 Journal-letter, 1 December 1912, W. Anthony Paddon Fonds.

37 HLP to JPL, 6 March [1913], Richard Paddon Papers.

38 Wallace, ed., *John McLean's Notes of a Twenty-Five Years' Service in the Hudson's Bay Territory*, 284.

39 Davies, "Notes on Esquimaux Bay and the Surrounding Country," 89.

40 Tremblay, ed., *Journal des voyages de Charles Arnaud, 1872–1873*, 13: "Someone who has spent a long time among them told me that not a single woman or girl was chaste; they are like that, and we can't do anything about it, poor Eskimos."

41 Mina had two older sisters and an older brother. See New Brunswick Census, 1871, 1881, 1891: Queen's County, Cambridge Parish; *McAlpine's New Brunswick Directory for 1896*, 1115; School Trustee's Returns, Sunbury County, New Brunswick, June 1897.

42 Student Records, Massachusetts General Hospital School of Nursing, 1873–1981: vol. S, 26; Boston Medical Library's Directory for Nurses, 1907–08, 194.

43 Reverby, *Ordered to Care*, 95–105.

44 Certificate of marriage dated 30 August 1915, Paddon and Van Sommer Family Papers.

45 Journal-letter, 9 June 1914, W. Anthony Paddon Fonds.

46 MGP to JPL, 14 June 1915, Richard Paddon Papers.

47 HLP to Richard Squires, 23 August 1917, Colonial Secretary's Correspondence.

48 "Report of an Official Visit to the Coast of Labrador," 362.

49 HLP to JPL, [December 1919], Richard Paddon Papers.

50 Gordon, "Labrador Teacher," 24.

51 HLP to Van Sommer family, 16 April 1927, Richard Paddon Papers.

52 HLP to JPL, 29 December 1928, Richard Paddon Papers.

53 HLP to JPL, 28 November 1928, Richard Paddon Papers.

54 HLP to JPL, 29 December 1928, Richard Paddon Papers.

55 HLP to JPL, 20 September 1930, Richard Paddon Papers.

56 HLP to Van Sommer family, 27 October 1932, Richard Paddon Papers.

57 Parsons to Fr O'Brien, 2 August 1933, Monsignor Edward Joseph O'Brien Letters and Papers. HLP also broached the subject of centralization in the Labrador souvenir supplement of the *St John's Daily News*, 19 October 1938.

58 Parsons to Fr O'Brien, 2 August 1933, Monsignor Edward Joseph O'Brien, Letters and Papers.

59 HLP to JPL, 22 June 1935, Richard Paddon Papers.

60 Ashdown and Green, "Report of the Commission Appointed by the Directors … to Confer with the Commission of Government," International Grenfell Association Fonds, 11. A financial shortfall was also reported by the consultancy firm of Tamblyn & Brown, Inc., in 1938.

61 Ashdown and Green, "Report of the Commission," 15, 17.

62 Ewbank, "The Bowater Agreement," in *Public Affairs in Newfoundland*, 10. See also Hiller, "The Politics of Newsprint," 34–6.

63 HLP to Van Sommer Family, 26 April 1938, W. Anthony Paddon Fonds.

64 Lady Grenfell to HLP, 21 April 1938, Wilfred T. Grenfell Papers.

65 H.L. Paddon, "North West River Jottings," 64.

66 HLP to Lady Grenfell, 16 June 1938, Wilfred T. Grenfell Papers.

67 MGP to Katie Spalding, 18 January 1940, Richard Paddon Papers. HLP's ashes were laid to rest in the cemetery at North West River. See photo of grave marked by a giant slab of Labradorite in Rev. G. Fowlow, "Labrador Voyage," 19.

68 MGP to Van Sommer family, 26 December 1939, Richard Paddon Papers.

69 Curtis to Ashdown, 20 February 1940, International Grenfell Association Fonds.

70 "Report of Commission on Public Health, 1911," 588–9.

71 Sontag, *Illness as Metaphor*, 14.

72 Leared, "On the Use of Cod-liver Oil Oleine," 58.

73 Macpherson, "The First Recognition of Beri-Beri in Canada," 278.

74 Little, "Beriberi Caused by Fine White Flour," 2029–30.

75 Little, "Beriberi," 1288.

76 Delatour, "Dr. John Mason Little," 11.

77 Appleton, "Observations on Deficiency Diseases in Labrador," 620.

78 Moseley, "The Third Year of Health Work," 106–9.

79 Aykroyd, "Vitamin a Deficiency in Newfoundland," 165.

80 Aykroyd, "Beriberi and Other Food-Deficiency Diseases in Newfoundland and Labrador," 367.

81 Mitchell, "Nutrition Survey in Labrador and Northern Newfoundland," 33.
82 Post Manager's journal, North West River, 31 October and 18 November 1918, Hudson's Bay Company Records.
83 Collier, *The Plague of the Spanish Lady*, 305.
84 Crosby, *Epidemic and Peace, 1918*, 189.
85 Billson, "The Memoir: New Perspectives on a Forgotten Genre," 264.
86 Neary, *Newfoundland in the North Atlantic World, 1929–1949*, 40.

THE LABRADOR MEMOIR OF DR HARRY PADDON

1 Major-General Charles George "Chinese" Gordon (1833–85) of the Royal Engineers, colonial administrator and Christian idealist, killed at the siege of Khartoum.
2 Sir Henry Tristram Holland (1875–1965), eye surgeon, joined the Church Missionary Society in the Punjab, where he remained for nearly fifty years.
3 Albert Schweitzer (1875–1965), German theologian, physician, and musician, established a hospital in French Equatorial Africa. Awarded the Nobel Peace Prize in 1952, he used the money to expand his hospital and build a leper colony.
4 C.T. Studd (1860–1931), outstanding British cricketer, devoted his life to Christianity after hearing the American evangelist Dwight L. Moody preach. Studd worked first in China, then in southern India and Africa. Wilfred Grenfell, while still a medical student, attended a Moody revival meeting in East London where Studd and his brother, J.E. Studd, were speaking and "stood up" for Christ, turning his life in the direction of practical Christianity. See Grenfell, *A Labrador Doctor*, 45.
5 Clarence Birdseye (1886–1956) of Brooklyn, New York, invented frozen foods as a result of his experience in Labrador. He first went to the coast with Grenfell in 1912 and returned to settle at Muddy Bay, where he started fur-trading and fox farming. Fishing through the ice, he noticed that freshly caught fish, when exposed to the icy wind and frigid temperatures, froze solid almost immediately and that when thawed and eaten they retained their fresh characteristics. He concluded that quick-freezing the fish prevented large crystals from forming, thus avoiding damage to their cellular structure.
6 SS *Tunisian*, 500 feet and 576 gross tons, a ship of the Allan Line built in 1900 at Linthouse, Scotland, and frequently used as an immigrant ship between Liverpool and Quebec City. She was scrapped at Genoa in 1928.
7 Thomas Barnardo (1845–1905) founded in the east end of London a mission for rescuing destitute children and in 1870 opened a boys' home in Stepney. His institutions sent thousands of children to British colonies and dependencies.

8 Gilbert Parker's *Seats of the Mighty* (1896), a romance set in eighteenth-century Quebec, captures the moment of British victory in 1759.

9 Thomas Gray, "An Elegy Wrote in a Country Church Yard" (1751), but HLP probably had in mind Gray's ruminations on lost youth in "An Ode on a Distant Prospect of Eton College" (1747), written from the perspective of the heights of Windsor.

10 The Government of Canada established the Intercolonial Railway in 1867 to fulfil one of the promises made to Nova Scotia and New Brunswick at Confederation: namely, to link the Maritime Provinces to central Canada and encourage industrialization. The railway was eventually absorbed into the Canadian National Railways system.

11 SS *Bruce*, 250 feet and 1,553 gross tons, built in Scotland in 1911 for the Reid Newfoundland Company, replaced the first *Bruce*, which was lost in the ice. These vessels provided a link between the railheads at North Sydney, Nova Scotia, and Port aux Basques, Newfoundland.

12 The Reid Newfoundland Company, which held a virtual monopoly on transportation, inaugurated a rail passenger service across the island of Newfoundland in 1898.

13 The Corner Brook mill was established in 1923, partly through the efforts of the prime minister, Sir Richard Squires, and the Newfoundland Power and Paper Company, Ltd. was formed. After two years of operation, the mill and its power station at Deer Lake were sold to a company that included the International Paper Company of New York. It was sold again in 1938 to the British company Bowater-Lloyd, at the time HLP completed his memoir.

14 HLP refers to Dillon Wallace, *The Lure of the Labrador Wild* (1905), an account of the tragic expedition conducted by Leonidas Hubbard, Jr.

15 SS *Prospero*, 205 feet and 978 gross tons, a coastal vessel of C.T. Bowering & Co. built at Port Glasgow, Scotland, with accommodation for 150 passengers.

16 James W. Wiltsie, medical assistant at Spotted Islands, and Alice Metcalfe, nurse at Battle Harbour, both from the state of New York.

17 SS *Clyde*, 155 feet and 439 gross tons, built at Glasgow in 1900 for the Reid Newfoundland Company.

18 Absurd tea party in Lewis Carroll, *Alice's Adventures in Wonderland* (1865).

19 The next section was first published as H.L. Paddon, "Ye Goode Olde Dayes," ADSF (July 1929): 51–7.

20 Alfred, first baron Tennyson (1809–1892), author of the ballad "The Revenge" (1880). Grenfell liked to claim kinship with Sir Richard but showed no evidence to support it.

21 Grenfell's ticket qualified him to take a yacht to sea but not to undertake overseas voyages.

22 Taylor, *A Manual of the Practice of Medicine*, 107: "It has been attributed to unsuitable food, e.g., mouldy rice; to bacilli found in the gastro-duodenal contents; and to toxins generated by organisms outside the body. But the cause is not yet really known."

23 Taylor, 108: "There is no specific for this disease. The essential thing is the removal to an uninfected locality; or failing that, to a well ventilated apartment high above the soil. Little more can be done in the early stages; in the later, iron and strychnine internally, and faradisation and massage to the limbs are recommended. For serious cardiac failure active purgatives, full doses of nitroglycerine or nitrite of amyl, and, if necessary, bleeding should be employed."

24 Vitamine: the first citation in the *Oxford English Dictionary* is dated 1912.

25 John Mason Little (1875–1926), a graduate of the Harvard Medical School who arrived in St Anthony in 1907, quickly became Grenfell's chief hospital administrator and surgeon. In 1917 Little returned to Boston with his wife, Ruth, a Mission teacher, and their four children. He died suddenly of pulmonary embolism combined with an inflammation of the heart muscle, and his ashes were returned to St Anthony, where they were sealed in a rock face on Fox Farm Hill, near those of Grenfell himself.

26 See Longfellow's translation of Friedrich von Langau, *Sinngedichte* (1653): "Though the mills of God grind slowly, yet they grind exceeding small;/Though with patience He stands waiting, with exactness grinds He all."

27 ss *Strathcona*, the first power-driven hospital vessel of the Royal National Mission to Deep Sea Fishermen, built by Philip and Sons, Dartmouth, and launched in 1899. This vessel, 97 feet long and 18 feet at the beam, displaced 130 tons and was fitted up with swinging cots and X-ray apparatus, perhaps the first so designed.

28 French Shore: the section of the north and west coasts of Newfoundland on which the French were granted seasonal fishing and drying privileges by the Treaty of Utrecht, 1713. The provenance of French place names is shown in Hollett and Kirwin, eds., *Place Names of the Northern Peninsula* (2000).

29 Pre-eclampsia and eclampsia: a convulsion or series of convulsions to which pregnant women are susceptible, often associated with hypertension. See also case of eclampsia, p. 156.

30 ss *Home*, 155 feet and 439 gross tons, built at Glasgow in 1900 for the Reid Newfoundland Company.

31 The Industrial Department of the Grenfell mission was inaugurated by Jessie Luther in 1906. See Rompkey, ed., *Jessie Luther at the Grenfell Mission* (2001).

32 According to the classification of the poor in Charles Booth's *Life and Labour of the People of London* (1889), Class B included those who because of shiftlessness, helplessness, idleness, or drink were inevitably poor, Class C those who worked by the job according to the season.

33 Charles Martyn Spencer (1887–1977), son of Grenfell's aunt, Evelyn Hutchison, and the Rev. Frederick Hamilton Spencer, a New Zealand missionary. Spencer trained at Macdonald College, McGill University, and during the summers helped establish gardens at St Anthony. Graduating with a degree in agriculture in 1911, he returned to New Zealand, where he developed a fruit orchard at Henderson, near Auckland.

34 Edgar "Ted" McNeill (1884–1970), formerly of Island Harbour, Labrador, had received some formal schooling at the Moravian boarding school at Makkovik and learned basic carpentry and drafting from the Rev. Hermann Jannasch. He later trained at the Pratt Institute and ultimately became designer and superintendent of the Grenfell Mission buildings. In 1955 he was elected mayor of St Anthony.

35 John Grieve, who received the MB and CHB (Edinburgh) in 1904, served at Battle Harbour at various times between 1906 and 1915 and at Harrington Harbour, 1913–14. He was appointed secretary and business manager of the Grenfell Mission office at St John's in 1918.

36 Baine, Johnston & Co. owned the property. For the events surrounding the establishment of this hospital, see Rompkey, ed., *Labrador Odyssey* (1996).

37 SS *Sagona*, 175 feet and 808 gross tons, built in 1912 at Dundee, Scotland, with accommodation for fifty saloon and forty steerage passengers. In 1923 *Sagona* was acquired by the Newfoundland government as a coastal steamer for the northern route as part of a larger deal with the Reid Newfoundland Company. As an icebreaker, she was also used in the seal fishery until 1938.

38 Plimsoll marks: gradation on a ship's side indicating the legal limits of submersion.

39 The Hawke Harbour whaling station, run by the Labrador Whaling and Manufacturing Company, incorporated in 1904, was the most successful of the twenty-one stations operated in Newfoundland and Labrador.

40 HLP conflates two Cartwrights engaged in the same Labrador enterprise: John Cartwright (1740–1824), social reformer and one-time major of militia, and George Cartwright (1739/40–1819), entrepreneur.

41 John Montagu, fourth earl of Sandwich (1718–92), first lord of the Admiralty, and political patron during George Cartwright's tenure. The bay, however, was more probably named by Captain James Cook, who surveyed it for the Admiralty and named it as he did the Sandwich Islands.

42 See George Cartwright, *Journal of Transactions and Events* (1792).

43 As part of a round-the-world tour, a squadron of U.S. Navy seaplanes landed there in August 1924.

44 General Italo Balbo (1896–1940), Italian fascist and minister of aviation, commanded a squadron of twenty-four hydroplanes which landed in Cartwright in 1933, in conjunction with the yacht *Alicia*, en route to the Chicago Century of Progress Exhibition. W.O. Douglas wrote, "The visitors were extremely kind to the Cartwright people and staged a reception to which all were invited. It was held in the Grenfell Association building. Catering was done by the yacht's chef and his staff, and wine flowed freely. A decorative archway built by the yacht's crew marked the entrance to the building and a large picture of Benito Mussolini hung on the wall. This painting was left in the building and was later destroyed when the building burned.

"There was a constant going and coming to and from the yacht, the shore, and the aircraft anchored in the bay. The local fishermen were plied with more wine than was good for them. The voluble, gesturing Italian airmen fascinated the local people who began to imitate them. So much wine was flowing that some of us had serious doubts as to whether or not this air armada would reach Chicago" (Douglas, "Memories of Muddy Bay," 46).

45 HLP refers to the effects of syphilis, as noted by the Moravian physician Dr S.K. Hutton, *Health Conditions and Disease among the Eskimos of Labrador*, 17: "The disease was brought to the coast by a party of Eskimos who had been exported for exhibition purposes by a speculator; two men are known to have had symptoms of syphilis at the time of their return from exhibition in 1902, and from this starting point the disease spread rapidly but insidiously." Hutton, who had worked directly with the Inuit population for seven years, argued that the incidence of syphilis had lowered the birth rate among the indigenous population and threatened its survival.

46 The HBC agent John McLean wrote in the mid-nineteenth century, "The Esquimaux half-breeds are both industrious and ingenious; they are at a loss for nothing. The men make their own boats, and the women prepare everything required for domestic convenience; almost every man is his own blacksmith and carpenter, and every woman a tailor and shoemaker. They seem to possess all the virtues of the different races from which they are sprung – except courage; they are generally allowed to be more timid than the natives" (Wallace, ed., *John McLean's Notes*, 285).

47 Like Shylock, the usurer in Shakespeare's *Merchant of Venice* (1600), I. iii. 144–52, who called for a forfeit of a pound of flesh if a loan were not repaid.

48 SS *Meigle*, 220 feet and 836 gross tons, built in 1881 at Lanark, Scotland, and owned by the Reid Newfoundland Company. *Meigle*

was used as a passenger and cargo vessel until the 1930s. In 1932, she was appropriated as an auxiliary jail and for that purpose was anchored in St John's harbour until 1933, when she was converted to a salt storage hulk, but in 1936 she was purchased by a Halifax company and taken back into service. *Meigle* was again pressed into service during the Second World War and survived until 1947, when she was wrecked at Marines Cove, Newfoundland.

49 Austin Bryant Reeve, Jr (1891–1968), son of a banker in Princeton, Illinois, educated at the University High School, Chicago, and the Hotchkiss School before entering the Sheffield Scientific School, Yale University, graduating in 1913. Reeve took a further degree in mechanical engineering from the Massachusetts Institute of Technology in 1916. He began an engineering career in New York with Westinghouse, Church, Kerr and Co. in 1917 but left to join the 311th Regiment, U.S. Army Engineers, attaining the rank of captain, and served in France. A Presbyterian, Reeve wrote in an alumni questionnaire that the most valuable thing he had obtained from his college career was the realization that the purpose of life was "to serve a devine [sic] master." He did not mention his experience in Labrador.

50 Charles A. Jerrett (1866–1935) entered his father's mercantile firm at Brigus, Newfoundland, at the age of fourteen and operated seasonally at Indian Harbour for twenty-three years. HLP explained to the family, "By last boat there came a Mr Jerrett, who owns the store here [sic], and does the biggest fish trade from here, buying up the season's catch from several lesser men outright. He supplies the hospital gratis with all the fish we need, and has done so for years, and, owning a motor launch, he saves us long rows over to the Marconi station from time to time, by sending for our messages when the signal flag shows there are such for us" (Journal Letter, 15 August 1912, W. Anthony Paddon Fonds).

51 The discarded surgical instruments, more prone to surgical infection, were probably donated. Such infection had been reduced considerably by Joseph Lister (1827–1912), who discovered antiseptics in 1865. At first Lister believed that infection was caused by airborne dust particles and sprayed the air with carbolic acid, but in 1865 he came upon the germ theory of Louis Pasteur, whose experiments revealed that fermentation and putrefaction were caused by micro-organisms brought into contact with organic material. Lister's discoveries met resistance at first, but by the 1880s they had become widely accepted.

52 Room: tract of waterfront land where fish is processed.

53 Planter: migratory Newfoundland fisherman conducting a summer fishery from a room in Labrador.

54 Kindle, *Geography and Geology of Lake Melville District*, 11: "The mountains of the plateau margin are composed of crystalline rocks of

Precambrian age and rise near the valleys as a rule from 800 to 2,000 feet A.T."

55 Väinö Tanner (1881–1948), Finnish geologist, anthropologist, geographer, and diplomat who produced the exhaustive study *Outlines of the Geography, Life and Customs of Newfoundland-Labrador* (1947). Tanner was awarded a doctorate in geology from Finland's Institute of Technology in 1914 for his ongoing studies of shoreline displacements in northern Europe after the Glacial Age. He became state geologist in 1918 but in the same year entered the foreign service as Finland's representative in the Balkan area, residing at Bucharest. In 1930 he took the chair of Geology at the University of Helsinki, and in 1936, in search of solutions to Fennoscandian problems in geography and geology on the other side of the Atlantic, he organized the Labrador expedition of 1937, which together with the expedition of 1939 resulted in the study published a year before he died.

56 Yale: forty-four foot ketch built by Rice Brothers, East Boothbay, Maine, and equipped with a ten-horsepower engine.

57 Revillon Frères Trading Co., Ltd., the Canadian fur-trading arm of the Paris-based Revillon Co., which first challenged the supremacy of the HBC in 1901. Revillon Frères offered competition until 1926, when HBC purchased 51 per cent of the Revillon stock. The two then operated ostensibly in competition until 1936, when HBC purchased the company outright.

58 RMS *Nascopie*, 286 feet and 2,476 gross tons, built in 1911 by Swan Hunter and Wigham Richardson, Neptune Works, Wallsend-on-Tyne.

59 Frank Lusk Babbott (1891–1970) arrived in Labrador at the end of his third year at Amherst College. After a year at medical school, he returned to Indian Harbour as assistant and helped establish the winter quarters at North West River. He was later president of the Long Island College of Medicine, where HLP's son Tony trained, and served on numerous boards and committees of Grenfell associations. He wrote to HLP later, "You have no idea how many times I look back on the summers of '12 and '14 which were without doubt one of the most powerful influences of my life" (Babbott to HLP, 13 January 1926, Richard Locke Paddon Papers).

60 HLP is not suggesting that scurvy is a consequence of club foot but that the case of club foot created circumstances of inactivity in which the patient's diet changed.

61 2 Thessalonians: 3:10: "For even when we were with you, this we commanded you, that if any would not work, neither should he eat."

62 Robert Edwin Peary (1856–1920), civil engineer of the U.S. Navy and arctic explorer, left New York on 6 July 1908 on his last attempt to reach the North Pole and passed through the Strait of Belle Isle, sending

a boat ashore at Point Amour lighthouse with telegrams before proceeding up the Labrador coast. He stopped at Indian Harbour on his return in the fall of 1909.

63 Donald Baxter Macmillan (1874–1970) accompanied Peary to the North Pole in 1908–9. He later designed the schooner *Bowdoin*, in which he engaged in twenty-six scientific voyages in various northern locations during the period 1921–54.

64 HLP applies army ranks to the RCMP, whose lowest commissioned rank is inspector. The rank of sergeant does exist, and below that corporal and constable.

65 Robert Abram Bartlett (1875–1946) accompanied Peary on three attempts to reach the North Pole, the second and third in command of the *Roosevelt*. In the *Effie M. Morrissey*, a two-masted schooner, 97 feet and 120 tons, donated by James B. Ford of New York in 1925, Bartlett sailed on numerous arctic expeditions during the period 1926–45.

66 Arthur W. Wakefield (1876–1949), son of William Wakefield of the Wakefield and Crewdson banking house, was educated at Sedbergh School, Yorkshire, and admitted a pensioner at Trinity College Cambridge in 1895, proceeding BA in 1898, MA, MB, and BChir in 1906, and MD in 1909. At Cambridge he won blues in boxing and cycling but interrupted his medical training to fight in the Boer War as a trooper, then qualified as MRCS and LRCP in 1904. That same year he won the United Hospitals heavyweight boxing championship, captained the London Hospital rugby team, and established a mountain-climbing record on Sca Fell Pike. He then studied surgery with Lister at the University of Edinburgh and subsequently at Heidelburgh, where he spoke fluent German, and served in the North Sea with the RNMDSF before coming to Labrador, 1908–14, as a voluntary medical officer. While working in Labrador, Wakefield disappeared in the summers to climb in the Rockies. Passing through Montreal, he met his future wife, whom he married in 1910, and their eldest son was born at Forteau. Wakefield had been a camping companion of HLP. From 1910 he had included him on the address list of the "diaries" he sent to the U.K., a practice HLP was to adopt himself. Wakefield left to serve in the RAMC, 1914–18, and was mentioned in despatches. He was a member of the Everest expedition of 1922, then settled at Keswick as a general practitioner.

67 Marjorie Wakefield (1886–1976) held a degree in French from McGill University. She took a year's training in dentistry before arriving on the Labrador coast.

68 HLP wrote to his sister from Mud Lake, "Miss Coates, the nurse, is rather a mis-fit, unfortunately, and as she and Mrs. Wakefield are both 'strong-minded females' the fur flies a bit occasionally – however it never lasts very long" (HLP to JPL, 6 March 1912, Richard Locke Paddon Papers).

69 Grey Owl: Canadian author and conservationist, born Archibald
   Stansfeld Belaney (1888–1938) at Hastings, the son of a Sussex doctor.
   Adopting the identity of Grey Owl, Belaney acquired international
   recognition in the 1930s for his writings and lectures on the north,
   but his contributions were somewhat diminished by the revelation of his
   true identity following his death in April 1938, after HLP had completed
   his manuscript.

70 Jack Miner (1865–1944), pioneer protector of migratory waterfowl,
   was born in Dover Center, Ohio, but moved to Ontario as a boy.
   In 1904 he founded the Jack Miner Bird Sanctuary for the conservation
   of migrating Canada geese and wild ducks. At his death he had banded
   over fifty thousand wild ducks and forty thousand migratory Canada
   geese and was ranked as the fifth best known man on the continent
   after Henry Ford, Thomas Edison, Charles Lindbergh, and Eddie
   Rickenbacker.

71 Flat: flat-bottomed, square-sterned boat about ten feet long, propelled
   by oars and used as a tender.

72 Anthony Mugford's family, who drowned in May 1928 while he was
   away at his traps: his wife, Mary Jane (Pottle) Mugford, 38; Elijah, 18;
   Sarah Elizabeth, 15; Freeman, 10; and Harriet Pottle, 14.

73 Kindle, 71: "The shape of Hamilton Inlet appears to justify its classification as a *ria*. This disposition or classification of Hamilton Inlet places it
   in a category of coast-line features which includes both river estuaries
   and indentations of the seacoast with sides which diverge seawards."

74 Marcel Raoul Thevenet (1875–1940) was something of an adventurer.
   Born in the historic town of Soissons, he spent four years in the French
   cavalry before coming to Canada in 1898 with the intention of doing
   farm work. But on 1 April he engaged at Regina as a constable of the
   North West Mounted Police in hopes of a posting in the north and
   remained on strength for two and a half years. In January 1900 he
   enlisted at Calgary for a year's service in the Boer War as a private
   soldier of the 2nd Battalion, Canadian Mounted Rifles, and was subsequently awarded the Queen's Medal with three clasps. (He was discharged
   from the NWMP on 4 February 1901.) Thevenet then decided to remain
   in South Africa with the Transvaal Constabulary before returning to
   Canada with Revillon Frères. He was a fur trader at Fort Chimo, where
   he entertained Dillon Wallace in 1905 (Wallace, *The Long Labrador
   Trail*, 204–5), then came to Labrador in 1909 with his wife, also French,
   and raised a daughter and four sons (Census of Newfoundland, 1935,
   75). J.M. Scott, who met him at North West River in 1928–29, wrote,
   "Now he was bringing up a family in this ideal playground for children.
   He spoke French to them, to us in perfect English and to the Indians
   in their own language" (Scott, *The Land That God Gave Cain*, 17).

75 Joseph Lescaudron (1883–1921), born at Kermoison, in the municipality of Batz. In 1917, while in the employ of Revillon Frères, he married Harriet Pardy at North West River and fathered two children. Four years later he died in a drowning accident while working for the same company at Fort Albany, Ontario.

76 José Mailhot shows in *The People of Sheshatshit*, 14–23, that the Labrador Innu were probably not baptized by the Jesuits, who concentrated their efforts in the southwestern part of Innu territory. Rather, their conversion took place during a long process beginning towards the end of the eighteenth century. There were two Indian Affairs agencies on the North Shore of the St Lawrence, situated at Betsiamites and Mingan.

77 The Grand River Company began logging operations on the Grand River around 1900 and built an establishment on Mud Lake Island, including a school and a Methodist church. When the mill closed after the winter of 1909–10, the Grenfell Mission established its hospital in the same buildings.

78 Malcolm McLean (d. 1935), of County Ross, Scotland, originally served the HBC as a labourer at North West River, 1872–77. See also p. 105.

79 Shareman: member of a fishing crew who receives a portion of the profits of a voyage rather than wages.

80 Dodd's Kidney Pills: a popular nostrum offered for the treatment of a variety of ailments, including backache. There was no scientific evidence for its effectiveness.

81 Dragon's blood: red resin obtained from the fruit of *Daemonorops propinquus* and commercially available in sticks or lumps.

82 Lady Constance Harris, wife of Governor Charles Alexander Harris, originated a system of medical aid for outport communities when she organized the Outport Nursing Committee in 1920. After it encountered a shortage of personnel, the wife of the next governor, Lady Elsie Allardyce, made the program self-supporting. In 1924 she formed NONIA and became its first president.

83 Shore fish: codfish prepared for market with a light application of salt and an extended drying period.

84 Bawn: expanse of rocks on which salted cod are spread.

85 The next section was first published as H.L. Paddon, "An October Sail around Hamilton Inlet and Southward Across Belle Isle Straits to Northern Newfoundland," *Yachting* 42, no. 2 (1927): 44–6.

86 Crackie: any small, noisy mongrel dog in Newfoundland and Labrador.

87 Mug-up: a casual cup of tea and snack.

88 SS *Solway*, 220 feet and 836 gross tons, built in 1881 at Whiteinch, Scotland, and owned by the Reid Newfoundland Company.

89 HLP thought Wakefield was insensitive to the Labrador community. He wrote to the nutrition worker in 1923, "He carried his own brown

bread on the steamer, to make converts. It was so soggy and unpalatable that I can well understand than many would stigmatize it as dog-feed, and it continued to be so throughout my association with him, nauseating the Lab. people who tried it just as it had Nflders on the steamer. His advocacy of fresh air was equally unfortunate in manner and effect. It is by long association with the people, and that alone, that we have undermined this prejudice (for which the Mission itself was responsible) to some extent" (HLP to Marion Moseley, 5 July 1923, International Grenfell Association Fonds.).

90 For Dr Wakefield's account of the winter's activities, see Wakefield, "The Winter's Work at Mud Lake," ADSF (October 1913): 7–13.

91 William E. Swaffield (1867–1952) of Westholme, Dorset, had been in Labrador with the HBC since 1891. He was in Cartwright, 1901–11, and served as district manager in Rigolet and Cartwright, 1911–18.

92 A group of Labrador Inuit were brought to Chicago during the World's Fair in 1893 to act as an attraction in the midway during the summer by exhibiting themselves in fur garments. At the conclusion, they were left to make their way home as best they could. See Rompkey, ed., *Jessie Luther at the Grenfell Mission*, 193–4; and for a wider discussion of this practice, Hinsley, "The World as Marketplace: Commodification of the Exotic at the World's Columbian Exposition, Chicago, 1893," 344–65.

93 Merrick, *True North*, 22: "A fur path in these parts is handed down from father to son. It consists mainly of a hazily defined territory. When a man has blazed his trails and built his little cabins (tilts), each a day's walk apart, and set out his two or three hundred traps, that land is his to hunt, and no one else's. Sometimes he farms out his paths to another hunter. In that case the owner must provide a canoe, and stoves for the tilts. The hunter gives him one-third of each haul."

94 Margaret Baikie, *Labrador Memories*, 12: "Mr Smith had twelve working at the post, some were Scotch, some English and one from Finland had a very hard name to speak so they called him Fred Hope. He hoped he would do well." Merrick writes in *True North*, 303, "I think the Hopes are part Norwegian. It is said Carl's father deserted from an English man-of-war in Nova Scotia and wandered 'down along' in fishing vessels. The name was impossible to pronounce. People said that they hoped to be able to twist their tongues around it some day. The Hope is all that has lasted."

95 William Seeley Mercer served in the Hamilton Inlet and Esquimaux Bay mission of the Methodist Church, 1912–16. He died in a snowstorm at Fogo, Newfoundland, in 1924.

96 Dr and Mrs Wakefield recalled, "Mrs. W. decorated the small Christmas tree – no one in the area had ever seen such a celebration in their lives – that graced the table. The Methodist minister, the only one in the area,

and Mr Learmonth, the Hudson Bay agent, a shy Scottish youth, a keen Frontiersman and very helpful to Dr. W. (he acted as an anaesthetist, satisfactorily, tho' he had never done it before). To celebrate Christmas they breakfasted at nine, a light lunch at 11[;] a long walk in the afternoon prompted ravenous appetites for a roast beef dinner in the evening, followed by singing. This was the staff Christmas.

"The next day at 1 p.m. the two doctors, dressed in Mrs. W's summer dresses, aprons, and with caps coquettishly affixed with adhesive tape, served as waitresses, and prompted much merriment among the diners – all the staff of the Mission. And in the evening a party for the children – 'He ain't never brought us nothin' before.' After a high tea served around the big tree, all the tables were cleared and the seats arranged to be ready for the arrival of Father Christmas" (Arthur Wakefield Diary No. 29, 19 December 1912).

97 Baikie, *Labrador Memories*, 13: "There were chairs all around the house. Mr Smith was standing at the table, and on the table were two decanters, one of wine and the other of rum and all around were wine glasses. There were three different kinds of cake. One sort was all shining with white icing and candies. There was a dish of raisins and one of candies. Mr Smith handed a glass of rum or wine to each man and as the last man took his, they all wished him a very happy New Year."

98 Frank Edmund Heath, born in Surrey in 1882, entered service with the HBC in 1911. He was clerk at Mud Lake outpost, 1912–15, and after military service, 1915–19, manager at Fort Chimo, returning to Labrador as post manager at North West River, 1922–25. After an interval as post manager at Pangnirtung, Baffin Land, he was post manager at Nain, 1928–32, then at Fort Hearne in the Eastern Arctic. In 1934 he retired in England, where the HBC assisted him in setting up a mink ranch.

99 The next section was first published as H.L. Paddon, "Ye Goode Olde Dayes [Concluded]," *ADSF* (January 1930): 155–63.

100 According to local lore, the name may also be related to the common experience of running out of supplies and being reduced to "butter and snow."

101 Baikie, *Labrador Memories*, 30.

102 Turn: as much wood, water, etc., as can be carried by a person at a time.

103 See Grenfell, "Notes on Clothing against Cold," 500–1. Following the Great War, Grenfell had the cloth manufactured by Walter Haythornthwaite, a Lancashire cotton manufacturer who marketed it as "Grenfell cloth." However, Grenfell never profited from the product that bore his name.

104 Kirkina (Jeffreys) Connuck, an Inuit, later spent two years in New York, where she was educated in the public schools. See *ADSF* (January 1904): 22–25; *ADSF* (January 1909): 10; Grenfell, *A Labrador Doctor*, 245.

105 In the ballad of "Bold Manan [sometimes Manning] the Pirate," pirates capture and ransack the *Fame* and murder the crew. To stop an argument among his men, Manan severs the head of a young lady on board whose fate they had been discussing. This song was never collected in print, and there is no other instance of its distribution in Newfoundland or Labrador. See Laws, *Native American Balladry*, vol. 1, 168.

106 "Rule Britannia," probably written by the Scottish poet James Thomson, first performed in the masque *Alfred* (1740). It concludes with the couplet, "Rule, Britannia, rule the waves;/Britons never will be slaves!"

107 Ballicater: ice formed by the action of spray and waves along the shoreline.

108 Quor: to choke flowing water with slush. Merrick, *True North*, 253: "At one point we had to climb a steep ice cliff formed by the seepage of water from above, 'quarr water' they call it."

109 Peter Galloway Smith (b. 1888) of Lumsden, Auchindoir, Aberdeenshire, where he had been a telegraph messenger. An apprentice clerk in Labrador, 1907–15, he then enlisted for the war. HLP would have known him as clerk at Cartwright and North West River, 1911–12.

110 2 Kings 2:11: "And it came to pass, as they still went on, and talked, that, behold, there appeared a chariot of fire, and horses of fire, and parted them both asunder; and Elijah went up by a whirlwind into heaven."

111 HLP refers to a common threat in Newfoundland and Labrador households whereby figures of authority were invoked to maintain peace and order among children. See Widdowson, *If You Don't Be Good*, 261–5.

112 The Lodge, also Lodge Bay, named by George Cartwright in 1770 at the location of his first winter quarters. See Cartwright, *Journal of Transactions and Events*, vol. 1, 38.

113 Scaffold: elevated platform for drying or storing nets or for protecting fish and meat.

114 2 Samuel: 23: "Saul and Jonathan were lovely and pleasant in their lives, and in their death they were not divided: they were swifter than eagles, they were stronger than lions."

115 Birket-Smith, *The Eskimos*, 21: "Russian fur traders had long plied their business on the far side of the Ural Mountains when the Tatar khanate Sibir, close to the Tobolsk of the present day, fell into the hands of the Cossacks in 1579. With this began the penetration of the Russians into Northern Asia."

116 Puerperal fever, or "childbed fever," was by far the most common cause of maternal mortality throughout the Western world until the late 1930s. After a successful delivery, a woman would develop an infection of the uterus that rapidly spread into the peritoneal cavity, causing agonizing peritonitis, and into the bloodstream, causing septicaemia, almost invariably fatal. The "raving insanity" referred to here arose from the

intensity of the pain, which caused the patient to emit a continuous cry of agony. (See Loudon, *The Tragedy of Childbed Fever*, 7.) It is now treated successfully with antibiotics.

117 The "wild man of the woods" is a familiar figure in folklore, and reports of the Abominable Snowman are regarded as modern variations on an ancient mythological theme. Edward Colpitts Robinson, *In an Unknown Land*, 133–9, discusses a sighting in Labrador, and Merrick writes in *True North*, 24, "Ghost stories are very real in this land of scattered, lonely homes and private fears. The Traverspine 'gorilla' is one of the creepiest."

118 The Legion of Frontiersmen was founded in London in 1904 by a former RCMP officer, Roger Pocock. Colonel D.P. Driscoll commanded the central headquarters.

119 SS *Kyle*, 220 feet and 1,055 gross tons, built in 1913 at Newcastle and owned by the Reid Newfoundland Company.

120 SS *Invermore*, 250 feet and 975 gross tons, built in 1881 at Glasgow and acquired by the Reid Newfoundland Company in 1909 to provide a fortnightly passenger, cargo, and mail service. She was lost on the Labrador coast in 1914. See p. 125.

121 See H.L. Paddon, "People Worth Knowing in Hamilton Inlet, Labrador, II, [John Groves]," ADSF (July 1920): 51–2; and Merrick, *True North*, 254: "Storms, weariness, nothing can swerve him from his purpose, and of all the men in the Inlet he still makes the best living. Some say that with trapping and trading he has made his fortune."

122 Luke 21: 19: "In your patience possess ye your souls."

123 Harry Louis Alexander (1887–1969), later to be a distinguished physician and teacher, was born in New York City and sent to Williams College, where he graduated in 1910. Alexander received the MD from Columbia University in 1914 and went overseas as a first lieutenant in the Medical Reserve Corps in 1918, publishing a series of medical monographs on service conditions. Returning to the United States, he was assistant resident at the Peter Bent Brigham Hospital, Boston, 1919–24, and after a period of allergy research at Cornell Medical School became associate professor of Medicine at Washington University, St. Louis, 1924–52. For some time, he was also general consultant to the Veterans Administration in Washington, D.C. He wrote *Bronchial Asthma* (1928), *Synopsis of Allergy* (1941), and *Reactions with Drug Therapy* (1955), edited the *Journal of Allergy* from its inception in 1929, and was co-editor of *Immunological Diseases* (1966). His work was recognized by numerous academic and civil honours.

124 By July HLP was short of basic equipment and drugs. He wrote the RNMDSF office in St John's, "I am sick of quackery and, if I am properly

staffed these up-to-date necessities will be used to great advantage. I could not order them until I was sure of scope for their use, but now I don't think we shall revert to the old nightmare" (HLP to Abram Sheard, 29 July 1913, RNMDSF Office Records, St John's).

125 Probably John Severy Hibben (1888–1956), who grew up in Pasadena, California, and attended Stanford University. He received the MD from the College of Physicians and Surgeons, Los Angeles, in 1914. After setting up practice in Pasadena, he was health officer for the city, 1917–22, and a founder of the Pasadena Women's Hospital. As a specialist in physical medicine and rehabilitation, he served as president of the American Congress of Physical Medicine and Rehabilitation. He also contributed numerous technical articles to professional journals and was a member of the editorial board of the journal *Archives of Physical Therapy, X-Ray and Radium*.

126 Ellen (Anderson) Morgan, daughter of the Norwegian settler Torsten (Kverna) Anderson.

127 Job Bros., the owners of the property, had neglected to make the mission's ownership legal. The mission wrote to HLP in June 1913, "There was a sign of reluctance at the time [6 June], but to go back on the understanding makes it very undesirable to spend money at Indian Harbour until the position is put right" (Abram Sheard to HLP, 25 June 1913, RNMDSF Office Records, St John's).

128 Hubert Kirby (1883–1959), born at King's Cove, Bonavista Bay, Newfoundland, the son of the Rev. William Kirby. Educated at Bishop Feild College and Queen's College, St John's, he was ordained a priest of the Church of England in 1908 and served as incumbent of Herring Neck, Newfoundland, before his appointment as incumbent of the mission of Sandwich Bay, 1911–15.

129 *Rigolet*: two-masted schooner, 51 feet and 27 gross tons, built in 1907 at North West Arm, Notre Dame Bay, Newfoundland, and owned by Augustus Goodridge, a St John's merchant.

130 Smyth Flinn, a native of South Carolina. HLP wrote to his sister, "Young Flinn, too, is a really nice boy in many ways & is throwing himself into everything very heartily. But he cannot say 'no' to anything in petticoats & Miss [Helen M.] Smith is not an ideal companion for him being a foolish, while harmless little creature (HLP to JPL, 3 April 1914, Richard Locke Paddon Papers). See Flinn, "The Humanness of the Liveyere," 137–8; Smith, "A Nurse's Experience on the Labrador Coast," 600–2.

131 James Alva Wilson (1854–1920), clerk-in-charge of the HBC district of Esquimaux Bay, 1892–1901.

132 Proverbs 31:10: "Who can find a virtuous woman? For her price is far above rubies."

133 John Cove and his wife, Theresa, the daughter of Lydia Tooktishina, sank in view of the older woman, who was then left to raise the remaining children.

134 The Rev. Berthold August Lenz (1873–1960) served in Labrador, 1899–1932, as missionary and trader in Nain, Hopedale, Okak, Killinek, and Makkovik. In 1900, he married Ingeborg Margarete Jannasch.

135 For an account of the Lenz household in Hopedale in 1910, see Rompkey, ed., *Jessie Luther at the Grenfell Mission*, 265–7.

136 Charles and Susan McNeill (eldest daughter of Torsten Andersen) and their son Jim.

137 The Rev. Paul Richard Hettasch (1873–1949) was born in South Africa but educated in Germany and England. He married Ellen Marie Koch in Neuwied in 1908, and that year the two came to Labrador. They first spent ten years at Hopedale. Then in 1909 Hettasch took a one-year furlough to receive medical training in Bonn, returning to take up duties at the Moravian hospital at Okak, where he replaced Dr S.K. Hutton and managed the hospital for two years until a fully qualified doctor was appointed. Hettasch was subsequently sent to Nain, where he remained until 1921. In 1927 he became superintendent of the Labrador mission, a position he held until 1941.

138 Freuchen, *Arctic Adventure*, 80: "A certain ritual has to be observed when arriving at any place in the Arctic. From the ice the visitors shout out:
    "'Sainak Sunai! Sainak Sunai! (Wonderful pleasure and happy to be here!)'
    "'Assukiak, assukiak! (Same to us, you are right!)' is the people's answer. They know immediately who is approaching."

139 Samuel King Hutton (1877–1961), a member of the English branch of the Moravian Church, practised medicine in Labrador for two periods between 1903 to 1913.

140 Francis Bowes Sayre (1885–1972) was recruited by Grenfell to work at St Anthony while still an undergraduate at Williams College. At his graduation in 1909, Sayre was valedictorian and Grenfell the recipient of an honorary degree. He then spent the summer in Labrador aboard *Strathcona* as Grenfell's secretary and general assistant, and in August Grenfell put him aboard the *Roosevelt* as Peary's secretary. In November Sayre acted as usher at Grenfell's wedding, and in 1913, when Sayre married Jessie Wilson, Grenfell was his best man. Sayre subsequently had a long career as lawyer, professor, author, and diplomat. He was, among other things, assistant secretary of state in the administration of Franklin D. Roosevelt, high commissioner to the Philippines, and chairman of the Trusteeship Council of the United Nations.

141 Reginald J.C. Handford, born in North Dakota in 1887 but living in England when he was hired by the HBC in 1908. Handford served

in Labrador as post manager, 1912–16, and retired in 1922 because
of ill health. He was appointed general manager of Revillon Frères
Trading Co. in 1932 and retired in 1936, when Revillon Frères sold
out to the HBC.

142 The Rev. Squire Joseph Townley (1865–1929), born at Dukinfield,
Cheshire. Trained as a weaver, he was ordained a deacon in 1891 for
service in Labrador and served at Hopedale, Hebron, Ramah, Okak,
Makkovik, and Nain, where in 1893 he married Mary Hannah Ridgway.
In 1909 he was ordained presbyter. He returned to England in 1924.

143 ss *Lintrose*, 255 feet and 1,616 gross tons, built at Newcastle in 1913
and owned by the Reid Newfoundland Company.

144 ss *Mongolian*, 400 feet and 4,838 gross tons, built in 1891 and owned
by the Allan Line.

145 *An Act for the Protection of Neglected, Dependent and Delinquent Children* provided a Newfoundland magistrate with wide-ranging powers for
taking children into custody; however, it was not passed until 1921.

146 Shakespeare, *Hamlet*, III. i. 60–3: "To die, to sleep – no more – and by
a sleep to say we end the heartache, and the thousand natural shocks
that flesh is heir to!"

147 Adam Smith (1723–90), Scottish philosopher and advocate of the free
market system who revolutionized economics with his *Wealth of
Nations* (1776).

148 G.K. Chesterton, *Charles Dickens* (1903) in *Collected Works* (1986–91),
vol. 15, 139: "When a group of superciliously benevolent economists
look down into the abyss for the surplus population, assuredly there is
only one answer that should be given to them; and that is to say, 'If
there is a surplus, you are a surplus.' And if any one were ever cut off,
they would be. If the barricades went up in our streets and the poor
became masters, I think the priests would escape, I fear the gentlemen
would; but I believe the gutters would be running with the blood of
philanthropists."

149 Cicero, *Phillipic*, III. xiv. 35: "*Nervos belli, pecuniam infinitam*"
(The sinews of war, unlimited money).

150 ss *Carthaginian*, 386 feet and 4,444 gross tons, built in 1884 at
Glasgow by the Govan Shipping Co. An immigrant ship of the Allan
Line, she hit a mine on 14 June 1917, near Inishtrahull, Ireland,
and sank.

151 The Rev. Henry Gordon (1887–1971) grew up in the Isle of Man, where
he learned seamanship, and was educated at King William's College.
After winning a scholarship to Keble College Oxford, he was ordained
a priest of the Church of England in 1911 and served in the diocese
of Liverpool before volunteering to go to Labrador as a missionary.
Following the Spanish Flu epidemic of 1919, he invited Clara Ashall

(1888–1976), a Montessori teacher educated at the Warrington Teacher Training College, to join him. They were married at Cartwright in 1921 by the Rev. C.A. Moulton of St Thomas's Church, St John's.

152 Church Militant: one of the tripartite forms of the Christian Church conceived since the Middle Ages – the visible body of the faithful striving to live the Christian life. Beyond the world was the invisible Church: the Church Expectant, containing the souls of the faithful departed, and the Church Triumphant of the saints.

153 Gilbert and Sullivan, *The Pirates of Penzance* (1879), II. 401–3: "When constabulary duty's to be done, / The policeman's lot is not a happy one."

154 Merrick, *Northern Nurse*, 113: "They always travelled so hard and fast on *Yale* that mighty little housekeeping ever got done, though they had to eat and sleep just the same. Those voyages up and down the bay were always ruthless and hardy and saga-like and wholly masculine. When the wind was fair, they didn't stop for storm or sickness or cold or hunger or any mortal thing. The minute they started they seemed to sink their individualities, pool them so to speak, in the boat and the success of the trip. Ordinarily the people who happened to be running *Yale* were as comfort-loving as anybody else, but when they were voyaging, all that was changed. They were different then, sterner, and they tried to believe that it made no difference whether they were cold and wet or warm and snug. The thing was to get there before a head wind came up."

155 Harold Thomas (1887–1967), a radiologist, graduated in 1915 with an MD from the Harvard Medical School. After working in Labrador from June to December that year, he was on the staff of the Hartford Hospital, 1916–18. He served at the Army Medical School in Washington and at Camp Devens, Massachusetts, during the Great War, then went to China as a staff member of the Hwa Mei Hospital, American Baptist Mission, Ningpo, until 1950. Returning to the U.S. in 1951, he spent five years in the Radiology Department of the Massachusetts General Hospital. He was later associate professor of Radiology, Albany Medical College, and chief of the Radiology Department, Veterans Administration Hospital, Albany, retiring from that hospital in 1963.

156 Merrick, *True North*, 177: "Willie never complained, never asked for help, though his broad laugh and joke for every one made it a pleasure to be allowed to do something for him. About seven years ago he developed tuberculosis in his lungs. His oldest boy was already dead of it. In a few months the father followed. I wish I might have known him. God, if there is one, gave him grit, and slowly broke him to pieces."

157 Lorenz Alexander Learmonth (1892–1985) of Stronsay, Orkney, began as an apprentice clerk of the HBC, 1911–14, then served in the army until 1919, when he returned as manager of various posts throughout the Arctic.

158 John Sheill Blackhall (1891–1963) of Leith, Scotland, an apprentice clerk at Rigolet, 1911–14, then clerk at North West River, 1914–15. In 1915 he enlisted in the Newfoundland Regiment and was taken prisoner in France. Returning to Labrador, he was post manager at Rigolet, 1919–22 before leaving for Fort Chimo and returned as post and section manager at Cartwright, 1931–37. After further appointments in the north, he retired to Peterhead, Aberdeenshire.

159 Murdoch McLean (1893–1966), youngest son of Malcolm McLean and Emily, Malcolm's first wife.

160 Merrick, *Northern Nurse*, 204: "Invalided back to Newfoundland just before the war ended, it was autumn when he reached there. No vessels were running north till spring. He'd have to spend the winter convalescing. He would eh? Instead, he got a motorboat to Battle Harbour at the southern tip of his own Labrador, gathered together makeshift gear, patched snowshoes, army rifle, toboggan hewed and whittled himself, and started home cross country. Four hundred miles or more through the hills and woods and lakes it is, nobody knows how far. No map, no Indian portage route, nothing. Day after day threading the long lakes, plodding through thick, dark woods, emerging on streams. By and by he struck the headwaters of the Traverspine." Michelin figures prominently as guide in Scott, *The Land That God Gave Cain* (1933). Goose Bay airport is supposed to have been built near his berry patch, located at the southeast corner. See also Carr, *Checkmate in the North*, 83.

161 Joseph Michelin, Jr (b. 1896), one of the few members of the Newfoundland Regiment to answer the roll call following its virtual destruction at the battle of Beaumont Hamel, 1 July 1916, moved to the United States after the war.

162 See Amy, "An Eskimo Patriot," 212–18.

163 John Blake (1881–1949), employed by the HBC as a carpenter and general servant at Rigolet in 1910 but retired in 1917. He was then employed aboard HBC vessels, notably as master of *Rigolet*. His daughter, Millicent (Blake) Loder, writes in *Daughter of Labrador*, 12: "When I was about two years old Pa had his right arm amputated, just below the elbow, due to tuberculosis of the bone. Since he had been right-handed, he had to learn to use his left hand for all his needs."

164 Thomas writes in "A Summer at Indian Harbor Hospital," ADSF (April 1916), 16, "How Dr. Paddon alone, in the summers past, has carried on this station is hard to imagine. I did not realize the situation until one Sunday when Dr. Paddon was 'in the Bay' I was left in charge. When 11 p.m. was striking we were rolling our last patient into bed – one with a septic hand who had arrived from 10 miles north. With the strains of 'A Perfect Day' in our ears we went to sleep realizing what Dr. Paddon has faced these last three years."

165 Ishpashtien Ashini (d. 1936), son of Shapatish and Manikanet Ashini, was baptized Ishpashtien (from French Bastien), but his name was anglicized as Pasteen, and thus he sometimes emerges as Pasteen Ashini. As often happened with Innu families, his family name was not transmitted to his children, but his anglicized Christian name was; thus, all the Pasteens in Sheshatshit, the Innu village opposite North West River, are his descendants. He died at the mouth of the Kenemu River, and his burial record shows that he was seventy-seven. In 1915, then, he would have been in his late fifties. Pasteen's wife was Shanut Pashtitshi, nicknamed Mishta-Shanut ("Big Charlotte"). She is buried in the Sheshatshit cemetery. Both Ishpashtien Ashini and his wife belonged to the southern division of the Sheshatshit band that hunted south of Lake Melville and had contacts with the Quebec Lower North Shore Innu. (Genealogical information provided by José Mailhot.)

166 The Rev. Edward Joseph O'Brien (1884–1986), born in Carbonear, Newfoundland, studied for the Roman Catholic priesthood in Dublin and was ordained in 1910. In 1914 he was appointed to the parish of Northern Bay, Newfoundland, which was then responsible for Labrador. He made his first visit to North West River in 1921 and thereafter spent more than twenty summers with the Innu of Sheshatshit and Davis Inlet, to whom he was affectionately known as "Father Whitehead" because of his prematurely grey hair. In 1946, Labrador was separated from his diocese, but O'Brien continued to serve at Northern Bay, retiring in 1970. Carr writes in *Checkmate in the North*, 179: "Father O'Brien has been spiritual adviser to these Indians for many years. Each year he comes up to Labrador on the s.s. *Kyle* or one of the other Newfoundland Government steamers which trade up and down the Labrador coasts during the summer season. He knows more about the Indians, their language, their tribal habits and their lives than any other living man. Obviously he is popular and highly respected by the Indians. They wouldn't think of failing to turn up at one or another of his calling-places each summer."

167 Erskine Childers, *The Riddle of the Sands: A Record of Secret Service Recently Achieved* (London: Smith, Elder, 1903), remarkable for its prescient narrative of a German invasion of England and the vividness of its yachting sequences.

168 Kedge off: move a boat off after going aground by means of a line attached to its kedge anchor.

169 2 Corinthians 5:1: "For we know that if our earthly house of this tabernacle were dissolved, we have a building of God, an house not made with hands, eternal in the heavens."

170 Harry Gordon Paddon (1915–1994), born at North West River on 20 December 1915, qualified as a forester in the U.S. in 1937, cruised

timber for Bowater-Lloyd during the negotiations mentioned at the end of this memoir, and later turned to trapping. For six years he operated a sawmill near the Allied air force base at Goose Bay and later joined Okanagan Helicopters, a supplier of northern radar sites, retiring in Vancouver. His recollections of the early years at North West River appear in *Green Woods and Blue Waters* (1989).

171 Goudie, *Woman of Labrador*, 13: "When he [HLP] would leave us he always shook our hands and said to us, 'Now children, eat all the meat and fish and red berries you can if you want to build strong bodies.'"

172 The huge "hospital city" at Étaples, France, deliberately bombed in 1918, when many nurses and orderlies were killed or wounded.

173 *Vaccinium vitis-idaea*: the mountain cranberry, known in Labrador as "red berry" and in Newfoundland as "partridge berry."

174 Psalm 16: 6: "The lines are fallen unto me in pleasant places; yea, I have a goodly heritage."

175 Carbou: Inuktitut for crow. Now Cape Caribou.

176 George Budgell (1887–1956) was engaged as HBC clerk at Rigolet in 1915. He passed his entire thirty-one years of service there.

177 Goudie, *Woman of Labrador*, 13: "Dr. Paddon was always busy. On his sick rounds he would also be preparing his songs for his yearly fair and concert. He was a good singer and a good actor. He always had one big sale about the twentieth of April. Everybody would gather in from around the Groswater Bay and join in the Grenfell Mission Spring Fair. The money was raised to help keep the Mission at work. The ladies would make handwork and the men would make pieces of furniture which would be put up for auction. Sometimes they would raise 700 dollars. Once they made 5,000 dollars. This was something the people looked forward to every year."

178 Seal finger occurs only among those who handle seals. The infection is thought to be transmitted through a small cut in the finger, after which an extremely painful swelling occurs within a few days. While the swollen flesh becomes soft, there is no pus, and consequently lancing provides no relief. The common treatment used to be amputation of the finger; however, nowadays the infection responds rapidly to antibiotics such as tetracycline, although it may recur.

179 Peter Heinbecker (1895–1967), born at Listowel, Ontario, received his undergraduate and medical education at McGill University, graduating in 1921 with an MD. After surgical training at the Johns Hopkins Hospital, the Royal Victoria Hospital, and the Presbyterian Hospital, New York, he arrived at St Louis, Missouri, to work in the physiology laboratories of Dr Joseph Erlanger at the Washington University School of Medicine. With Dr Erlanger, Dr Herbert S. Gasser, and Dr George H. Bishop, he participated extensively in the analysis of nerve fibre

conduction and function which resulted in the awarding of the Nobel Prize to Erlanger and Gasser in 1944. Heinbecker himself was the author of numerous publications in neurophysiology, endocrinology, and metabolism. He obtained the first reliable measurements of the speed of conduction in human nerves, including the discovery of the significant disparities that exist in the velocity of nerve fibres directed to the viscera and skin. During his work on poison ivy, his request to HLP and the extract of poison ivy were sent by the Harvard Medical School physiologist Dr Alexander Forbes. (Copy of HLP's letter to Forbes, 2 September 1937, provided by Mrs June Clark.)

180 The prophylactic treatment of poison ivy, or *Rhus* dermatitis, was attempted in the United States in the 1920s and 1930s through numerous sensitization studies using creams and extracts of poison ivy and poison oak. One such sequence arose from the myth that American Indians developed a resistance to poison ivy because they chewed the leaves. In an experiment involving 227 Navajo, Pueblo, and Apache, a resinous extract of poison ivy leaves was applied to the surface of the skin, but it showed only a slightly different response to the same test applied to white subjects (Deibert, Menger, and Wigglesworth, 289). Heinbecker attempted a similar test on sixty-five Inuit of the south coast of Baffin Island during the Putnam Baffin Island Expedition of 1927, based on the assumption that the Inuit were of similar racial origins, and concluded that the lack of susceptibility of the Baffin Island Inuit was due to a lack of contact rather than a lack of racial characteristics essential to the development of susceptibility (Heinbecker, 367).

181 There are two kinds of beri-beri. "Dry" beri-beri is associated with energy deprivation and inactivity characterized by mental confusion, muscular wasting, loss of function, or paralysis of the lower extremities. "Wet" beri-beri is the result of high carbohydrate intake, along with strenuous exercise characterized by edema, tachycardia, pulmonary congestion, and enlarged heart.

182 Sir Walter Edward Davidson (1859–1923), governor of Newfoundland, 1913–17.

183 Grenfell's account of his survival in the spring of 1908 is recorded in *Adrift on an Icepan* (1909).

184 Job 16: 2: "I have heard many such things: miserable comforters are ye all."

185 The next section was first published as H.L. Paddon, "Emily Beaver Chamberlin Hospital, Winter 1918–19," ADSF (July 1919): 80–3.

186 Selma V. Carlson (1888–1968), head nurse at Indian Harbour, 1915–18, then at St Anthony, 1928–46. HLP wrote, "Miss Carlson is full of energy, & very capable. She is very keen on dog driving, can handle an axe well, teaches cooking, needlework, is secretary to the club,

takes a class in Sunday School, can crochet, spin & weave" (Journal-Letter, 15 December 1917, W. Anthony Paddon Fonds.). Her ashes were buried at St Anthony, alongside those of Grenfell.

187 Smallpox is a viral disease passed by inhalation of air droplets, or aerosols. Following infection, the patient typically develops fever, severe aching pains, and prostration. A rash develops over the face and spreads to the extremities, soon becoming blisters, and gradually scabs form which eventually separate and leave pitted scars. Death may occur during the second week. In this case HLP may have diagnosed one of two milder epidemiologic types: alastrim or chickenpox.

188 The Rev. Henry Gordon reported, however, that they were both buried and the two survivors taken away. See Gordon, *The Labrador Parson*, 140.

189 Rev. Henry Gordon, *A Winter in Labrador, 1918–1919* [New York, 1920].

190 Like John the Baptist in John 3:3: "For this is he that was spoken of by the prophet Esaias, saying, The voice of one crying in the wilderness, Prepare ye the way of the Lord, make his paths straight."

191 Dante Alighieri (1265–1321), whose *Divina Commedia* begins with a description of hell conceived as a succession of circles to which the various categories of sinners are assigned.

192 *Harmony*, 150 feet and 403 registered tons, the fifth and last Moravian supply vessel so named, was originally the barque *Lorna Doone*, built at Dundee in 1876 and subsequently fitted with auxiliary steam power. The ship was purchased in 1901 but sold to the HBC in 1926, when the Moravian Church leased its trading stations to the HBC for twenty-one years. She was then registered as *Bayharmony* but sold for scrap in 1927.

193 Psalm 90: 10: "The days of our years are threescore years and ten; and if by reason of strength they be fourscore years, yet is their strength labour and sorrow; for it is soon cut off, and we fly away."

194 Milda, Clarence and Adeline, children of Joshua and Ellen (McLean) Michelin.

195 Charles S. Curtis (1887–1964), a graduate of the Harvard Medical School, arrived at St Anthony in 1915. Following Grenfell's retirement, he was made medical superintendent and remained so until his own retirement in 1959.

196 Philip Place (1882–1955), born at Concord, Massachusetts, received the MD from Tufts College Medical School in 1909 and served in the Great War before coming to Indian Harbour in 1921. HLP did not regard him highly as an administrator or surgeon, however, but valued his mechanical skills. He wrote in 1921, "he is a genius with marine or stationary engines, plumbing, glazing, etc., & has really won the people's hearts. He repaired over 70 guns last winter, & some 30 motor engines this spring & summer, & that is real Good Samaritan work in this country" (HLP to Ambrose Lloyd, 31 August 1921, Richard Locke Paddon

Papers). See also Place, "A Winter Medical Trip, North West River, 1921," 5–7.

197 Sir Charles Alexander Harris (1855–1947), who though born in Wales was educated at St John's, where he accompanied his father, the Rev. G. Poulett Harris. After spending a career in the public service, Harris was created a knight in 1917 and appointed governor of Newfoundland, a position he held until 1922.

198 ss *Seal*, 175 feet and 608 gross tons, built in 1911 by Napier and Miller, Ltd., Old Kilpatrick, Scotland, and owned by Baine, Johnston & Co., St John's. The *Seal* was lost after an explosion on 9 June 1926 east of Baccalieu Island, Newfoundland, on the way to the seal fishery.

199 Gilbert Blake accompanied Mina Hubbard on this journey, but the actual guide was George Elson of Moose Factory. See Hubbard, *A Woman's Way through Unknown Labrador* (1908); and H.L. Paddon, "People Worth Knowing in Hamilton Inlet, Labrador," ADSF (April 1920): 15–16.

200 The next section is condensed from Grenfell, "Above the Big Falls," in *Northern Neighbours*, 243–60.

201 A treatment for gastric ulcer devised by Hermann Albert Dietrich Lenhartz (1854–1910), a Hamburg physician, involving neutralization of the gastric juice by the administration of protein food. Eggs were the main staple: one on the first day, two on the second, three on the third, and so on, up to eight. Milk was also given, beginning with eight ounces a day, increasing to thirty-six. The food was administered in small quantities every hour, combined with subnitrate of bismuth in large doses, all of which continued for three to four weeks, the patient remaining in bed throughout.

202 The family of Robert Best: his wife Elsie (Blake) Best and their children, Claris, Armenius, Judson, Barbara, and Elsie.

203 The terms for submission of evidence to the judicial committee of the Privy Council of the United Kingdom were not worked out and signed until 1920 and modified in 1922. The final decision, however, was not made until 1927.

204 Tidal surveys conducted by the Government of Canada in 1923 are collected in *Great Britain, Labrador Boundary Case: Oral Argument*, 6, Part 14: "Reports and Documents Relating to the Locations of the Seacoast Line with Relation to the Estuary of the Hamilton River System."

205 Merrick, *Northern Nurse*, 104: "From the very first I had been surprised at the size of the hospital, a white, frame three-story building. In many respects it was amazingly modern, with hardwood floors, roller beds, linoleum in the kitchen. The big difficulty was that the ward was on the second floor and no bathroom was there, no sink, no water facilities of any kind. In the huge cellar was a broken hand pump, but the water

wasn't good. 'Do you mean to say,' I asked Doctor Paddon, 'that you built a $4,000 hospital here, and no water?'"

206 The next section was first published as H.L. Paddon, "A Winter Afternoon in Labrador," ADSF (January 1919): 155–6.

207 Varick Frissell (1903–31) volunteered in 1922, while a student at Yale, to work in Labrador, driving a dog-team in winter and working aboard *Strathcona* in summer. At St Anthony he was instrumental in creating a water supply for the community. In 1925 he and fellow student and mission volunteer Jim Hillier, along with two guides, set out to explore the Hamilton River to the Grand Falls and shot the first film of the waterfall. They also discovered the Unknown River, renaming it the Grenfell River, and are reputed to have discovered Twin Falls. However, in an account of his explorations written for the *Financial Post*, 19 October 1928, Frissell mentions only McLean Falls, "where John McLean stood eighty-eight years before." He also wrote an account of his trip for the *Geographical Journal* entitled "Explorations in the Grand Falls Region of Labrador," which earned him membership in the Royal Geographical Society; and in 1926 he completed a film from his Hamilton River footage, *The Lure of Labrador*. Graduating from Yale the following year, he finished in 1928 a second film, *The Swilin' Racket* (later renamed *The Great Arctic Seal Hunt*), compiled from film he had shot aboard the ss *Beothic*. In February 1930 he began work on *The Viking*, reputedly the first sound film shot in Canada and one of the first sound-synchronized films shot on location. Filmed during the annual Newfoundland seal hunt, it took its title from the ss *Viking*, captained by Bob Bartlett, who also played a major role in it. *The Viking* was first shown at the Nickle Theatre, St John's, on 5 March 1931, but Frissell needed more footage of icebergs, seals, and heavy weather and set out a few days later on *Viking*'s annual sealing voyage. On 15 March, while the ship was caught in ice off the Horse Islands, an explosion in the powder room blew out the stern section, claiming twenty-seven lives. Frissell's body was never recovered.

208 Stuck, *A Winter Circuit of Our Arctic Coast*, 36–7: "Here was a youth of twenty, mission-bred for ten years, well-grown, well-appearing, polite-spoken, with a fair English education and a good deal of general infor-mation, who had been used for a long time as Eskimo interpreter. But he had never made a sled, or a pair of snowshoes, or a canoe, in his life, and was unpractised in the wilderness arts by which he must make a living unless he were to be dependent upon mission employment. What was true of him was true in lesser degree of other bright boys at the place, and I found the same tendency admitted – and deplored – not only at mission stations but at places where there was only a govern-ment school, along the coast. I make no doubt that it might be found

at missions in Africa or the Philippines or wherever else education in the common sense of the term has been taken to a primitive people."

209 The next section was first published as H.L. Paddon, "The Last Voyage of the *Thistle*: An Incident in the Career of the Auxiliary Ketch *Yale*," *Yachting* 51, no. 4 (1932): 68–9; 110.

210 *Thistle*, two-masted schooner, 63 feet and 40 gross tons, built in 1904 at Liverpool, Nova Scotia.

211 *Fort Rigolet*, single-masted, steam-driven sailing vessel, 46 feet and 20 gross tons, built in 1927 at Monroe, Trinity Bay, Newfoundland.

212 Jack Watts (1902–75), born at Brigus, Newfoundland, began with summer work for the Brigus firm of J.W. Hiscock at Smokey, near Indian Harbour. In 1923 he joined the Canadian Marconi Co. as a wireless operator and was sent to Makkovik and Smokey. Talked into doing wireless work for the Grenfell Mission at North West River, he remained in 1928 as general foreman and served as HLP's indispensable technical man and supervisor of construction. HLP wrote in 1930, "Jack Watts is another valuable member, a 'Newfoundlander in whom is no guile'. Honest, with a tremendous 'drive' in work, and outspoken in defence of righteousness, again with a genuine religious conviction" (HLP to Van Sommer family, 18 January 1930, Richard Locke Paddon Papers). Following HLP's death, Watts continued his support of the mission in cooperation with Mina Paddon and ultimately Dr Tony Paddon.

213 Although the name Peter Lewis Brook appears on the map, it was often referred to in the oral tradition as "Peter Lucy's Brook," after a Peter Lucy, who lived there.

214 The next section was first published as H.L. Paddon, "Log of a Komatik Trip," ADSF (July 1931): 64–73.

215 In Matthew 8: 32, Jesus casts out devils from two men of Gadara: "And he said unto them, Go, and when they were come out, they went into the herd of swine: and, behold, the whole herd of swine ran violently down a steep place into the sea, and perished in the waters."

216 William Joseph Cobb (1909–87), born at Barred Islands, Newfoundland, joined the HBC in 1928 as an apprentice clerk at Rigolet. In 1933 he became post manager at Hopedale and managed several other posts in the Canadian north, retiring as deputy general manager of the HBC's Northern Stores Department in 1965.

217 George Borrow, *Lavengro* (1851), ch. 92: "I often think I should like to have another rally – one more rally, and then – but there's a time for all things – youth will be served, every dog has his day, and mine has been a fine one – let me be content."

218 The Suttons were friends of HLP's family near Reading, and he could order from them directly. See Sutton & Sons, *The Culture of Vegetable and Flowers*, 14th ed. (London: Simpskin, Marshall & Co., 1919).

219 HLP describes here a type of supernatural or ghostlike figure acknowledged the world over and invoked also in Newfoundland for purposes
of social control, as documented in John Widdowson, *If You Don't
Be Good* (1977). In this case HLP relates the Labrador legend of Old
Smoker, based on the life of James Smoker, who lived in the early 1800s
south of Cartwright. According to this legend, Old Smoker is a
"helpful" apparition. See Burdett, "Some Smoker Stories," 5; Kennedy,
Labrador Village, 89–90.

220 For further discussion of aboriginal beliefs in Labrador, see Ferguson,
"The Book of Black Hearts," 107–21.

221 There were now two brothers besides Tony and Harry. Richard
(1920–99) was born at Malet's Bay, Vermont, and educated at the
Lenox School and Trinity College, Hartford, Connecticut. During World
War II he enlisted in the Royal Canadian Naval Volunteer Reserve and
served on loan to the Royal Navy, after which he entered the shipping
business in New York with the firm of Hansen, Tiedeman & Dalton as
charter manager in the ships division and later became a partner. He
married Lydia, the daughter of Frank Babbott, his father's assistant at
Indian Harbour. John Gilchrist Paddon (1927–) was born at Pittsfield,
Massachusetts, and educated at the Grenfell Mission school, North West
River, before being sent to the United States and graduated from Proctor
Academy, Andover, New Hampshire, in 1944. Enlisting immediately in
the Royal Canadian Naval Volunteer Reserve, he was discharged in
March 1945, and after studying at Trinity College for two and a half
years he returned to Labrador to open a lumber milling operation in
partnership with Harry. He then worked in the airline industry in British
Columbia and eventually retired in 1993 after sixteen years with the
Canada Post Corp.

222 Kate Austen (1885–1989), of Campsie, New South Wales, received
the certificate of the Australian Trained Nurses Association in 1920
and one in obstetrics from the Royal Hospital for Women, Paddington.
In 1927 she nursed briefly at the American Hospital of Paris before
answering an advertisement of the Grenfell Mission for a nurse at Indian
Harbour and North West River, 1927–30. There she met and married
the mission teacher Elliott Merrick (1906–97), an American who
subsequently published three volumes and several short stories based
on his Labrador experiences. In *Northern Nurse* (1942), where Merrick
recounts Austen's nursing exploits from her point of view, he writes
of HLP's period of absence, "So instead of being helper-nurse to a
veteran doctor who had spent twenty years in this forest-rimmed trapper
settlement, I suddenly became, at the beginning of our long isolated
winter season, head of the station and the only medical authority on
the eastern edge of this continent between Belle Isle Strait and the North

Pole. I would have to make the doctor's dogteam trips" (Merrick, *Northern Nurse*, 120).

223 Harry Telford Roy Mount (1896–1986) of Aurora, Ontario, fought as a sapper with the Canadian Engineers, 1916–19, at Passchendaele and Vimy Ridge and was awarded the Military Medal. He received the MB from the University of Toronto in 1924 and in 1925 began postgraduate training in surgery and neurosurgery at the Mayo Clinic, but in 1926 he interrupted his training for three years when he was invited by Grenfell to join him at St Anthony. Mount next received the MS in neurosurgery from the University of Minnesota in 1931 and opened a practice in Ottawa in 1933. Merrick, *Northern Nurse*, 56: "Doctor Mount had time for everything and was never busy. This was his 'vacation.' The most difficult cases along the coast, or operations so big one surgeon couldn't handle them, were saved for him. A dozen tonsils here, a thoractomy there and he breezed on north. A day or two ashore catching salmon, and then a stop to mend up another six or eight broken lives. It sounds debonair."

224 The next section was first published as H.L. Paddon, "Log of the *Maraval*," ADSF (January 1931): 147–58.

225 The Rev. Walter Whatley Perrett (1869–1950) was born into a Moravian family at Malmesbury, Wiltshire. He trained as a tailor, then prepared for missionary service at Fairfield College. After his ordination as deacon in June 1892, he left for Okak, and in September 1895 he married Helen Ridgway, who served with him in various Labrador locations. See biography of Perrett by S.K. Hutton, *A Shepherd of the Snow* (1936).

226 Frank Douglas Phinney (1873–1938) earned a BA from the University of New Brunswick in 1895 and an MD from the University of Pennsylvania in 1899. He practiced as an oculist and aurist in Cincinnati and was on the staff of the Bethesda Hospital and St Anthony's Hospital. See Frank D. Phinney, "The Eye Doctor," ADSF (January 1929): 152–5; and Merrick, *Northern Nurse*, 57: "Dr. Phinney came to Indian Harbour on a pleasure yacht named *Zavorah*, lent him by the mission, a slim white craft very different in build from the boats we usually saw. He did six eye operations, three of them being cataract removals, on Eskimo women Sabina Muktilik, Barbara Mugasuk, and Lin Tupin, whom Doctor Paddon had brought from the north. From them Doctor Phinney, who was making a study of eskimo snowglasses, plants and a number of other things, learned the Eskimo words *atsuk* (I don't understand [know]), and *auction eye*, a greeting which seemed to connote 'be strong,' or something similar."

227 Herman Moret (1890–1971) of Lausanne, Switzerland, attended McGill University in 1914–15 and again in 1920–21. He graduated with the

degrees MD, CM, in 1922. Moret was at Battle Harbour during the summers 1922 and 1930 and served at St Mary's River, 1931–32.

228 Charles Hogarth Forsyth (1905–63), who trained at the London Hospital Medical College, received the joint qualification MRCS, LRCP, in 1929. Forsyth was medical officer at St Anthony in 1936, while still attached to the London Hospital, and in 1937 medical officer in charge of St Mary's River hospital. He subsequently entered into practice at Fort Walton Beach, Florida, and remained there until his death.

229 C. Denley Clark (1908–2001), born of missionary parents in what is now Thailand, was sent to be educated in England and qualified MB, ChB, from the University of Leeds in 1933. After obtaining the FRCS in 1936, he spent the following year at St Mary's River and returned in 1938 to the Woolwich Memorial Hospital, where he remained throughout the Blitz. In 1943 he joined the RAMC and was in France on D-Day but was sent to Burma as the war closed. Released from the army in the rank of lieutenant-colonel, he obtained a second FRCS in England in 1947 and was appointed consultant surgeon to the Pinderfields Hospital Group, Wakefield, West Yorkshire, in 1950. Throughout these years he maintained his connection with the Grenfell Association of Great Britain.

230 The next section was first published as H.L. Paddon, "Cruise of the *Maraval*, Summer of 1931," ADSF (April 1932): 11–15.

231 *Pauline C. Winters*, two-masted schooner, 121 feet and 140 gross tons, built in 1923 at Lunenburg, Nova Scotia, and bought in 1932 by G & A. Buffett, Ltd., Grand Bank, Newfoundland. She survived until 1963, when she sank off Boat Harbour, in the Strait of Belle Isle.

232 HLP alludes to "The Mouse and the Lion," a fable attributed to Aesop.

233 See also H.L. Paddon, "*Vale*, Indian Harbour," ADSF (October 1929): 108–11.

234 Strangulation: a hernia is said to be "strangulated" when the contents are constricted in such a way as to obstruct and arrest the flow of blood.

235 Andrew L. Banyai, "Topical Application of Codliver Oil in Tuberculosis," *American Review of Tuberculosis* 36 (1937): 250–8.

236 Robert Hancock Goodwin (1903–88) graduated from Princeton with an AB in 1925 and from the Harvard Medical School with an MD in 1929 with a specialization in obstetrics and gynaecology, after which time he was on the staff of the Boston City Hospital, 1929–31, and the Boston Lying-in Hospital, 1931–32. Goodwin substituted for Dr Charles Curtis at St Anthony hospital in the spring of 1933, then spent the summer at Cartwright and Twillingate, Newfoundland. He returned again in the summer of 1934 but spent most of his subsequent career in New Bedford, Massachusetts. He served as a naval reservist with the rank of commander at the Department of the Navy, Washington, D.C., from 1942 to 1946 and subsequently at the U.S. Army Parachute School

and did isolated work on horseback with Chinese guerillas in Inner Mongolia, 1943–45.

237 Gadoment, a preparation marketed by E.L. Patch & Co., was alleged to contain 70 per cent cod liver oil in a wax base with zinc oxide benzoin and phenol and proposed for the treatment of burns, cuts, and minor skin irritations. However, in 1936 the council of the American Medical Association declared it unacceptable as a new and non-official remedy because of its insufficiently declared composition and unwarranted therapeutic claims. See "Gadoment Not Acceptable for N.N.R.," 1384. Other experiments at this time reported the favourable healing action of cod liver oil in tuberculous ulcers. See, for example, Horace R. Getz, "Cod Liver Oil Therapy in Experimental Tuberculosis," 543–5.

238 The *British Medical Journal* featured a variety of treatments associated with cod liver oil throughout the 1930s, including a leading article in *BMJ* I (1931): 853–4. HLP refers here to "Crude Cod-liver Oil in Treatment of Wounds," *BMJ* I (1937): 169.

239 T.J. Smith & Nephew produced Elastoplast in 1933 and released the booklet *Elastoplast Technique* (1933). By the time the third edition was published in 1935, thirty thousand copies had been distributed to medical practitioners. HLP refers here to Surg. Lt. P.K. Fraser, RN, "A Note on the Treatment of Boils and Carbuncles," 894–5; and a letter from a Birmingham practitioner in *BMJ* I (1935): 1249, who employed it successfully in the treatment of impetigo and who observed that children so treated needed no longer be absent from school.

240 Parke, Davis & Co., the pharmaceutical company which invented gelatin capsules, manufactured vaccines, serums, and hormones.

241 Guy Bousfield (1893–1974) studied at St Thomas's Hospital and qualified MB, BS, in 1918. He subsequently turned to medical research and received the MD from the University of London in 1929. Bousfield was later director of the Public Health Laboratory, Camberwell, and immunological specialist to the London and Middlesex county councils. Throughout his career he was primarily concerned with problems of immunization and the investigation of vaccines, and he published extensively on infectious diseases, notably on the Schick test and on diphtheria and scarlet fever immunization.

242 Fred Coleman Sears (1866–1949), professor of Pomology, Massachusetts Agricultural College, who advised Grenfell on agricultural matters during the summers 1928–39.

243 The Labrador Development Company, a timber export business started in 1934 by J.O. Williams of Cardiff, who secured a loan from the Commission of Government. In the first year of operation, six hundred people were hired to cut wood at Alexis Bay, St Michael's Bay, and Lewis Bay. A townsite was started near Alexis Bay, where the company built

houses, a community hall, and a hospital. In 1941, the settlement was renamed Port Hope Simpson after the commissioner for Natural Resources, Sir John Hope Simpson.

244 William D. Timmons of Pennsgrove, New Jersey, dentist in Labrador, 1937–38.

245 The final sentence was amended by Mina Paddon to read, "But whatever befalls the country, the Grenfell Mission has had a large share in the steady improvements which are leading up to the developments which we foresee."

Bibliography

SELECTED WRITINGS OF DR HARRY PADDON

1 *Toilers of the Deep: A Monthly Record of Work amongst Them.* Publication of the Royal National Mission to Deep Sea Fishermen, *vol. 1 (1886) – 78 (1994).*
"Forty Days with Fleeters and Single-boaters." *Toilers* 21 (1906): 236–7.
"A Trip to the Great Northern Fleet." *Toilers* 22 (1907): 167.
"North Sea Wanderings in August and September." *Toilers* 22 (1907): 256.
"North Sea Jottings." *Toilers* 24 (1909): 132.
"Adrift in a Fish-Carrier." *Toilers* 25 (1910): 303.
"Jottings from Labrador." *Toilers* 27 (1912): 273–4.
"Indian Harbour Work." *Toilers* 28 (1913): 237.
"Indian Harbour." *Toilers* 29 (1914): 237.
"Work at Indian Harbour." *Toilers* 30 (1915): 170–1.
"Our Work in Labrador." *Toilers* 31 (1916): 111.
"North West River Cottage Hospital, Winter 1918–19." *Toilers* 34 (1919): 120–2.
"Ye Good Olde Dayes." *Toilers* 44 (1929): 161–3, 230–1, 258–9.
"The Log of a Winter Cruise." *Toilers* 45 (1930): 364–8.

2 *Among the Deep Sea Fishers.* Publication of the International Grenfell Association, Toronto and Boston, *vol. 1 (1903) – 78 (1981).*
"Items from Indian Harbour." ADSF (July 1913): 18.
"Indian Harbour Items." ADSF (October 1913): 25–6.
"Indian Harbour Hospital." ADSF (January 1914): 13–5.

"Mud Lake Hospital." *ADSF* (July 1914): 50–5.

"Indian Harbour Hospital." *ADSF* (October 1914): 107–8.

"Indian Harbour Hospital." *ADSF* (January 1915): 138–40.

"Indian Harbour, Labrador." *ADSF* (October 1915): 91–3.

"Christmas at North West River." *ADSF* (July 1916): 54–5.

"Emily Beaver Chamberlin Memorial Hospital." *ADSF* (October 1916): 103–5.

"Emily Beaver Chamberlin Memorial Hospital." *ADSF* (October 1917): 104–5.

"The 'Fish Crew's Venture' in Groswater Bay." *ADSF* (January 1918): 137–9.

"Indian Harbour, Labrador." *ADSF* (January 1918): 147–9.

"Indian Harbour Hospital." *ADSF* (July 1918): 57.

"Emily Beaver Chamberlin Memorial Hospital." *ADSF* (July 1918): 58–9.

"Indian Harbour Hospital." *ADSF* (October 1918): 102–3.

"A Tale of Three Pups." *ADSF* (October 1918): 116–7.

"A Winter Afternoon in Labrador." *ADSF* (January 1919): 155–6.

"Emily Beaver Chamberlin Memorial Hospital." *ADSF* (July 1919): 80–3.

"The Orphan Children of Labrador and Their Prospects." *ADSF* (July 1919): 94–5.

"Central Labrador Today." *ADSF* (January 1920): 107–11.

"People Worth Knowing in Hamilton Inlet, Labrador [Bert Blake]." *ADSF* (April 1920): 15–6.

"People Worth Knowing in Hamilton Inlet II – John Groves." *ADSF* (July 1920): 51–2.

"Indian Harbour." *ADSF* (October 1920): 109–11.

"Progress and Ambition 'Down North.'" *ADSF* (January 1921): 160–1.

"Indian Harbour Hospital." *ADSF* (October 1921): 84–6.

"Labrador Public Schools, Ltd." *ADSF* (October 1921): 93–5.

"North West River Hospital." *ADSF* (October 1922): 70–2.

"Indian Harbour Hospital." *ADSF* (October 1922): 72.

"Christmas at North West River." *ADSF* (July 1923): 48–50.

"Winter Season at North West River." *ADSF* (October 1923): 92–4.

"Side Lights on Medical Mission Work." *ADSF* (January 1924): 122–3.

"Wanted: Transmitting Apparatus for North West River." *ADSF* (January 1924): 123.

"Fire Destroys Emily Beaver Chamberlin Memorial Hospital." *ADSF* (April 1924): 3–5.

"Labrador and Its Prospects." *ADSF* (July 1924): 48–9.

"Indian Harbour, Labrador." *ADSF* (October 1924): 103–4.

"Madame X." *ADSF* (January 1925): 171.

"People and Things and the Future of Labrador." *ADSF* (July 1925): 66–70.

"The Mission's Most Northerly Out-Posts." *ADSF* (January 1926): 152–6.

"Events in Dr Paddon's Districts." *ADSF* (October 1926): 95.

"Why Work in the Labrador is Worth While." *ADSF* (April 1927): 8–10.

"A Great Acquisition." *ADSF* (July 1927): 63.

"On Furlough." *ADSF* (July 1927): 76–7.

"A Gallon of Gas Fund." *ADSF* (October 1927): 134–5.

"The Breaking of a Long Silence." *ADSF* (January 1928): 157–8.

"The Thousand Natural Shocks That Flesh Is Heir To." *ADSF* (January 1928): 172–3.

"Christmas at North West River." *ADSF* (April 1928): 31–3.

"News from North West River." *ADSF* (July 1928): 62–4.

"An Easter Letter from Labrador." *ADSF* (July 1928): 64–5.

"The I.G.A. Spring Fair, North West River." *ADSF* (July 1928): 86–7.

"A Letter from Dr Paddon." *ADSF* (January 1929): 170–1.

"Ye Good Olde Dayes." *ADSF* (July 1929): 51–7.

"*Vale*, Indian Harbour." *ADSF* (October 1929): 108–11.

"The Coming of the New *Maraval*." *ADSF* (October 1929): 134.

"Aftercare of Sufferers from Tuberculosis." *ADSF* (October 1929): 130–1.

"Ye Good Olde Dayes [Concluded]." *ADSF* (January 1930): 155–63.

"Crossing the Bar." *ADSF* (January 1930): 181.

"Dr Paddon Reviews Last Summer's Work." *ADSF* (January 1930): 178–81.

"The Log of a Winter Cruise." *ADSF* (July 1930): 69–77.

"North West River District Medical and Surgical Report." *ADSF* (July 1930): 81–2.

"Log of the *Maraval*." *ADSF* (January 1931): 147–58.

"Summer Work at Indian Harbour and North West River, 1930." *ADSF* (January 1931): 183–5.

"Log of a Komatik Trip." *ADSF* (July 1931): 64–73.

"Darkness and Dawn." *ADSF* (July 1931): 88.

"Cruise of the *Maraval*, Summer of 1931." *ADSF* (April 1932): 11–15.

"The Cartwright Pipeline." *ADSF* (July 1932): 65–9.

"Activities in the North West River District." *ADSF* (January 1933): 151–6.

"News and Comments from the Northernmost District." *ADSF* (July 1933): 66–72.

"Cruise of the *Jessie Goldthwait*." *ADSF* (October 1933): 130–5.

"Early Winter on Hamilton Inlet." *ADSF* (April 1934): 19–21.

"A Thousand Miles by Komatik." *ADSF* (July 1934): 55–66.

"Last Summer in the North West River District." *ADSF* (October 1934): 105–7.

"Dr Paddon's Winter Itinerary." *ADSF* (April 1935): 18–23.

"Letter from Dr Paddon." *ADSF* (July 1935): 54–7.

"Summer Itinerant Service in 1935: Log of the *Maraval* and *Strathcona II*." *ADSF* (October 1935): 107–14.

"With the Trappers to Muskrat Falls." *ADSF* (January 1936): 145–7.

"North West River in the Year 1935." *ADSF* (January 1936): 150–2.

"Dr Paddon on Vacation." *ADSF* (April 1936): 8–10.

"Dr Paddon as Special Deputy." *ADSF* (July 1936): 58–60.

"Log of the Mission Yacht *Maraval*." *ADSF* (October 1936): 91–4.

"Log of the Mission Yacht *Maraval*." *ADSF* (January 1937): 146–51.

"A Winter Medical Patrol." *ADSF* (April 1937): 14–8.

"North West River Comes of Age." *ADSF* (July 1937): 61–5.
"Log of the *Maraval*." *ADSF* (October 1937): 107–13.
"Log of the *Maraval*." *ADSF* January 1938): 147–54.
"North West River Jottings." *ADSF* (July 1938): 64–6.
"The *Maraval* in Service." *ADSF* (October 1938): 87–95.
"The *Maraval* in Service." *ADSF* (January 1939): 146–55.
"By Winter Mail from North West River." *ADSF* (July 1939): 46–50.
"Log of the *Maraval*." *ADSF* (October 1939): 92–4.
"Of North West River." *ADSF* (January 1940): 136–8.
"Medical Control." *ADSF* (April 1940): 7–8.

3 *Other*
"Some Labrador Cruises." *Yachting* 42, no. 2 (1927): 44–6.
"The Last Voyage of the *Thistle*." *Yachting* 51, no. 4 (1932): 68–9, 110.
"Labrador To-day: A Lecture to the Medical and Physical Society." *St Thomas' Hospital Gazette* 35 (1936): 283–7.
"Labrador: Its People and Its Problems." *St John's Daily News*, 19 October 1938.

RELATED WORKS

Manuscripts

Ashdown, Cecil S., and T.A. Greene. Report of the Commission Appointed by the Directors of the International Grenfell Association, April 13th, 1935, to Confer with the Commission of Government for Newfoundland and Survey Conditions on the Coast of Newfoundland & Labrador. [New York, 1935].
Boston Medical Library's Directory for Nurses. Countway Library of Medicine, Boston Massachusetts.
Catalogus der Missionare. Moravian Archives, Bethlehem, Pennsylvania. Microfilm copies at the Centre for Newfoundland Studies, Memorial University, and at the National Archives of Canada, Ottawa.
Census of Newfoundland, 1935. Provincial Archives of Newfoundland and Labrador, St John's.
Colonial Secretary's Correspondence. Provincial Archives of Newfoundland and Labrador, St John's.
Dienerblatt. Unitaetsarchiv Herrnhut, Germany. Microfilm copies at the Centre for Newfoundland Studies, Memorial University, and at the National Archives of Canada, Ottawa.
Fonds Revillon Frères. National Archives of Canada, Ottawa.
Frissell, Varick. Papers. Library of Congress, Washington, D.C.
Gordon, Clara. "Labrador Teacher: Journal of Clara Gordon, 1919–1925." Unpublished typescript in the possession of Philip Gordon, Postwick, Norwich.

Grenfell Association of Great Britain and Ireland Fonds. Provincial Archives of Newfoundland and Labrador, St John's.

Grenfell, Wilfred T. Papers. Stirling Library, Yale University, New Haven, Connecticut.

Hudson's Bay Company Records. Hudson's Bay Company Archives, Winnipeg, Manitoba.

International Grenfell Association Fonds. Provincial Archives of Newfoundland and Labrador, St John's.

International Grenfell Association Staff Records. Grenfell Regional Health Services, St Anthony, Labrador.

Linder, L. "Chronologisches Verzeichnis der Missionare der Brüdergemeine." Unitäts–Archiv Herrnhut.

[Lloyd], Jessie M. Paddon. [Narrative of her early life, 1883–1902.] Unpublished manuscript, 1947–54, in the possession of Raymond Lloyd, Tetbury, Gloucestershire.

Lloyd, Raymond. "Jessie Marian Paddon, 1877–1958: The Story of Her Forebears, Background and Early Life." Unpublished manuscript, 1986, in the possession of Raymond Lloyd, Tetbury, Gloucestershire.

Merrick, Elliott. Merrick Collection. Centre for Newfoundland Studies Archives, Memorial University.

New Brunswick Census, 1871, 1881, 1891. National Archives of Canada, Ottawa.

North West River Births and Marriages, 1884–1950. United Church Archives, St John's.

O'Brien, Monsignor Edward Joseph. Letters and Papers, 1923–47. Centre for Newfoundland Studies Archives, Memorial University.

Paddon, Richard. Papers. Family of Richard Locke Paddon, Jr.

Paddon, W. Anthony. Fonds. Provincial Archives of Newfoundland and Labrador, St John's.

Paddon Family Papers. Sheila Paddon, North West River, Labrador.

Paddon and Van Sommer Family Papers. Richard Lloyd, Twyford, Berkshire.

[Paton, J.L.] "Education on the Labrador." Report submitted to the Department of Education, Newfoundland, May 1929. Board of Governors Records, Memorial University.

Records of the Guest Hospital, Dudley. Dudley Archives and Local History Service, Coseley, West Midlands.

Registrar General of Shipping and Seamen, Certificates of Vessel Registry. Maritime History Archive, Memorial University.

RNMDSF Committee Minutes and Records. Royal National Mission to Deep Sea Fishermen, London.

RNMDSF Office Records, St John's, Newfoundland. Yale University Library, New Haven, Connecticut.

Roberts, Dr Kenneth B. Fonds. Faculty of Medicine Founders' Archive, Memorial University.

Royal Canadian Mounted Police Personnel Records, 1873–1974. National Archives of Canada, Ottawa.
School Trustee's Returns, Sunbury County, New Brunswick, 1896–1902. Provincial Archives of New Brunswick, Fredericton.
Student Records, Massachusetts General Hospital School of Nursing, 1873–1981. Countway Library of Medicine, Boston, Massachusetts.
University College, Oxford. Admissions Register, 1863–1940.
– Tutorial Lists, 1896–1914.
Wakefield, Arthur and Marjorie. Papers. R.W. Wakefield, Montreal.

Published Works

Amy, Lacey. "An Eskimo Patriot [John Shiwak]." *Canadian Magazine* 51 (1918): 212–18.
Andersen, Joan. *Makkovik: 100 Years Plus*. Makkovik: Joan Andersen/ Robinson-Blackmore 1996.
Annual Report of Dudley Guest Hospital, 30 September 1910–30 September 1911. Dudley: Herald Free Press, 1911.
Apple, Rima D. *Vitamania: Vitamins in American Culture*. New Brunswick, N.J.: Rutgers University Press 1996.
Appleton, V.B. "Observations on Deficiency Diseases in Labrador." *American Journal of Public Health* 11 (1921): 617–21.
Armitage, Peter. *The Innu (The Montagnais-Naskapi)*. New York: Chelsea House 1991.
Arnold, David, ed. *Imperial Medicine and Indigenous Societies*. Manchester: Manchester University Press 1988.
Ashford, L.J. *The History of the Borough of High Wycombe from Its Origins to 1880*. London: Routledge & Kegan Paul 1960.
Aykroyd, W.R. "Vitamin A Deficiency in Newfoundland." *Irish Journal of Medical Science* 28 (1928): 161–5.
– "Berberi and Other Food-Deficiency Diseases in Newfoundland and Labrador." *Journal of Hygiene* 30 (1930): 357–86.
Baikie, Leslie D., comp. *Up and Down the Bay: The Baikie Family of Esquimaux Bay*. N.p., n.d. [1989].
Baikie, Margaret. *Labrador Memories: Reflections at Mulligan*. Happy Valley-Goose Bay: Them Days, [1984].
Banyai, Andrew L. "Topical Application of Codliver Oil in Tuberculosis." *American Review of Tuberculosis* 36 (1937): 250–8.
– "Cod-Liver Oil as Local Treatment for Tuberculous Lesions." *British Journal of Tuberculosis* 34 (1940): 107–16.
Bebbington, D.W. *Evangelicalism in Modern Britain: A History from the 1730s to the 1980s*. London: Unwin Hyman 1989.
Billson, Marcus. "The Memoir: New Perspectives on a Forgotten Genre." *Genre* 10 (1977): 259–82.

Binney, George. *The Eskimo Book of Knowledge*. Rendered into the Labrador dialect by Rev. W.W. Perret with Dr S.K. Hutton. London: Hudson's Bay Co. 1931.

Birket-Smith, Kaj. "The Question of the Origin of Eskimo Culture: A Rejoinder." *American Anthropologist* n.s. 32 (1930): 608–24.

– *The Eskimos*. London: Methuen 1936.

Bishop, Theresa Lynn. "Public Health and Welfare in Newfoundland, 1929–1939." MA thesis, Queen's University, 1984.

Black, W.A. "Population Distribution of the Labrador Coast, Newfoundland." *Geographical Bulletin* no. 9 (1957): 53–74.

Bradley, Ian, ed. *The Complete Annotated Gilbert and Sullivan*. Oxford: Oxford University Press 1996.

Brice-Bennett, Carol. "Two Opinions: Inuit and Moravian Missionaries in Labrador, 1804–1860. MA thesis, Memorial University, 1981.

– ed. *Remembering the Years of My Life: Journeys of a Labrador Inuit Hunter.* St John's: ISER Books 1999.

Buckle, Francis. *The Anglican Church in Labrador, 1848–1998*. Labrador City: Archdeaconry of Labrador 1998.

Budgel, Richard. *A Survey of Labrador Material in Newfoundland & Labrador Archives*. Happy Valley–Goose Bay: Labrador Institute of Northern Studies [1985].

Budgel, Richard, and Michael Staveley. *The Labrador Boundary*. Happy Valley–Goose Bay: Labrador Institute of Northern Studies, 1987.

Bulgin, Iona. "Mapping the Self in the 'Utmost Purple Rim': Published Labrador Memoirs of Four Grenfell Nurses." PhD thesis, Memorial University, 2001.

Burdett, James. "Some Smoker Stories." *Them Days* 4, no. 4 (1979): 5.

Burry, L. "Reminiscences of a Clergyman in Labrador." *Newfoundland Medical Association Newsletter* 16 (1974): 20–2.

Campbell, Lydia. *Sketches of Labrador Life*. Happy Valley–Goose Bay: Them Days 1980.

Carpenter, Kenneth J. *Beriberi, White Rice, and Vitamin B: A Disease, a Cause, and a Cure*. Berkeley: University of California Press 2000.

Carr, William Guy. *Checkmate in the North: The Axis Planned to Invade America*. Toronto: Macmillan 1944.

Cartwright, George. *Journal of Transactions and Events, during a Residence of Nearly Sixteen Years on the Coast of Labrador; Containing Many Interesting Particulars, Both of the Country and Its Inhabitants, Not Hitherto Known*. 3 vols. Newark 1792.

Cemetery Inscriptions from the Labrador. Happy Valley–Goose Bay: Newfoundland and Labrador Genealogical Society and Them Days 1985.

"Cod-Liver Oils and Irradiated Preparations." *British Medical Journal* 1 (1931): 653–4.

Collier, Richard. *The Plague of the Spanish Lady: The Influenza Pandemic of 1918–1919*. New York: Atheneum 1974.

Cooke, Alan, and Fabien Caron, comps. *Bibliographie de la Péninsule du Québec-Labrador.* 2 vols. Boston: G.K. Hall 1968.

Cordia, Maylean. *Nurses at Little Bay.* Sydney: Prince Henry Trained Nurses' Association 1990.

Cornelsen, Richard Zerbe. "Moravian Communities in Labrador, 1850–1920: A Theocracy Undermined." MA thesis, Associated Mennonite Biblical Seminaries, 1991.

Corner, George W. "Hospital Work of the Labrador Mission." *Modern Hospital* 3 (1914): 72–8.

Crellin, John K. *Home Medicine: The Newfoundland Experience.* Montreal: McGill-Queen's University Press 1994.

Crosby, Alfred W., Jr. *Epidemic and Peace, 1918.* Westport, Conn.: Greenwood Press 1976.

Cuthbertson, D.P. *Report on Nutrition in Newfoundland.* London: His Majesty's Stationery Office 1947.

Davies, D. James. *Cod Liver Oil.* St John's: Government of Newfoundland 1930

Davies, K.G., ed. *Northern Quebec and Labrador Journals and Correspondence, 1819–35.* London: Hudson's Bay Record Society 1963.

Davies, W.H.A. "Notes on Esquimaux Bay and the Surrounding Country." *Transactions of the Literary and Historical Society of Quebec* 4, pt. 1 (1843): 70–94.

Deibert, Olin, E.F. Menger, and A.M. Wigglesworth. "Relative Susceptibility of the American Indian Race and the White Race to Poison Ivy." *Journal of Immunology* 8 (1923): 287–9.

Delatour, Beeckman J. "Dr John Mason Little." ADSF (July 1973): 10–12.

Douglas, W.O. "Memories of Muddy Bay." *Beaver* (Summer 1978): 42–7.

Elastoplast Technique: A Classified Reference to the Applications of Elastoplast. Hull: T.J. Smith & Nephew 1933.

Ewbank, R.B. *Public Affairs in Newfoundland: Addresses, 1936–1939.* Cardiff: William Lewis 1939.

Ferguson, Mark. "The Book of Black Hearts: Readdressing the Meaning and Relevance of Supernatural Materials." *Journal of Canadian Studies* 29, no. 1 (1994): 107–21.

Fitzhugh, Lynne D. *The Labradorians: Voices from the Land of Cain.* St John's: Breakwater Books 1999.

Fitzhugh, William W. *Environmental Archaeology and Cultural Systems in Hamilton Inlet, Labrador: A Survey of the Central Labrador Coast From 3000 B.C. to the Present.* Washington: Smithsonian Institution Press 1972.

Flinn, T. Smyth, "The Humanness of the Liveyere." ADSF (January 1915): 137–8.

Forbes, Alexander. *Northernmost Labrador Mapped From the Air.* New York: American Geographical Society 1938.

Forsyth, C. Hogarth. "Life and Work in Labrador." *Medical Press and Circular* 204 (1940): 398–402.

Forty-sixth Annual Report of the McLean Hospital School of Nursing. Boston: T.O. Metcalf Co. 1928.

Foster, Joseph, ed. *Alumni Oxonienses: The Members of the University of Oxford, 1500–1886.* 8 vols. Oxford: Parker & Co. 1888.

Fowlow, Rev. G. "Labrador Voyage." *Diocesan Magazine* 62 (1952): 14–19, 51–60.

Fraser, Surg. Lt. P.K., RN. "A Note on the Treatment of Boils and Carbuncles." *British Medical Journal* 2 (1935): 894–5.

Freuchen, Peter. *Eskimo.* Trans. A. Paul Maerker–Branden and Elsa Branden. New York: Horace Liveright 1931.

– *Arctic Adventure: My Life in the Frozen North.* New York: Farrar & Rinehart 1935.

Frissell, Varick. "Explorations in the Grand Falls Region of Labrador." *Geographical Journal* 69 (1927): 332–40.

Fuller, Elizabeth F. "Nutrition Classes at St Anthony." ADSF (January 1921): 151–8.

Fyfe, Betty P. "A Labrador Children's Home." ADSF (January 1940): 127–31.

"Gadoment Not Acceptable for N.N.R." *Journal of the American Medical Association* 107 (1936): 1384.

Getz, Horace R. "Cod Liver Oil Therapy in Experimental Tuberculosis." *Proceedings of the Society for Experimental Biology and Medicine* 38 (1938): 543–5.

Gordon, Alexander. *What Cheer O? Or, the Story of the Mission to Deep Sea Fishermen.* London: James Nisbet & Co. 1890.

Gordon, Rev. Henry. *A Winter in Labrador, 1918–1919.* Preface by the Governor of Newfoundland. [New York, 1920].

– "Life in Labrador." *United Empire* 14 (1923): 285–8.

– "Dr Paddon." ADSF (April 1940): 5–6.

– *A Servant of Christ: A Study of the Religious Outlook of Sir Wilfred Grenfell.* London: Grenfell Association of Great Britain and Ireland 1966.

– *The Labrador Parson: Journal of the Reverend Henry Gordon, 1915–1925.* St John's: Provincial Archives of Newfoundland and Labrador [1972].

[Gordon, Rev. Henry?] "Dr H.L. Paddon. By One Who Knows Him." *Toilers* (May 1919): 45–6.

Goudie, Elizabeth. *Woman of Labrador.* Toronto: Peter Martin Associates 1973.

Goudie, Horace. *Trails to Remember.* St John's: Jesperson Press 1991.

Gray, Doug. *R.M.S. Nascopie: Ship of the North.* Ottawa: Golden Dog 1997.

Gray, James T. "Glacial History of the Eastern Mealy Mountains, Southern Labrador." *Arctic* 22 (1969): 106–11.

Great Britain. Privy Council. Judicial Committee. *Labrador Boundary Case: Oral Argument.* 10 vols. London 1927.

– *In the Matter of the Boundary between the Dominion of Canada and the Colony of Newfoundland in the Labrador Peninsula: Between the Dominion of Canada of the One Part and the Colony of Newfoundland of the Other Part; Report of the Lords of the Judicial Committee of the Privy Council, Delivered the 1st March, 1927.* London: Harrison & Sons 1927.

Grenfell, Wilfred T. *Northern Neighbours.* London: Hodder & Stoughton 1906.

– *Adrift on an Icepan.* Boston and New York: Houghton Mifflin 1909.

– "Notes on Clothing against Cold." *British Medical Journal* 1 (1916): 500–1.

– *A Labrador Doctor: The Autobiography of Wilfred Thomas Grenfell, M.D. (Oxon.), C.M.G.* Boston and New York: Houghton Mifflin 1919.

– "Medical Pioneering in Labrador." *British Medical Journal* 1 (1930): 122–3.

– ed. *Labrador: The Country and the People.* New York: Macmillian 1910.

Groves, Lt.-Col. Percy. *Historical Records of the 7th or Royal Regiment of Fusiliers.* Guernsey: Frederick B. Guerin 1903.

Grygier, Pat Sandiford. *A Long Way from Home: The Tuberculosis Epidemic among the Inuit.* Montreal: McGill-Queen's University Press 1994.

The Guest Hospital Dudley, 1871–1971. Dudley: Guest Hospital 1971.

Gwynn, Robin D. *Huguenot Heritage: The History and Contribution of the Huguenots in Britain.* London: Routledge & Kegan Paul 1985.

Haberman, J. Victor. "The Lenhartz Treatment of Gastric Ulcer at the Eppen-dorfer Krankenhaus, Hamburg." *Lancet* 2 (1906): 25–6.

Hamelin, Louis-Edmond. *Canadian Nordicity: It's Your North, Too.* Trans. William Barr. Montreal: Harvest House 1978.

Harris, Lynda. *Revillon Frères Trading Company Limited: Fur Traders of the North, 1901–1936.* 2 vols. [Toronto]: Ministry of Culture and Recreation 1976.

Heinbecker, Peter. "The Susceptibility of Eskimos to an Extract from *Toxicodendron Radicans* (L.)." *Journal of Immunology* 15 (1928): 365–7.

Henrikson. Georg. *Hunters of the Barrens: The Naskapi on the Edge of the White Man's World.* St John's: Institute of Social and Economic Research 1973.

Hiller, James K. "The Foundation and the Early Years of the Moravian Mission in Labrador, 1752–1805." MA thesis, Memorial University, 1967.

– "The Politics of Newsprint: The Newfoundland Pulp and Paper Industry, 1915–1939." *Acadiensis* 19, no. 2 (1990): 3–39.

Himmelfarb, Gertrude. *Poverty and Compassion: The Moral Imagination of the Late Victorians.* New York: Knopf 1991.

Hind, Henry Youle. *Explorations in the Interior of the Labrador Peninsula, the Country of the Montagnais and Nasquapee Indians.* 2 vols. London: Longman, Green, Longman, Roberts & Green, 1863.

Hinsley, Curtis M. "The World as Marketplace: Commodification of the Exotic at the World's Columbian Exposition, Chicago, 1893." In Ivan Karp and Steven D. Lavine, eds., *Exhibiting Cultures: The Poetics and Politics of Museum Display* (Washington: Smithsonian Institution Press, 1991), 344–65.

Hollett, Robert, and William J. Kirwin, eds. *Place Names of the Northern Peninsula.* New edition. St John's: ISER Books 2000.

Holmes, Arthur D. "Modern Cod Liver Oil as a Source of Fat Soluble Vitamins." *Boston Medical and Surgical Journal* 194 (1926): 714–16.

House, Edgar. *The Way Out: The Story of Nonia, 1920–1990.* St John's: Creative Printers 1990.

Hubbard, [Mina]. *A Woman's Way through Unknown Labrador.* New York: McClure 1908.

Hunter, Isabel, and Shelagh Wotherspoon. *A Bibliography of Health Care in Newfoundland.* St John's: Faculty of Medicine, Memorial University 1986.

Hustich, Ilmari. *Notes on the Coniferous Forest and Tree Limit on the East Coast of Newfoundland-Labrador.* Acta Geographica 7, no. 1. (Helsinki, 1939).

[–]"To the Memory of Väinö Tanner." *Terra* 75 (1963): 31–2.

Hutton, S.K. *Among the Eskimos of Labrador: A Record of Five Years' Intercourse with the Eskimo Tribes of Labrador.* London: Seeley, Service 1912.

– *Health Conditions and Disease among the Eskimos of Labrador.* Poole: J. Looker [1925].

– *By Eskimo Dog-Sled and Kayak.* London: Seeley, Service 1925.

– *A Shepherd of the Snow: The Life Story of Walter Perrett of Labrador.* London: Hodder & Stoughton 1936.

Innis, Harold A. *The Fur Trade in Canada.* Introduction by Arthur J. Ray. Toronto: University of Toronto Press 1999.

Jenness, Diamond. *Eskimo Administration: III. Labrador.* Montreal: Arctic Institute of North America 1965.

Kennedy, John C. "The Impact of the Grenfell Mission on Southwestern Labrador." *Polar Record* 24 (1988): 199–206.

– *People of the Bays and Headlands: Anthropological History and the Fate of Communities in the Unknown Labrador.* Toronto: University of Toronto Press 1995.

– *Labrador Village.* Prospect Heights, Illinois: Waveland Press 1996.

– "Labrador Métis Ethnogenesis." *Ethnos* 62, 3–4 (1997): 5–23.

Kindl, Rita. "Change and Continuity: Three Generations of Women's Work in North West River, Labrador." MA thesis, Memorial University, 1999.

Kindle, E.M. *Geography and Geology of Lake Melville District, Labrador Peninsula.* Geological Survey Memoir 141. Ottawa: King's Printer 1924.

Kirk-Greene, Anthony. *Britain's Imperial Administrators, 1858–1966.* London: Macmillan 2000.

Kleivan, Helge. *The Eskimos of Northeast Labrador: A History of Eskimo-White Relations, 1771–1955.* Oslo: Norsk Polarinstitutt 1966.

Knowling, William R. "Ignorant, Dirty and Poor: The Perception of Tuberculosis in Newfoundland, 1908–1912." MA thesis, Memorial University, 1997.

Kranck, E.H. *Bedrock Geology of the Seaboard Region of Newfoundland Labrador.* Newfoundland Geological Survey Bulletin no. 19. St John's 1939.

Labrador. Ottawa: Department of Mines 1933.

Laws, G. Malcolm. *Native American Balladry: A Descriptive Study and a Bibliographical Syllabus.* 2 vols. Philadelphia: American Folklore Society 1964.

Leacock, Eleanor. *The Montagnais "Hunting Territory" and the Fur Trade.* Memoir no. 78. Menasha, Wisc.: American Anthropological Association [1954].

Leared, Arthur. "On the Use of Cod-liver Oil Oleine." *Medical Times and Gazette* 2 (1855): 58–9.

Le Bourdais, D.M. "North West River." *Beaver* (Spring 1963): 14–21.

Linking the Generations: A Collection of Oral Histories Excerpts from the Battle Harbour Region. Mary's Harbour: Battle Harbour Literacy Council 1998.

Little, J.M. "Medical Conditions on the Labrador Coast and North Newfoundland." *Journal of the American Medical Association* 50 (1908): 1037–9.

– "Berberi Caused by Fine White Flour." *Journal of the American Medical Association* 58 (1912): 2029–30.

– "Beriberi." *Journal of the American Medical Association* 63 (1914): 1287–90.

Loder, Millicent Blake. *Daughter of Labrador.* St John's: Harry Cuff Publications 1989.

Loudon, Irvine. *The Tragedy of Childbed Fever.* Oxford: Oxford University Press 2000.

Lush, Gail. "Health, Education and Dietary Reform: Gendering the 'New Science' at the Grenfell Mission, 1912–1933." MA thesis, Memorial University, 2003.

McAlpine's New Brunswick Directory for 1896. St John: McAlpine Publishing Co. [1896].

Mailhot, José. *The People of Sheshatshit: The Land of the Innu.* Trans. Axel Harvey. St John's: ISER Books, 1997.

Mailhot, José, and Andrée Michaud. *North West River: Étude ethnographique.* Québec: Institut de géographie, Université Laval 1965.

Macdonald, Alec. *A Short History of Repton.* London: Ernest Benn 1929.

McDonald, Donna. *Lord Strathcona: A Biography of Donald Alexander Smith.* Toronto: Dundurn Press 1996.

McGee, John T. *Cultural Stability and Change among the Montagnais Indians of the Lake Melville Region of Labrador.* Washington: Catholic University of America Press 1961.

McGhee, Robert. *Ancient People of the Arctic.* Vancouver: UBC Press 1996.

McInnes, E.M. *St Thomas' Hospital.* London: George Allen & Unwin 1963.

MacLeod, Roy, and Milton Lewis, eds. *Disease, Medicine, and Empire: Perspectives on Western Medicine and the Experience of European Expansion.* London: Routledge 1988.

Macpherson, Cluny. "The First Recognition of Beri-Beri in Canada?" *Canadian Medical Association Journal* 95 (1966): 278–9.

Mason, J.C.S *The Moravian Church and the Missionary Awakening in England, 1760–1800.* London: Royal Historic Society 2001.

Mathiasson, Therkel. "The Question of the Origin of Eskimo Culture." *American Anthropologist* n.s. 32 (1930): 591–607.

Meacham, Standish. *Lord Bishop: The Life of Samuel Wilberforce*. Cambridge, Mass.: Harvard University Press 1970.

The Medical Directory 1936. London: J. & A. Churchill 1936.

Mercantile Navy List. London: Spottiswoode 1857-present.

Merrick, Elliott. *True North*. New York: Scribner's 1933.

– *Frost and Fire*. New York: Scribner's 1939.

– *Northern Nurse*. New York: Scribner's 1942.

Messiter, Mina, ed. *Repton School Register, 1557–1910*. Repton: A.J. Lawrence 1910.

Milward, Richard. *A New Short History of Wimbledon*. Wimbledon: Wimbledon Society 1989.

Mitchell, H.S. "Nutritional Survey in Labrador and Northern Newfoundland." *Journal of the American Dietetic Association* 6 (1930): 29–35.

Mosdell. H.M. *Commission on Health and Public Charities: First Interim Report*. St John's: King's Printer 1930.

Moseley, Marion R. "The Third Year of Health Work." ADSF (January 1923): 106–9,

Neary, Peter. "The Diplomatic Background to the Canada-Newfoundland Goose Bay Agreement of October 10, 1944." *Newfoundland Studies* 2 (1986): 39–61.

– *Newfoundland in the North Atlantic World, 1929–1949*. Montreal: McGill-Queen's University Press 1988.

– ed. *White Tie and Decorations: Sir John and Lady Hope Simpson in Newfoundland, 1934–1936*. Toronto: University of Toronto Press 1996.

Newfoundland. *Census of Newfoundland and Labrador, 1911*. St John's: King's Printer 1914.

– *Acts of the General Assembly of Newfoundland*. St John's: Office of the Royal Gazette 1922.

– *The Health and Public Welfare Act, 1931*. St John's: King's Printer [1931].

– *Tenth Census of Newfoundland and Labrador, 1935*. 2 vols. St John's: Evening Telegram 1937.

– *Acts of the Honourable Commission of Government of Newfoundland, 1938*. St John's: King's Printer 1938.

– *Acts of the Honourable Commission of Government of Newfoundland, 1939*. St John's: King's Printer 1939

Newfoundland Royal Commission Report, 1933. London: HMSO 1933.

Ohler, W. Richard. "Effects of Exclusive Diet of Wheat Flour, in the Form of Ordinary Bread, on Fowls." *Journal of Medical Research* 31 (1914): 239–46.

Overton, James. "Brown Flour and Beriberi: The Politics of Dietary and Health Reform in Newfoundland in the First Half of the Twentieth Century." *Newfoundland Studies* 14 (1998): 1–27.

Oxford University Calendar for the Year 1907. Oxford: Clarendon Press 1907.

Paddon, Rev. H. *A Sermon Preached at Loudwater Chapel ... on the Death of ... Edward Arnold.* Wycombe [1865].
- *Thoughts on the Evangelical Preaching of the Present Day.* 4th ed. London: William MacIntosh 1872.
- *Thoughts for the Christian Laity.* 2nd ed. London: William MacIntosh 1873.
- *Court Dress; or, The Bride of Christ Ready and Waiting to be Presented.* 2nd ed. London: William MacIntosh 1874.
- *Death Abolished; or, The Saint's Deliverance from the Fear of Death.* 2nd ed. London: William MacIntosh 1875.
Paddon, Harold [sic] G. *Green Woods and Blue Waters: Memories of Labrador.* St John's: Breakwater Books 1989.
Paddon, W.A. "Tuberculosis Control in Northern Labrador." Dip. Public Health thesis, London School of Hygiene and Tropical Medicine 1957.
- "The Grenfell Mission of Labrador." *Dalhousie Medical Journal* 18 (1965): 17–20.
- "The Forgotten Years, 1912–1945." ADSF (July 1981): 6–12.
- *Labrador Doctor: My Life with the Grenfell Mission.* Toronto: James Lorimer 1989.
Parker, Gilbert: *The Seats of the Mighty, Being the Memoirs of Captain Robert Moray, Sometime an Officer in the Virginia Regiment, and Afterwards of Amherst's Regiment.* New York: D. Appleton & Co. 1896.
Parsons, F.G. *The History of St Thomas's Hospital.* 2 vols. London: Methuen 1932–34.
Parsons, John, and Burton K. Janes. *The King of Baffin Land: The Story of William Ralph Parsons, Last Fur Trade Commissioner of the Hudson's Bay Company.* St John's: Creative Publishers 1996.
Peacock, F.W. *Reflections from a Snowhouse.* With Lawrence Jackson. St John's: Jesperson Press 1986.
Perry, Jill Samfya. "Nursing for the Grenfell Mission: Maternalism and Moral Reform in Northern Newfoundland and Labrador, 1894–1938." MA thesis, Memorial University, 1997.
[Peters, Andrew]. "Codliver Oil and Fat-Soluble Vitamins." *American Review of Tuberculosis* 15 (1927): 100–1.
Phinney, Frank. "The Eye Doctor." ADSF (January 1929): 152–5.
Place, Philip W. "A Winter Medical Trip, North West River, 1921." ADSF (July 1922): 5–7.
Plaice, Evelyn. *The Native Game: Settler Perceptions of Indian/Settler Relations in Central Labrador.* St John's: ISER Books 1990.
"The Practice of Medicine in Labrador." *Radiology* 26 (1936): 243–6.
Pringle, George C.F. *In Great Waters: The Story of the United Church Marine Mission.* Toronto: United Church of Canada 1928.
Rasmussen, Knud. *Eskimo Folk-Tales.* London: Gyldendal; Copenhagen: Christiana 1921.

Ray, Arthur J. *The Canadian Fur Trade in the Industrial Age.* Toronto: University of Toronto Press 1990.

"Report of an Official Visit to the Coast of Labrador by the Governor of Newfoundland, during the Month of August, 1906," *Journal of the House of Assembly* (St John's: *Evening Telegram* 1907), 300–79.

"Report of Commission on Public Health, 1911," *Journal of the House of Assembly* (St John's: *Evening Chronicle* 1912), 585–628.

Reptonian. Vol. 1 (1866) to the present.

Reverby, Susan M. *Ordered to Care: The Dilemma of American Nursing, 1850–1945.* Cambridge: Cambridge University Press 1987.

Revillon, Victor. *Aventures d'un gentleman trappeur au nouveau monde.* [Paris]: Hachette 1980.

Robinson, Edward Colpitts. *In an Unknown Land: A Journey through the Wastes of Labrador in Search of Gold.* London: Elliot Stock 1909.

Rolleston, Sir Humphrey. *The British Encyclopaedia of Medical Practice.* 13 vols. London: Butterworth & Co., Ltd. 1937.

Rompkey, Ronald. "Elements of Spiritual Autobiography in Sir Wilfred Grenfell's *A Labrador Doctor.*" *Newfoundland Studies* 1 (1985): 17–28.

– "Heroic Biography and the Life of Sir Wilfred Grenfell." *Prose Studies* 12 (1989): 159–73.

– *Grenfell of Labrador: A Biography.* Toronto: University of Toronto Press 1991.

– Introduction to Elliott Merrick, *The Long Crossing and Other Labrador Stories* (Orono: University of Maine Press 1992), xi–xx.

– "'The Land That God Gave Cain' and the Representation of Labrador." *Canadian Issues/Thèmes canadiens* 20 (1998): 155–63.

– ed. *Labrador Odyssey: The Journal and Photographs of Eliot Curwen on the Second Voyage of Wilfred Grenfell, 1893.* Montreal: McGill-Queen's University Press 1996.

– ed. *Jessie Luther at the Grenfell Mission.* Montreal: McGill-Queen's University Press 2001.

Sailing Directions for Lake Melville and Approaches, Coast of Labrador. Ottawa: King's Printer 1931.

St Thomas' Hospital Gazette 1 (1891) to the present.

St Thomas's Hospital Medical School: Prospectus for the Year Commencing October, 1911. London: W.P. Griffith & Sons 1911, 1912.

Saunders, Gillian, comp. *Snowblind and Seal Finger: Stories of Early Labrador Medicine.* Happy Valley–Goose Bay: Them Days, 1998.

Scott, J.M. *The Land That God Gave Cain: An Account of H.G. Watkins's Expedition to Labrador, 1928–1929.* London: Chatto and Windus 1933.

– *Gino Watkins.* London: Hodder & Stoughton 1935.

Scott, Peter J. *Edible Fruits and Herbs of Newfoundland.* St John's: Memorial University 1975.

Sears, Fred C. "The Agricultural Possibilities in Labrador." *ADSF* (January 1929): 144–7.
- "Farming in Labrador." *Better Crops with Plant Food* 16, no. 4 (1931): 43–4, 47–8.
- "The Labrador Garden Campaign." *ADSF* (January 1933): 167–71.
- "Some Interesting Characters of the Labrador." *ADSF* (April 1933): 6–10.
- "The 1933 Labrador Garden Campaign." *ADSF* (April 1934): 8–12.
Sexé, Marcel. *Two Centuries of Fur-Trading, 1723–1923: The Romance of the Revillon Family.* Paris 1923.
Smillie, W.G. "An Epidemic of Influenza in an Isolated Community: Northwest River, Labrador." *American Journal of Hygiene* 11 (1930): 392–8.
Smith, Helen. "A Nurse's Experience on the Labrador Coast." *American Journal of Nursing* 17 (1917): 600–2.
Smith, Henry Fly. *The Handbook for Midwives.* London: Longmans, Green 1872.
Sontag, Susan. *Illness as Metaphor.* New York: Vintage 1979.
Speck, Frank G. *Naskapi: The Savage Hunters of the Labrador Peninsula.* Norman: University of Oklahoma Press 1935.
Spufford, Francis. *I May Be Some Time: Ice and the English Imagination.* New York: St Martin's Press 1997.
Stedman, Thomas Lathrop. *A Practical Medical Dictionary.* New York: William Wood 1926.
Steele, J.D. "Medicine in Labrador." *Milwaukee Medical Times* 13 (1940): 15–18.
Steven, David, and George Wald. "Vitamin A Deficiency: A Field Study in Newfoundland and Labrador." *Journal of Nutrition* 21 (1941): 461–76.
Story, G.M., W.J. Kirwin, and J.D.A. Widdowson, eds. *Dictionary of Newfoundland English.* Toronto: University of Toronto Press 1982.
Strong, William Duncan. "A Stone Culture from Northern Labrador and Its Relation to the Eskimo-Like Cultures of the Northeast." *American Anthropologist* n.s. 32 (1930): 126–44.
- *Anthropometric Observations on the Eskimos and Indians of Labrador.* Chicago: Field Museum of Natural History 1939.
- *Labrador Winter: The Ethnographic Journals of William Duncan Strong, 1927–1928.* Ed. Eleanor B. Leacock and Nan A. Rothschild. Washington: Smithsonian Institution Press 1994.
Stuck, Hudson. *A Winter Circuit of Our Arctic Coast: A Narrative of a Journey with Dog-Sleds around the Entire Arctic Coast of Alaska.* New York: Scribner's 1920.
Suk, V. *On the Occurrence of Syphilis and Tuberculosis amongst the Eskimos and Mixed Breeds of the North Coast of Labrador: A Contribution to the Question of the Extermination of Aboriginal Races.* Brno 1927.
Swain, Hector. *Lester Leeland Burry: Labrador Pastor and Father of Confederation.* St John's: Harry Cuff Publications 1983.

Tanner, Väinö. *Outlines of the Geography, Life and Customs of Newfoundland-Labrador (The Eastern Part of the Labrador Peninsula)*. 2 vols. Cambridge: Cambridge University Press 1947.

Taylor, Frederick. *A Manual of the Practice of Medicine*, 8th ed. London: J. & A. Churchill 1908.

Taylor, Garth. "Indian-Inuit Relations in Eastern Labrador, 1600–1976." *Arctic Anthropology* 16, no. 2 (1979): 49–58.

Taylor, William E. *La préhistoire de la péninsule du Labrador*. Études anthropologiques, no. 7. Ottawa: Secrétariat d'état 1964.

Thomas, Bernard, ed. *Repton, 1557 to 1957*. London: B.T. Batsford 1957.

Thomas, Harold. "A Summer at Indian Harbor Hospital." *ADSF* (April 1916), 16.

Thomson, James. *The Plays of James Thomson*. Ed. Percy G. Adams. New York: Garland 1979.

Todd, W.E. Clyde. *Birds of the Labrador Peninsula and Adjacent Areas*. Toronto: University of Toronto Press/Carnegie Museum 1963.

Tremblay, Huguette, ed. *Journal des voyages de Charles Arnaud, 1872–1873*. Montréal: Les Presses de l'Université du Québec 1977.

Van der Linden, Willem, Richard H. Fillon, and David Monahan. *Hamilton Bank, Labrador Margin: Origin and Evolution of a Glaciated Shelf*. Ottawa: Canadian Hydrographic Service and Geological Survey of Canada 1976.

Van Sommer, Annie, and Samuel M. Zwemer, eds. *Our Moslem Sisters: A Cry of Need from Lands of Darkness Interpreted by Those Who Heard It*. London: Fleming H. Revell Co. 1907.

[Van Sommer, James.] *Practical Suggestions on the Use of Scripture in Extempore Prayer*. London: Morgan & Chase [1869].

– *Sunday*. 2nd ed. London: John F. Shaw & Co., n.d.

– *Lay Service: Its Nurseries and its Spheres*. London: John F. Shaw & Co., n.d.

– *The Grace of God That Bringeth Salvation: Its Sevenfold Elementary Lessons*. London: Morgan and Scott, n.d.

– *Outlines of Scriptural Facts: Past, Present, and Prophetic*. London: John F. Shaw & Co., n.d.

– *The Parable of the Prodigal Son*. London: James Nisbet & Co. [1878].

– *Prayer Meetings: Practical Suggestions*. London: Morgan & Chase [1869].

– *Extempore Prayer*. 3rd ed. London: John F. Shaw & Co., n.d.

– *"The Kingdom of God;" The Central Idea in the New Testament Scriptures*. Privately printed 1900.

[Van Sommer, James, Jr.] *Rewards of the Van Sommer Family*. Bath: Ralph Allen Press 1945.

Van Sommer, William. "The Family of Van Sommer and Its Connexions." *Proceedings of the Huguenot Society of London* 15 (1936): 141–4.

Vaughn, Margery, and Helen S. Mitchell. "A Continuation of the Nutrition Project in Northern Newfoundland." *Journal of the American Dietetic Association* 8 (1933): 526–31.

Vigne, Randolphe. "The Van Sommers – A Huguenot Tradition." *Proceedings of the Huguenot Society of London* 24 (1986): 285–95.

Wakefield, A.W. "The Winter's Work at Mud Lake." *ADSF* (October 1913): 7–13.

Wakeley, Cecil P.G., and John B. Hunter. *Rose & Carless Manual of Surgery for Students and Practitioners.* 15th ed. 2 vols. London: Baillière, Tindall & Cox 1937.

Wallace, Dillon. *The Lure of the Labrador Wild.* New York: Fleming H. Revell 1905.

– *The Long Labrador Trail.* New York: Outing 1907.

Wallace, W.S., ed. *John McLean's Notes of a Twenty-Five Years' Service in the Hudson's Bay Territory.* Toronto: Champlain Society 1932.

Waugh, L.M. "Nutrition and Health of the Labrador Eskimo, with Special Reference to the Mouth and Teeth." *Journal of Dental Research* 8 (1928): 428–9.

Wheeler, E.P. *Labrador Eskimo Place Names.* National Museum of Canada Bulletin no. 131. Ottawa: Minister of Resources and Development 1953.

[White, James]. *Forts and Trading Posts in Labrador Peninsula and Adjoining Territory.* Ottawa: King's Printer 1926.

Who's Who In and From Newfoundland, 1930. St John's: R. Hibbs [1930].

Widdowson, John. *If You Don't Be Good: Verbal Social Control in Newfoundland.* St John's: ISER Books 1977.

Young, Arminius. *A Methodist Missionary in Labrador.* Toronto: S. and A. Young 1916.

– *One Hundred Years of Mission Work in the Wilds of Labrador.* London: Arthur H. Stockwell [1931].

Zimmerly, David William. *Cain's Land Revisited: Culture Change in Central Labrador, 1775–1972.* St John's: ISER Books 1975.

Index